CONCEPTS OF
PHYSICAL FITNESS
WITH LABORATORIES

FIFTH EDITION

CONCEPTS OF
PHYSICAL FITNESS
WITH LABORATORIES

CHARLES B. CORBIN
Arizona State University

RUTH LINDSEY
California State University, Long Beach

ꟼcb
Wm. C. Brown Publishers
Dubuque, Iowa

Book Team
Edward G. Jaffe *Senior Editor*
Lynne M. Meyers *Associate Editor*
Mary Jean Gregory *Production Editor*
Geri Wolfe *Designer*
Mavis M. Oeth *Permissions Editor*
Shirley M. Charley *Visual Research Editor*

Wm. C. Brown *Chairman of the Board*
Mark C. Falb *President and Chief Executive Officer*

wcb

Wm. C. Brown Publishers, College Division
Lawrence E. Cremer *President*
James L. Romig *Vice-President, Product Development*
David A. Corona *Vice-President, Production and Design*
E. F. Jogerst *Vice-President, Cost Analyst*
Bob McLaughlin *National Sales Manager*
Marcia H. Stout *Marketing Manager*
Craig S. Marty *Director of Marketing Research*
Eugenia M. Collins *Production Editorial Manager*
Marilyn A. Phelps *Manager of Design*
Mary M. Heller *Visual Research Manager*

Consulting Editor: Aileene Lockhart (Texas Woman's University)

Cover photo by S. B. Productions/The Image Bank

New illustrations rendered for this text by Ruth Krabach;
Stephen G. Moon, M.S.; and Laurel S. Antler.

Figure 6.3a and page 42 (right): © David Corona. Figure 6.3b, Figure 6.4, and
page 42 (left): © Tom Ballard/EKM-Nepenthe.

Library of Congress Catalog Card Number: 84-71636

ISBN: 0-697-07232-0

Printed in the United States of America
10 9 8 7 6 5 4 3

TABLE OF CONTENTS

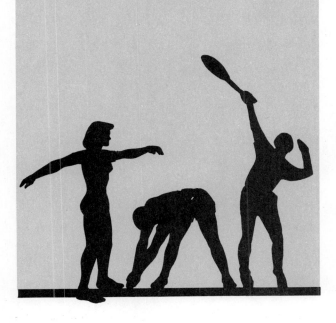

Preface   vii
A Note to the Reader   viii
A Note to the Instructor   viii

Section One
PHYSICAL FITNESS

1 Introduction   2
2 Physical Fitness   8
3 Hypokinetic Disease   16
4 Preparing for Exercise   26
5 Threshold of Training and Target Zones for
      Health-Related Physical Fitness   33
6 Cardiovascular Fitness   36
7 Strength   46
8 Muscular Endurance   56
9 Flexibility   60
10 Body Composition/Weight Control   69
11 Skill-Related Physical Fitness   82

Section Two
PROGRAMS OF EXERCISE

12 Aerobic Exercise   88
13 Strength and Endurance Exercises   94
14 Stretching Exercises   111
15 Sports, Preplanned, and Anaerobic Exercise
       Programs   117
16 Exercises for Care of the Back and Good
       Posture   126

Section Three
IMPORTANT FITNESS FACTORS

17 Exercise Cautions   136
18 Exercise and Nutrition   143
19 Stress, Tension, and Relaxation   149
20 Body Mechanics   156
21 Hypokinetic Disease Risk Factors   162
22 Exercise for a Lifetime   166

Section Four
PLANNING FOR FITNESS

23 Enjoying Exercise   172
24 Planning Your Exercise Program   177
25 Exercise and the Consumer   180

THE LABS

1	A Physical Activity Questionnaire	187
2	Physical Fitness	189
3	Hypokinetic Diseases and Conditions	191
4A	Physical Activity Readiness	193
4B	The Warm-Up and Cool Down	195
5	No laboratory	
6A	Counting the Pulse (Heart Rate)	197
6B	The Cardiovascular Threshold of Training	199
6C	Evaluating Cardiovascular Fitness	201
7A	Evaluating Isotonic Strength	203
7B	Evaluating Isometric Strength	205
8	Evaluating Muscular Endurance	207
9	Evaluating Flexibility	209
10A	Evaluating Body Fatness	211
10B	Determining "Desirable" Body Weight	213
11	Evaluating Skill-Related Physical Fitness	215
12A	Jogging/Running	217
12B	Aerobic Exercise	219
13	Weight Training for Strength	221
14	Stretching Exercises	223
15A	Sports for Physical Fitness	225
15B	Preplanned and Anaerobic Exercise Programs	227
16A	Care of the Back	229
16B	Posture	231
17	Contraindicated Exercises	233
18A	Nutrition and Activity Assessment	235
18B	Exercise for Caloric Expenditure	237
19A	Evaluating Your Stress Level	239
19B	Response to Stress	241
19C	Evaluating Neuromuscular Tension	243
19D	Relaxing Tense Muscles	245
20	No laboratory	
21	Assessing Heart Disease Risk Factors	247
22	Physical Activity for a Lifetime	249
23	A Physical Activity Questionnaire: A Reevaluation	251
24	Planning Your Personal Exercise Program	253
25	Exercise and the Consumer	257

APPENDIXES

A	PAR-X Questionnaire	259
B	Calorie Guide to Common Foods	261
C	Calories Per Minute in Activity	264
Index		265

PREFACE

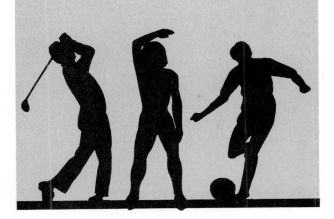

Concepts of Physical Fitness is designed primarily for an introductory course at the college level. In it we have attempted to provide the reader with the best scientific evidence in physical fitness—particularly in the area of health-related physical fitness. The text is appropriate for both men and women.

An outline format is used to give the reader a concise and factual presentation with regard to the *why, how,* and *what* of exercise and physical activity for fitness. Discussion is kept to a minimum; references and suggested readings are provided for the reader who wishes to pursue a specific topic.

The title of the fifth edition has been changed to more accurately reflect the content of the text. It is divided into four sections. The first section, entitled "Physical Fitness," includes eleven concepts (chapters) that elaborate on the need for fitness, distinguish between health-related and skill-related fitness, and present the various components of fitness, including warm-up, cool down, and target zones. Section 2, "Programs of Exercise," includes five concepts that describe exercises, activities, sports, and special programs for developing each of the health-related fitness components discussed in the first section, as well as exercises to prevent backaches and inefficient postures.

The third section, "Important Fitness Factors," contains six concepts involving factors that must be considered in any health-related fitness program. These include facts about dangerous exercises, the importance of good nutrition, the relief of stress and tension, the avoidance of risk factors (especially for cardiovascular disease), and the role of fitness programs in daily life—"from the cradle to the grave." Section 4, "Planning for Fitness," puts it all together in three concepts that include strategies for motivation and getting more enjoyment out of exercise. This section also includes what is perhaps the most important concept in the text: how to plan an individualized program for yourself based upon your needs and interests. The program you plan is based on the self-tests you perform in the laboratory experiences. Finally, the last concept in Section 4 tells the reader how to avoid the rip-offs and quackery so frequently found in the fitness industry.

There are a total of twenty-five concepts and thirty-seven accompanying laboratories. The labs are numbered to correspond with the concepts that they supplement.

The laboratories are done on tear-out pages so that they can be completed and handed into the instructor. Much of the Lab Resource Materials necessary to complete the tear-out lab sheets is included in the Concept section of the text. This was done so that important information would not be torn from the book and so would be available for future reference. When possible, charts and rating scales are presented in both the Lab Resource Materials and in the tear-out lab sheets. An understanding and appreciation of the information presented in these pages should provide the foundation for an intelligent selection of activities and health practices to aid you in leading a useful and productive life.

A NOTE TO THE READER

Concepts of Physical Fitness is unlike other textbooks you may have used in the past. To make the book as easy to use as possible, we have organized it in a unique way.

First, the text has an outline format. For this reason, it does not read like most texts. However, the information is useful and precise. Secondly, references are listed to support the facts presented in the text. While we do not expect you to look up each reference, we do want you to know where to look for more information. Two or three references in each concept are designated as "suggested readings" by an asterisk(*).

Another important feature of *Concepts of Physical Fitness* is the tear-out lab sheets. These sheets have been perforated so that you can hand them in to your instructor if requested to do so. Important testing or exercise information is included in the concept to which each lab pertains. This section of the concept, Lab Resource Materials, has been positioned here because we feel certain that you will want to keep this information for future use. And as an added convenience, rating charts and scales are presented in both the tear-out labs and the Lab Resource Materials. Finally, special tables are included in the appendixes at the end of the book.

Concepts of Physical Fitness is intended to help you make important decisions about your personal exercise program and your personal physical fitness both now and during the rest of your life. We trust that you will find the book interesting and useful.

A NOTE TO THE INSTRUCTOR

A comprehensive instructor's manual is available to teachers who adopt *Concepts of Physical Fitness*. This manual includes suggestions for organizing the classes, grading, lecture outlines, and laboratory instructions, as well as suggested supplementary activities. It explains how to use only the part of these concepts in the text that fit your particular course. A master set of illustrations suitable for transparencies is available to accompany the lectures, and computer software is available from Wm. C. Brown Publishers to help you with testing and to help students with self-testing and program planning.

If you have used any of the four previous editions, you will note that we have discontinued documenting each statement. This makes the book more readable. However, the references for all facts are included and are now placed at the end of each concept. Every concept includes the most up-to-date scientific information available. Each concept and lab has been rewritten from previous editions. Also, several new concepts have been added.

The arrangement of the concepts into four sections is designed to give the text a more logical format. We have adopted some new terminology in Concept 9 (Flexibility) to more nearly fit the clinical model, while still attempting to keep it in simple enough terms for nonprofessionals. We feel the introduction of color in the book and the illustration of muscles involved in each exercise will be a great help to the student. Finally, you will note that there are only two authors involved in this edition. Our proven ability to work together on other books and the greater ease of coordinating and blending the work of two (as opposed to four) authors should result in a better text.

We extend special thanks to those reviewers who gave us suggestions for this fifth edition, and to those users who made this edition possible because they had adopted our book in its previous editions.

James B. Angel — Samford University
Stanely R. Brown — University of British Columbia
Jeanne A. Ashley — Greenfield Community College
James R. Marett — Northern Illinois University
Sister Janice Iverson — South Dakota State University
Al Leister — Mercer County Community College
David Laurie — Kansas State University
Bo Fernhall — Northern Illinois University

Section One
PHYSICAL FITNESS

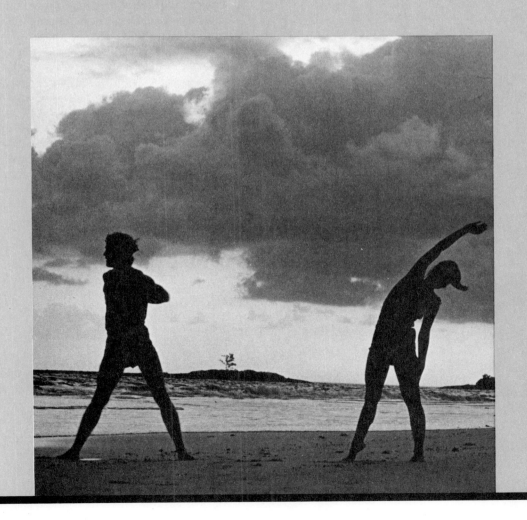

1
INTRODUCTION

CONCEPT 1

Regular exercise is important for all people.

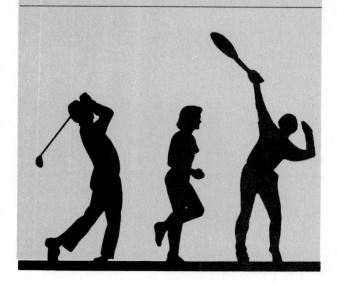

INTRODUCTION

The human organism was designed to be active. Anthropologists indicate that the need to be active is associated with the "fight or flight" response. In search of food, primitive people sometimes had to fight with other predators, or in some cases, to flee for safety. In either case, the response was often vigorous activity. Even our more recent ancestors were required to do vigorous activity as a relatively major part of their normal daily routine. However, automation and technology have freed modern civilization from the exhausting physical labor required of earlier generations. The heavy physical work of the farmer and manual laborer is less and less likely to be a part of the normal daily routine of the average North American. Statistics indicate that in the past 100 years, the average workweek has been greatly reduced, thereby netting the average person many hours of free time annually.

Even though exercise has become less necessary as a part of the normal work of many adults, the need for regular exercise has not decreased. If anything, it has increased. Though we do not have to flee from saber-toothed tigers or fight wild animals for our food, our bodies still respond with the fight or flight response. The business person's stomach "churns" before the important meeting and the anxious sports fan's heartbeat increases during the close contest. The body is readied for activity, but the activity never comes. As a result, many Americans lack physical fitness and suffer from hypokinetic disease, or diseases associated with inactivity.

The need for good physical fitness and accompanying mental and physical health is vital for everyone. The human's need for regular exercise is critical in modern society. We have the necessary free time to be active, and given adequate information, all of us can learn to make intelligent decisions about lifetime health, physical fitness, and exercise. ↑ Conclusion

TERMS

Exercise—Exercise, as used in *Concepts of Physical Fitness,* means human movement or physical activity. This term includes such formal activities as calisthenics, movements done in sports, dance, and games, as well as less formal activities, such as walking, jogging, and swimming. In this book, exercise, physical activity, and human movement are used interchangeably, and in general, are used to describe large muscle activities rather than highly specific, relatively nontaxing movements of small muscle groups.

Hypokinetic Disease or Condition—"Hypo" means under or too little, and "kinetic" means energy or activity. Thus, hypokinetic means "too little activity." A hypokinetic disease or condition is associated with lack of physical activity or too little regular exercise. Examples of such conditions include heart disease, low back pain, diabetes, and obesity.

Physical Fitness—Physical fitness is the entire human organism's ability to function efficiently and effectively. It is made up of at least eleven different components, each of which contributes to the ability to work effectively, to enjoy leisure time, to be healthy, to resist hypokinetic diseases, and to meet emergency situations. Though the development of physical fitness is the result of many things, optimal physical fitness is not possible without regular exercise.

SOME DISCOURAGING FACTS (THE BAD NEWS)

Too many North American adults are not as active as they should be.

Recent statistics indicate that only 15 to 20 percent of all adults exercise regularly enough to build optimal fitness. We often think that younger people are more active than adults, but even among individuals as young as fourteen, only 19 percent are considered avid exercisers.

Many North American children are not as fit as they should be.

The results of recent studies reveal that more than one-half of school-age children are not as fit as they should be. This affects their health and their functioning for work and play.

Teenagers are especially likely to lack good fitness.

Of all groups studied, teenagers are more apt than any other to be unfit. Too many teens decrease, rather than increase, in fitness following elementary school. During this time, proper exercise and a healthy lifestyle can result in exceptional fitness gains. Instead, lack of exercise and improper nutrition often result in a fitness decline at this age.

Adult women are often less active than adult men.

Adult women are often less active than adult men even though all evidence indicates that the benefits of exercise for women are similar to those for men. Nevertheless, recent studies indicate that considerably more men are involved in regular physical activity than are women.

Too many adults suffer from hypokinetic diseases.

In 1961, Kraus and Raab coined the term "hypokinetic disease." They pointed out that recent advances in modern medicine had been quite effective in eliminating infectious diseases, but that degenerative diseases, characterized by sedentary or "take-it-easy" living, had increased in recent decades. In fact, heart disease is the leading cause of death in western society; high blood pressure afflicts an estimated 37 million adults; stroke kills nearly 200,000; and atherosclerosis causes more than 500,000 heart attacks each year. The leading medical complaint in the United States is low back pain, and nearly one-half of all North Americans are considered to be obese. Studies now show that the symptoms of hypokinetic disease begin in youth. This fact, plus the relatively low fitness levels of children, suggests that the incidence of hypokinetic disease in our culture will not be reduced without considerable lifestyle change in people of all ages.

Many people are ignorant of the facts about exercise and physical fitness.

Unfortunately, many American adults hold misconceptions about health, fitness, and exercise. For example, 57 percent of inactive adults feel such sports as baseball and bowling provide enough exercise to develop good health and physical fitness. And although the facts indicate otherwise, those who do not exercise regularly believe that they get all the exercise they need. Interestingly, those who report that they participate in regular exercise are also the ones who are likely to feel that they do not get enough exercise for their own good. Other common misconceptions involve exercise and nutrition, the value of specific exercises, water replacement during exercise, and exercise in high temperature, to name but a few.

SOME ENCOURAGING FACTS (THE GOOD NEWS)

North Americans are becoming more active in recent years.

Surveys taken in the 1960s indicated that only about 24 percent of all adults exercise in some form during their free time. Recent statistics indicate that as many as 50 to 60 percent of Americans are now active on a regular basis, though as previously noted, too many are not active enough to promote optimal fitness. In Canada, 56 percent of the total population over the age of ten is active for at least three hours per week on a regular basis.

Most adults realize the value of exercise and physical fitness.

Current findings show that the interest in fitness and exercise generated among large numbers of North Americans in the 1960s and 1970s is still prevalent today. Almost all adults believe that exercise is important for good health and fitness, and that regular activity and sports are valuable for their children.

Increasing numbers of women are getting involved in regular exercise.

It is true that women are less likely than men to be active, but it is also true that they are becoming active in sports and physical activities at a distinctly more rapid rate than men. Also, activities previously considered to be "for men only" are gaining in popularity among women.

Adults who learn the facts about exercise tend to be more active and have better attitudes than those who hold misconceptions.

Though too many adults are inactive and uninformed of the facts about fitness and exercise, those adults who have learned the facts tend to persist in activity over the years. Those who are well informed are able to make intelligent decisions about exercise, including the ultimate decision to participate in adequate regular exercise for developing optimal fitness.

Industry has recognized the importance of exercise programs to employee fitness and productivity.

Realizing that many jobs are not as active as they were prior to automation, industry has taken steps to provide on-the-job exercise and fitness programs for their employees. Because medical costs are skyrocketing; because hypokinetic diseases such as back pain account for a billion dollar annual loss in production; and because absenteeism can be reduced considerably by offering employees an exercise and fitness program, company officials endorsed the fitness-in-industry movement. Evidence indicates that such programs are cost-effective as well as popular among employees. One company official notes, "It's the best fringe benefit we've offered."

The United States Army has recently implemented a program to teach the fitness facts to supplement physical training programs.

For years, the military has had physical training programs designed to "get people fit." Unfortunately, these programs sometimes resulted in only short-term fitness gains because they taught participants to "hate exercise." The new program recognizes the importance of learning the facts about fitness and the need for each person to develop a personalized fitness program that can be used for a lifetime.

FACTS ABOUT WHY PEOPLE DO NOT EXERCISE

The number one reason people give for not exercising is, "I don't have the time."

More than one-half of those who do not exercise regularly reason that, "I don't have the time." Often in the same breath the person says, "I am too busy." Young people state that they will soon be established and able to take the time to exercise. Older people state that they wish they had taken the time when they were younger.

Another major reason people do not exercise is, "It's too inconvenient."

Many people who avoid exercise do so because it is inconvenient. They are exercise procrastinators. Specific reasons for procrastinating include, "It makes me sweaty," "It messes up my hair," and "I just can't find the energy." (It is interesting, though, that people who do exercise regularly report improvements in their appearance and a feeling of increased energy.)

Large numbers of adults are not active because they "just don't enjoy exercise."

The reasons some people do not enjoy exercise include "people might laugh at me," "sports make me nervous," and "I am not good at physical activities." These people often lack confidence in their own abilities. In some cases, this is because of their past experiences in physical education or in athletics. With properly selected activities, even those who have never enjoyed exercise can get "hooked."

Poor health is a reason some people avoid exercise.

Some people avoid exercise because of health reasons. While it is true that there are good medical reasons for not exercising, many people with such problems can benefit from exercise if it is properly designed for them.

Lack of facilities and bad weather are reasons some do not exercise regularly.

Regular exercise is much more convenient if facilities are easy to reach and the weather is good. Still, recreational opportunities have increased considerably in recent years. Furthermore, some of the most popular activities for building fitness require very little equipment, can be done in or near the home, and are inexpensive.

FACTS ABOUT WHY PEOPLE DO EXERCISE

The number one reason people exercise regularly is "for health and physical fitness."

Ninety percent of all adults recognize the importance of exercise to good health and fitness. More than one national survey has shown that health and fitness is the single most important reason why people engage in regular exercise. Unfortunately, many adults say that a "doctor's order to exercise" would be the most likely reason to get them to begin a regular program. For some, however, waiting for a doctor's order may be too late.

Enjoyment is a major reason people exercise regularly.

A majority of adults say that "enjoyment" would be of paramount importance in deciding to exercise. This is not surprising, given statements from joggers that they began exercising for fitness but continue for such reasons as the "peak experience," the "runner's high," and "spinning free." In fact, movement can be an end in itself. Satisfaction can be derived from the mere involvement in the movement activity. The sense of fun, the feeling of well-being, and the general enjoyment associated with physical activity is well documented.

Relaxation and release from tension are important reasons given for doing regular exercise.

Relaxation and release from tension rank high as important reasons for doing regular exercise. Exercise, such as walking, jogging, or cycling, is a way of getting some "quiet time" away from the stress of the job. For years, it has been recognized that exercise in the form of sports and games provides a "catharsis," or outlet, for the frustrations of normal daily activities. There is even evidence that for some people, regular exercise can help reduce depression, a common symptom in western culture.

Physical activity can provide a way of meeting a challenge and developing a sense of personal accomplishment.

A sense of personal accomplishment associated with performing various physical activities is frequently a reason people exercise. In some cases, it is merely learning a new skill, such as racquetball or tennis; in other cases, it is running a mile or doing a certain number of sit-ups that provides this feeling of accomplishment. The challenge of doing something never done before is apparently a very powerful experience. Physical activities provide opportunities not readily available in other aspects of life.

An important reason many people exercise is the social experience of involvement.

Physical activity often provides the opportunity to be with other people. It is this social experience that many appreciate most about exercise. Frequent answers to the question, "Why do you exercise?" include: "It is a good way to spend time with other members of the

family;" "It is a good way to spend time with close friends;" and "Being part of the team is a satisfying feeling." Physical activity settings can also provide an opportunity for making new friends.

The competitive experience is an important reason people participate in sports and physical activities.

"The thrill of victory" and "sports competition" are two reasons often given for participation in physical activities. For many people, the competitive experiences can be very satisfying.

Physical appearance is a reason given by many for doing regular exercise.

People indicate that an important reason for exercising is improving physical appearance. In our society, "looking good" is highly valued, thus physical attractiveness is another major reason for participating in regular exercise.

OTHER IMPORTANT FACTS

The most popular forms of exercise among adults require very little skill or equipment and are easily accessible.

Surveys consistently show that the most popular activities among adults are walking, swimming, bicycling, calisthenics, and jogging/running. All of these can be done in or near the home for little or no cost. None requires a high degree of physical skill to be successful or to enjoy the benefits associated with regular involvement. These activities are not often those that people value for their children, nor those in which they themselves were involved as children. And although football, baseball, basketball, gymnastics, and boxing are the activities adults most enjoy watching, they often are not the ones in which these adults participate.

Exercise can be important for many reasons, but it is not a cure-all, and if done improperly, can be dangerous.

The many benefits of exercise are well documented in this book. As is pointed out in later sections of *Concepts of Physical Fitness,* however, certain types of exercise are contraindicated for certain people. Doing too much too soon can be dangerous for those who have not been involved in exercise on a regular basis. Those who exercise irregularly, such as the "weekend athlete" who exercises vigorously only on weekends or other "special occasions," may be asking for trouble. There is some evidence that even avid exercisers can become overly involved with their commitment to physical activity and develop an "activity neurosis." This condition can develop if an individual becomes irrationally concerned about his or her need for involvement in exercise.

There is no single best form of exercise for all people.

Different people participate in different types of exercise for different reasons, as has been previously discussed. This is as it should be. There is evidence that each person has his or her own unique movement personality: no two people move in the same way. Because movement personalities differ, there is a wide variety of leisure activities selected by different individuals. The choice of exercise and physical activities should be made only after carrying out the following steps:

1. Assess your current health and physical fitness status to determine your individual needs.
2. Examine your current interests. (Exercise should be enjoyable.)
3. Acquire a knowledge and an understanding of the values of different activities.
4. Determine which activities will best meet your needs and interests.
5. Acquire skill and knowledge in the selected activities.

Exercise is for virtually everyone.

Exercise, whether it be sports or some other form of physical activity, should not be limited to those with good athletic ability. Regardless of your age, sex, or athletic ability (if there is no serious medical limitation), there is some form of activity that you will find enjoyable and in which you can succeed.

LAB RESOURCE MATERIALS (FOR USE WITH LAB 1, PAGE 187)

CHART 1.1 The Physical Activity Questionnaire

The term "physical activity" in the following statements refers to all kinds of activities, including sports, formal exercises, and informal activities, such as jogging and cycling. Check your answers first, and then read the directions for scoring at the end of the questionnaire.

	Strongly Agree	Agree	Undecided	Disagree	Strongly Disagree	Score
1. Doing regular physical activity can be as harmful to health as it is helpful.	☐	☐	☒	☐	☐	3
2. One of the main reasons I do regular physical activity is because it is fun.	☐	☒	☐	☐	☐	4
3. Participating in physical activities makes me tense and nervous.	☐	☐	☐	☐	☒	5
4. The challenge of physical training is one reason why I participate in physical activity.	☐	☐	☒	☐	☐	3
5. One of the things I like about physical activity is the participation with other people.	☐	☒	☐	☐	☐	4
6. Doing regular physical activity does little to make me more physically attractive.	☐	☐	☐	☐	☒	5
7. Competition is a good way to keep a game from being fun.	☐	☐	☐	☐	☒	5
8. I should exercise regularly for my own good health and physical fitness.	☒	☐	☐	☐	☐	5
9. Doing exercise and playing sports is boring.	☐	☐	☐	☐	☒	5
10. I enjoy taking part in physical activity because it helps me to relax and get away from the pressures of daily living.	☒	☐	☐	☐	☐	5
11. Most sports and physical activities are too difficult for me to enjoy.	☐	☐	☐	☐	☒	5
12. I do not enjoy physical activities that require the participation of other people.	☐	☐	☐	☐	☒	5
13. Regular exercise helps me look my best.	☒	☐	☐	☐	☐	5
14. Competing against others in physical activities makes them enjoyable.	☐	☐	☒	☐	☐	3

Score the physical activity questionnaire as follows:

1. For items 1, 3, 6, 7, 9, 11, and 12, give one point for strongly agree, two for agree, three for undecided, four for disagree, and five for strongly disagree. Put the correct number in the blank to the right of the statements.
2. For items 2, 4, 5, 8, 10, 13, and 14, give five points for strongly agree, four for agree, three for undecided, two for disagree, and one for strongly disagree. Put the correct number in the blank to the right of the statements.
3. Determine each of the following seven scores by adding the numbers to the right of the items as indicated (two numbers for each score).

Health and fitness score	Item 1 __3__	+Item 8 __5__	= __8__
Fun and enjoyment score	Item 2 __4__	+Item 9 __5__	= __9__
Relaxation and tension release score	Item 3 __5__	+Item 10 __5__	= __10__
Challenge and achievement score	Item 4 __3__	+Item 11 __5__	= __8__
Social score	Item 5 __4__	+Item 12 __5__	= __9__
Appearance score	Item 6 __5__	+Item 13 __5__	= __10__
Competition score	Item 7 __5__	+Item 14 __3__	= __8__

Total score __62__

4. Determine your total score by adding each of the seven scores. Write your total score in the bottom blank.
5. Use Chart 1.2 to determine your rating on each score.

CHART 1.2 Physical Activity Questionnaire Rating Scale

Classification	Each of Seven Scores	Total Score
Excellent	9–10	63–70
Good	7–8	50–62
Fair	6	42–49
Poor	4–5	30–41
Very poor	3 or less	29 or less

REFERENCES

American Heart Association. *1983 Heart Facts Reference Sheet.* Dallas: American Heart Association, 1983.

Condon, J. "Executive Sweat." *Women in Sports* (October 1977):20.

Corbin, C. B. "Self-Confidence of Women in Sports." In *Clinics in Sports Medicine: Women in Sports,* edited by W. M. Walsh. Philadelphia: W. B. Saunders Co., 1984.

*Corbin, C. B., and R. Lindsey. *The Ultimate Fitness Book.* New York: Leisure Press, 1984.

Csikzentmihaly, M. *Beyond Boredom and Anxiety.* San Francisco: Jarsey-Bass, 1977.

Department of the Army. *The Individual's Handbook on Physical Fitness.* Washington: Department of the Army, 1983.

Fast, J. *Body Language.* New York: Pocket Books, 1971.

Fitness Canada. *Canada Fitness Survey—Highlights.* Ottawa, Ontario: Government of Canada, 1983.

Gilliam, T. B., et al. "Exercise Programs for Children: A Way to Prevent Heart Disease?" *Physician and Sportsmedicine* 10(1982):96.

Greist, J. H., et al. "Running Through Your Mind." In *Psychology of Running,* edited by M. H. Sacks and M. L. Sachs. Champaign, IL: Human Kinetics, 1981.

Harris, L., and Associates. *The Perrier Study: Fitness in America.* New York: Great Waters of France, 1979.

Hodgson, J. D. "Leisure and the American Worker." *Journal of Health, Physical Education, and Recreation* 43 (1972):38.

Kenyon, G. S. "Six Scales for Assessing Attitudes Toward Physical Activity." *Research Quarterly* 39(1968):566.

Kostrubala, T. *Joy of Running.* New York: J. B. Lippencott, 1976.

*Kraus, H., and W. Raab. *Hypokinetic Disease.* Springfield, IL: C. C. Thomas, 1961.

Little, J. C. "The Athlete's Neurosis—A Deprivation Crisis." In Sacks, M. H. and M. L. Sachs, *Psychology of Running.* Champaign, IL: Human Kinetics, 1981.

Nabisco/AAU. *Toasted Wheat and Raisins/AAU Fitness Profile of American Youth.* Chicago: Golin-Harris, 1983.

Pollock, M. L., J. H. Wilmore, and S. M. Fox. *Health and Fitness through Physical Activity.* New York: John Wiley and Sons, 1978.

President's Council on Physical Fitness and Sports. *President's Council on Physical Fitness and Sports Newsletter,* Special Edition (May 1973):1.

Research and Forecasts, Inc. *The Miller Lite Report on American Attitudes toward Sports.* Milwaukee: Miller Brewing Co., 1983.

Simon, D. G., and J. G. Travell. "Myofascial Origins of Low Back Pain." *Postgraduate Medicine* 73(1983):66.

Slava, S., D. R. Laurie, and C. B. Corbin. "The Long-Term Effects of a Conceptual Physical Education Program." *Research Quarterly for Exercise and Sports* 55 (1984):161.

Snyder, E. E., and E. Spreitzer. "Adult Perceptions of Physical Education in the Schools and Community Sports Programs for Youth." *The Physical Educator* 40(1983):88.

Stone, W. J. "Exercise and Long-Term CV Risk Reduction in Corporate Executives." *Health Education* 14(1983):26.

Thorland, W. G., and T. B. Gilliam. "Comparison of Serum Lipids between Habitually High and Low Active Pre-Adolescent Males." *Medicine and Science in Sports and Exercise* 13(1981):316.

Villeneuve, K., et al. "Employee Fitness: A Bottom Line Payoff," *Journal of Physical Education, Recreation and Dance* 54(1983):35.

Wicks, B. "Physical Fitness Programs in Business and Industry." *National Intramural and Recreational Sports Association* 7(1983):31.

2
PHYSICAL FITNESS

CONCEPT 2

Physical fitness is not only one
of the most important keys to a healthy body;
it is also the basis for dynamic
and creative activity.
— President John F. Kennedy, 1960

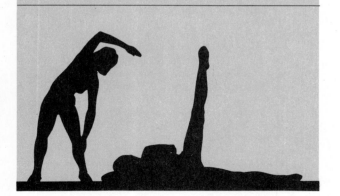

INTRODUCTION

Some people associate "good physical fitness" with being good at sports and games. It does take a certain degree of fitness to excell in these activities, but being able to perform specific sports skills may not be a good indicator of total physical fitness as some sports require only specific aspects of fitness.

Historically, physical fitness has often been misrepresented, at times identified exclusively with skill in sports, or at other times identified too closely with only one of the many aspects of physical fitness. For example, in previous decades, fitness for men was often associated with muscle strength. This is evidenced by the popularity of programs such as Charles Atlas' Dynamic Tension Program advertised widely in magazines and comic books. In the 1960s and 1970s, with the popularity of jogging and other forms of aerobic exercise, many people associated physical fitness almost exclusively with cardiovascular fitness. Recently, research and popular literature has brought considerable attention to flexibility as an important component of fitness. It is true that each of these is important, but it cannot be overemphasized that physical fitness is not a single entity, but consists of a number of different characteristics of which strength, cardiovascular fitness, and flexibility are only three. The possession of each of the specific components of fitness is critical to the development of optimal physical fitness and to achieving the benefits associated with being optimally fit.

HEALTH-RELATED FITNESS TERMS

Body Composition—The relative percentage of muscle, fat, bone, and other tissue of which the body is composed. A fit person has a relatively low percentage of body fat (body fatness).

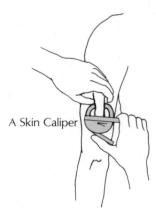

A Skin Caliper

Body Composition
(Fatness)

Cardiovascular Fitness—The ability of the heart, blood vessels, blood, and respiratory system to supply fuel, especially oxygen, to the muscles during sustained exercise. A fit person can persist in physical activity for relatively long periods of time without undue stress.

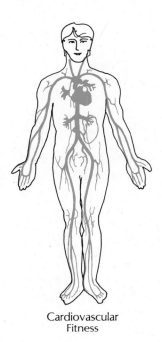

Cardiovascular
Fitness

Muscular Endurance—The ability of the muscles to repeatedly exert themselves. A fit person can repeat strength performances without undue fatigue.

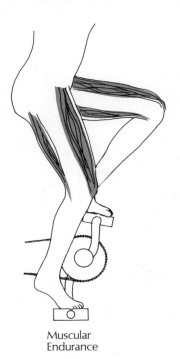

Muscular
Endurance

Flexibility—The range of motion available in a joint. It is affected by muscle length, joint structure, and other factors. A fit person can move the body joints through a full range of motion in work and in play.

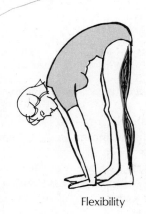

Flexibility

Strength—The ability to exert an external force or to lift a heavy weight. A fit person can do work or play that involves exerting force, such as lifting or controlling one's own body weight.

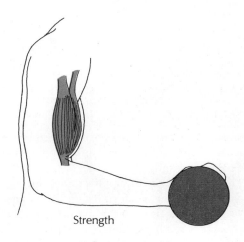

Strength

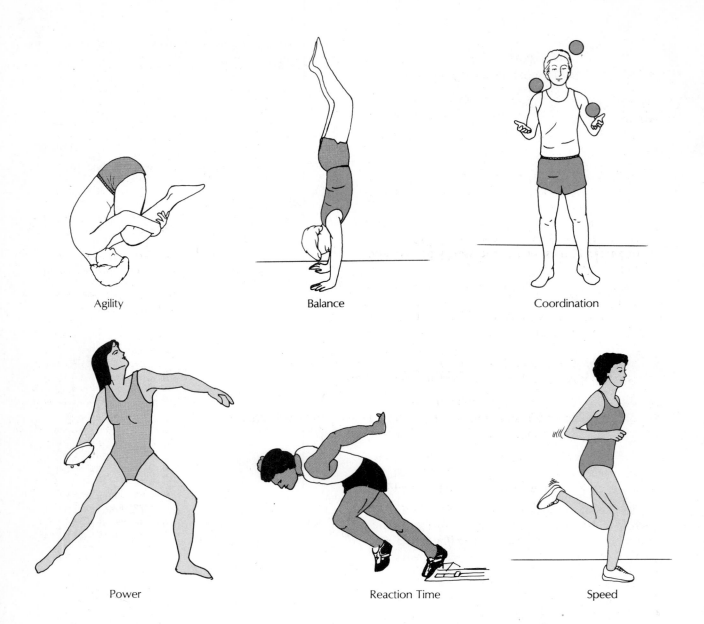

Agility

Balance

Coordination

Power

Reaction Time

Speed

SKILL-RELATED FITNESS TERMS

Agility—The ability to rapidly and accurately change the position of the entire body in space. Springboard diving and wrestling are examples of activities that require exceptional agility.

Balance—The maintenance of equilibrium while stationary or while moving. Performing on the balance beam or working as a riveter on a high-rise building are activities that require exceptional balance.

Coordination—The ability to use the senses, with the body parts to perform motor tasks smoothly and accurately. Juggling, batting a baseball, or kicking a soccer ball are examples of activities requiring good coordination.

Power—The ability to transfer energy into force at a fast rate. Throwing the discus and putting the shot are activities that require power.

Reaction Time—The time elapsed between stimulation and the beginning of reaction to that stimulation. Driving a racing car and starting a sprint race require good reaction time.

Speed—The ability to perform a movement in a short period of time. A runner on a track team or a wide receiver on a football team needs good foot and leg speed.

THE FACTS

Physical fitness is a part of total fitness.

Aspects of total fitness include emotional, social, spiritual, and mental fitness as well as physical fitness.

Physical fitness consists of many components, each of which is specific in nature.

Physical fitness is a combination of several aspects rather than a single characteristic. A fit person possesses at least adequate levels of each of the five health-related fitness components, and each of the six skill-related fitness components. People who possess one aspect of physical fitness do not necessarily possess all of the other aspects.

Each of the eleven components of physical fitness is separate and different from each of the others. There is some relationship between different fitness characteristics, but, for example, people who possess exceptional strength do not necessarily have good cardiovascular fitness, and those who have good coordination do not necessarily possess good flexibility.

Body composition, cardiovascular fitness, flexibility, muscular endurance, and strength are the health-related components of physical fitness.

Because each fitness characteristic has a direct relationship to good health and lessened risk of hypokinetic disease, each is considered to be a part of health-related physical fitness.

Agility, balance, coordination, power, reaction time, and speed comprise the skill-related components of physical fitness.

Because each of the fitness characteristics is related to performing motor skills such as those required in sports and in specific types of jobs, each is considered to be a part of skill-related physical fitness. Skill-related fitness is sometimes called "sports fitness" or "motor fitness."

Good physical fitness, particularly health-related fitness, is important to optimal health.

Optimal health is more than freedom from disease. According to the World Health Organization, health is "a state of complete physical, mental, and social well-being and not merely the absence of disease and infirmity." Good fitness can contribute to buoyant health including feeling good, looking good, and enjoying life, as well as having a reduced risk of certain disease.

TABLE 2.1 The Physical Health Benefits of Activity

Major Benefit	Related Benefits
Improved cardiovascular fitness	• Stronger heart muscle • Lower heart rate • Possible reduction in blood pressure • Reduced blood fat, including low density lipids (LDL) • Possible resistance to atherosclerosis • Possible improved peripheral circulation • Improved coronary circulation • Resistance to "emotional storm" • Less chance of heart attack • Greater chance of surviving a heart attack • Increased protective high density lipids (HDL) • Increased oxygen carrying capacity of the blood
Greater lean body mass and lesser body fat	• Greater work efficiency • Less susceptibility to disease • Improved appearance • Less incidence of self-concept problems related to obesity
Improved strength and muscular endurance	• Greater work efficiency • Less chance of muscle injury • Decreased chance of low back problems • Improved performance in sports • Improved ability to meet emergencies
Improved flexibility	• Greater work efficiency • Less chance of muscle injury • Less chance of joint injury • Decreased chance of low back problems • Improved sports performance
Other health benefits of exercise and physical activity	• Increased ability to use oxygen • Quicker recovery after hard work

Good health-related physical fitness contributes to positive physical health, including a reduced risk of hypokinetic diseases.

Many of the contributions of health-related physical fitness are described in more detail later in this book. However, the physical health benefits associated with involvement in regular, properly planned exercises are summarized in Table 2.1. Physical fitness also contributes to positive mental health. Mental illness is now

TABLE 2.2 The Mental Health Benefits of Activity

Major Benefit	Related Benefits
Reduction in mental tension	• Relief of depression • Improper sleep habits • Fewer stress symptoms • Ability to enjoy leisure • Possible work improvement
Opportunity for social interactions	• Improved quality of life
Resistance to fatigue	• Ability to enjoy leisure • Improved quality of life • Improved ability to meet some stressors
Opportunity for successful experience	• Improved self-concept • Opportunity to recognize and accept personal limitations
Improved physical fitness	• Improved sense of well-being • Improved self-concept • Improved appearance

recognized as a health problem, not a personal weakness or a reason for social disgrace. The serious nature of mental health problems is illustrated by the following facts: approximately 25,000 suicides occur in the United States each year; doctors estimate that as many as 70 percent of all illnesses are psychosomatic, or emotionally related. Some of the mental health benefits that are derived from regular physical activity and good physical fitness are summarized in Table 2.2.

Good physical fitness can help an individual enjoy his or her free time.

A person who is not too fat, has no back problems, does not have to worry about high blood pressure, and has reasonable skills in different lifetime sports is more likely to get involved and stay regularly involved in leisure time activities than one who does not have these characteristics. It is said that enjoying your leisure time may not add years to your life, but it can add life to your years.

Good physical fitness can help an individual work effectively and efficiently.

A person who can resist fatigue, muscle soreness, back problems and other symptoms associated with poor health-related fitness is capable of working productively and having energy left over at the end of the day. Surveys of employees who have the opportunity to improve fitness through involvement in employee fitness programs indicate that 75 percent have an improved sense of well-being. Employers indicate that absen-

teeism is decreased by up to 50 percent among program participants. These people, with good skill-related fitness, may be more effective and efficient in performing specific motor skills required for certain jobs.

Good physical fitness is essential to effective living.

Although the need for each component of physical fitness is specific to each individual, every person requires enough fitness to be able to perform normal daily activities without undue fatigue. Whether it be for walking, performing household chores, or merely feeling good and enjoying the "simple things in life" without pain or fear of injury, good fitness is important to all people.

Good physical fitness may help you function safely and assist you in meeting unexpected emergencies.

Emergencies are never expected, but when they do arise, they often demand performance that requires good fitness. For example, flood victims may need to fill sandbags for hours without rest, and accident victims may be required to walk or run long distances for help. Also, good fitness is required for such simple tasks as safely changing a spare tire or loading a moving van without injury.

Physical fitness is the basis for dynamic and creative activity.

Though the following quotation is now over twenty years old, it clearly points out the importance of physical fitness. "The relationship between the soundness of the body and the activity of the mind is subtle and complex. Much is not yet understood, but we know what the Greeks knew: that intelligence and skill can only function at the peak of their capacity when the body is healthy and strong, and that hardy spirits and tough minds usually inhabit sound bodies." President John F. Kennedy stated it well when he said, "Physical fitness is the basis of all activities in our society; if our bodies grow soft and inactive, if we fail to encourage physical development and prowess, we will undermine our capacity for thought, for work, and for the use for those skills vital to an expanding and complex America."

There is no substitute for regular exercise for building physical fitness.

There is no doubt that heredity, nutrition, and other aspects of positive lifestyles all contribute to good physical fitness. Nevertheless, regular, properly done exercise is essential for the development of optimal physical fitness.

CHART 2.1 Physical Fitness Stunts

Item	Fitness Aspect	Pass	
1. *One foot balance*. Stand on one foot; press up so that the weight is on the ball of the foot with the heel off the floor. Hold the hands out in front and the other leg straight.	Balance (10 sec.)	Yes ☐	
2. *Long jump*. Stand with the toes behind a line; using no run or hop step, jump as far as possible. To pass, men must jump their height plus six inches. Women must jump their height only.	Power	Yes ☐	
3. *Jack spring*. From a standing position, jump into the air, kick the legs up and out and touch the feet with the hands. Repeat 2 times, touching the floor once between jumps.	Agility	Yes ☐	
4. *Paper drop*. Have a partner hold a piece of paper so that the side edge is between your thumb and index finger about the width of your hand from the top of the page. When your partner drops the paper, catch it before it slips through the thumb and finger. Do not move your hand lower to catch the paper.	Reaction time	Yes ☐	

CHART 2.1 *continued*

Item	Fitness Aspect	Pass	
5. *Double heel click*. With the feet apart, jump into the air and tap the heels together twice before you hit the ground. You must land with your feet at least 3 inches apart.	Speed	Yes ☐	
6. *Paper ball bounce*. Wad up a sheet of notebook paper into a ball. Bounce the ball back and forth between the right and left hands. Keep the hands open and palms up. Bounce the ball three times with each hand (6 total). Alternate hands for each bounce.	Coordination	Yes ☐	
7. *Run in place*. Run in place for 1 and ½ minutes (120 steps per minute). Rest for 1 minute and count the heart rate for 30 seconds. A heart rate of 60 or lower passes.	Cardiovascular fitness	Yes ☐	
8. *Toe touch*. Sit on the floor with your feet against a wall. Keep the feet together and the knees straight. Bend forward at the hips. Reach forward and touch your closed fists to the wall. Bend forward slowly, do not bounce.	Flexibility	Yes ☐	

CHART 2.1 *continued*

Item	Fitness Aspect	Pass
9. *The pinch.* Have a partner pinch a fold of skin on the back of your upper arm halfway between the tip of the elbow and the tip of the shoulder. Use your textbook to measure the skinfold width. Men: No greater than thickness of textbook. Women: No greater than one and one-half the thickness of the textbook.	Body composition (body fatness)	Yes ☐
10. *High leg press up.* Start in the push-up position with a partner holding the legs off the ground. Keep the body straight, press off the floor until the arms are fully extended. Women repeat once, men three times.	Strength	Yes ☐
11. *Four-minute hop.* With the hands behind the head, pogo hop over a line as many times as possible in four minutes. Five hundred jumps over the line passes.	Muscular endurance and cardiovascular fitness	Yes ☐

REFERENCES

"Children Who Want to Die." *Time* (September 25, 1978):82.

*Corbin, C. B., and R. Lindsey. *The Ultimate Fitness Book.* New York: Leisure Press, 1984.

Corbin, C. B., ed. *A Textbook of Motor Development.* Dubuque, IA: Wm. C. Brown Publishers, 1980.

Kennedy, J. F. "The Soft American." *Sports Illustrated* 13 (December 1960):15.

La Place, J. *Health.* 3d ed. Englewood Cliffs, NJ: Prentice-Hall, 1980.

*Paffenbarger, R. S., and R. T. Hyde. "Exercise as Protection Against Heart Attack." *New England Journal of Medicine* 302 (1980):1026.

Physician and Sportsmedicine. Published monthly, contains articles of all kinds on exercise, sports, and fitness.

Pollack, M. B., C. O. Purdy, and C. R. Carroll. *Health: A Way of Life.* Glenview, IL: Scott Foresman and Co., 1979.

Sherin, K. "Aerobic Exercise: Can You Answer the Question Patients Ask?" *Postgraduate Medicine* 73(1983):157.

Wicks, B. "Physical Fitness Programs in Business and Industry." *National Intramural and Recreational Sports Association Journal* 7(1983):31.

3
HYPOKINETIC DISEASE

CONCEPT 3

In many cases,
hypokinetic disease can be prevented or
treated with proper exercise.

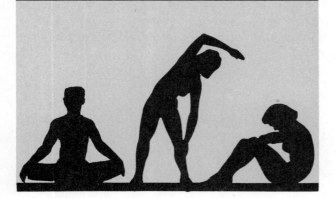

INTRODUCTION

One of the ways that exercise, and the resulting health-related physical fitness, contributes to optimal health is by helping to reduce the risk of hypokinetic disease and related conditions. Given the epidemic proportions of heart disease, the prevalence of back pain as a major adult complaint, the high incidence of overfatness among children as well as adults, and the dangers associated with the widespread existence of high blood pressure, ulcers, and mental disorders, the reduction of hypokinetic disease is a priority health concern for western culture.

TERMS

Angina Pectoris—Chest pain resulting from reduced oxygen supply to the heart muscle.

Arteriosclerosis—Conditions that cause the arterial walls to become thick, hard, and nonelastic; hardening of the arteries.

Atherosclerosis—The deposition of materials along the arterial walls; a type of arteriosclerosis.

Collateral Circulation—Development of auxiliary blood vessels that may take over normal coronary blood circulation to obstructed vessels in the event of diminished blood flow.

Congestive Heart Failure—The inability of the heart muscle to pump the blood at a life-sustaining rate.

Coronary Occlusion—The blocking of the coronary blood vessels.

Coronary Thrombosis—The formation of a clot that occludes, or blocks, a coronary artery.

Emotional Storm—A traumatic emotional experience that is likely to physiologically affect the human organism.

Fibrin—The substance that, in combination with blood cells, forms a blood clot.

Hypertension—Another word for high blood pressure.

Lipid—All fats and fatty substances.

Lipoprotein—Fat-carrying proteins in the blood.

Lordosis—Excessive lowback curve; swayback.

Parasympathetic Nervous System—Branch of the autonomic nervous system that slows the heart rate.

Referred Pain—Pain resulting from a problem in one part of the body, but felt at a different location.

Risk Factor—Any of the factors that increase the risk of hypokinetic diseases or conditions.

Sympathetic Nervous System—Branch of the autonomic nervous system that prepares the body for activity by speeding up the heart rate.

THE FACTS

The link between regular physical activity and good health is now well documented.

Based on the results of long-term research on large numbers of people, medical researchers have reached the following conclusion: "Evidence mounts that the relationship between exercise and good health is more than circumstantial. If some questions are not yet answered, they are far less important than those that have been" (Paffenbarger and Hyde, 1981). These researchers add that the true role of exercise has been known for centuries. In fact, several hundred years ago, John Dryden noted: "Better to hunt in fields, for health unbought, than fee the doctor for nauseous draught; the wise, for cure, on exercise depend; God never made his work for man to mend."

FACTS ABOUT EXERCISE, CARDIOVASCULAR FITNESS, AND HEART DISEASE

There are many different types of heart disease.

Hypertension (high blood pressure), atherosclerosis, arteriosclerosis, coronary occlusion, angina pectoris, and congestive heart failure are among the more prevalent forms of heart disease. Evidence indicates that inactivity may relate in some way to each of these types of heart disease.

A wealth of statistical evidence indicates that active people are less likely to have coronary heart disease than inactive people.

Much of the research relating inactivity to heart disease has come from occupational studies that show a high incidence of heart disease for people in occupations involving only sedentary work. Even with the limitations inherent in these types of studies, the findings of more and more occupational studies present convincing evidence that the inactive individual has an increased risk of coronary heart disease.

Studies also indicate that people who are physically active in their leisure time have a reduced risk of coronary heart disease if the exercise they choose is done above the cardiovascular threshold of training and in the cardiovascular fitness target zones.

Regular exercise is one effective means of rehabilitation for a person who has coronary heart disease or who has had a heart attack.

Not only does regular exercise seem to reduce the risk of developing coronary heart disease, there is also evidence that those who already have the condition may reduce the symptoms of the disease through regular exercise. For those who have had heart attacks, regular and progressive exercise can be an effective prescription when carried out under the supervision of a physician. It should be pointed out, however, that exercise is not the treatment of preference for all heart attack victims. In some cases, it may be contraindicated.

Recent decreases in the incidence of heart disease in the United States may be, in part, due to recent increases in activity levels of American adults.

In 1961, only 24 percent of Americans participated in regular physical activity. By 1980, more than twice as many American adults reported involvement in regular physical activity. During this same period of time, the incidence of heart disease decreased by 14 percent. While heart disease is still present in epidemic proportions (one in three males will have a heart attack by age sixty), many experts feel that the increase in regular exercise by previously sedentary Americans is one reason for the modest decreases in heart disease in the last two decades.

Contrary to popular belief, exercise does not cause "athlete's heart" nor does it injure the hearts of children.

The term *athlete's heart* is a misnomer. While some investigators have found increases in heart size as a result of training, this is not the pathological increase in size associated with heart disease. There is no evidence that heavy exercise injures a normal heart.

Many parents suggest that strenuous exercise is harmful to their children. To be sure, overstrenuous activity for long periods of time may have deleterious effects, but regular activity has no harmful effect on children's hearts.

There are many theories that attempt to explain the causes of coronary heart disease and the reasons regular exercise reduces the risk of this disease.

Six of the most plausible theories of heart disease are the Oxygen Pump Theory, the Lipid Deposit Theory, the Protective Protein Theory, the Fibrin Deposit Theory, the Coronary Collateral Circulation Theory, and the Loafer's Heart Theory. There is evidence that regular exercise relates in some way to each of these theories.

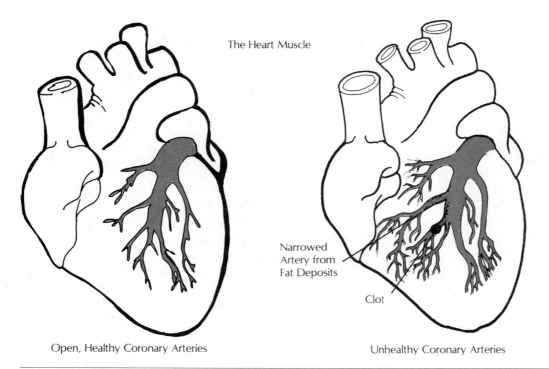

The Heart Muscle

Narrowed
Artery from
Fat Deposits

Clot

Open, Healthy Coronary Arteries

Unhealthy Coronary Arteries

FIGURE 3.1 Atherosclerosis

THE OXYGEN PUMP THEORY

There is evidence that regular exercise will increase the ability of the heart muscle to pump blood as well as oxygen.

The Oxygen Pump Theory suggests that a fit heart muscle is one that is able to handle any *extra* demands placed on it. Through regular exercise, the heart muscle gets stronger and therefore pumps more blood with each beat, resulting in a lessened heart rate and a greater heart efficiency. Of importance is the fact that the heart is just like any other muscle—it must be exercised regularly if it is to stay fit. The fit heart pumps more blood, thus supplying more oxygen during physical exertion and times of emotional stress.

THE LIPID DEPOSIT THEORY

There is evidence that exercise can reduce lipid deposit atherosclerosis and thus help to reduce the risk of heart disease.

The heart has its own arteries that supply blood to the heart muscle. If these vessels become clogged, there is danger of a heart attack. The Lipid Deposit Theory of heart disease suggests that one of the causes of heart disease may be the narrowing of the artery within the heart resulting from fat or lipid deposits on the walls of these arteries (atherosclerosis). If the deposits on the inner walls of the arteries become excessive, there is a diminished blood flow to the heart. Also, there is increased danger of a heart attack as a result of a clot

lodging in the already narrowed coronary artery (coronary thrombosis). (Refer to Figure 3.1.)

There are several kinds of fats in the bloodstream, including lipoproteins, phospholipids, triglycerides, and cholesterol. Whereas cholesterol is the most well-known fat, it may be no more a culprit than the other fats. Many blood fats are manufactured by the body itself, while others are ingested in high fat foods, particularly saturated fats (fats that are solid at room temperature). Whatever the source of the fat and the type of fat involved, the following two conclusions are justified by recent research.

1. Exercise can reduce blood fat levels, particularly for individuals who have above normal blood fat levels.
2. There is an increased risk of coronary heart disease with increased blood fat levels.

THE PROTECTIVE PROTEIN THEORY

There is evidence that exercise can increase levels of protective proteins in the blood and thus help reduce the risk of heart disease.

The Lipid Deposit Theory suggests that excess fats in the blood may result in atherosclerosis and may contribute to coronary heart disease. The Protective Protein Theory suggests that the levels of fat-carrying proteins (called lipoproteins) in the blood may be related to the incidence of coronary heart disease. Lipoproteins are of several sizes including large or very low

The Heart Muscle

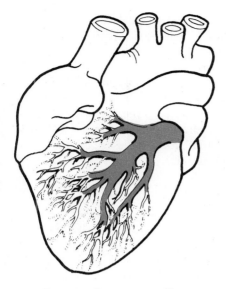

Dormant Coronary Arteries

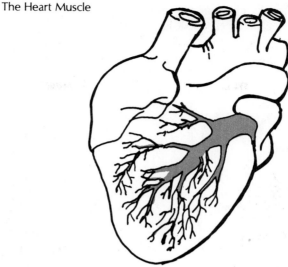

Open Coronary Collateral Arteries

FIGURE 3.2 Coronary Collateral Circulation

density (VLDL), medium or low density (LDL), and small or high density (HDL). It appears that the medium-sized lipoproteins (LDL) are undesirable because they may be deposited on the wall of the artery just as other fats described in the Lipid Deposit Theory. It also appears that the small lipoproteins (HDL) are protective proteins. People who have high levels of the small lipoproteins (HDL) in the blood have a lessened risk of coronary heart disease.

At this time, the best evidence suggests that high density lipoproteins (HDL), or protective blood proteins, pick up excess fats in the bloodstream and carry them to the liver where they are eliminated from the body. There is evidence that those who exercise regularly have higher levels of these proteins in the blood.

THE FIBRIN DEPOSIT THEORY

There is evidence that regular exercise can reduce fibrin deposit atherosclerosis and thus help reduce the risk of heart disease.

Fibrin is a sticky, threadlike substance in the bloodstream that is important to the blood-clotting process. The Fibrin Deposit Theory of heart disease suggests that the narrowing of the wall of the artery (atherosclerosis) may result from fibrin deposits. A heart attack may result from the diminished flow of blood to the heart caused by the fibrin deposits or by a clot lodged in the *now* narrowed artery.

The fibrin and lipid deposit theories are compatible, since it may be the deposits of both the sticky fibrin and fat that are responsible for atherosclerosis. If

this is correct, exercise may help prevent a heart attack. The following research findings form the basis for this statement:

1. Exercise causes the breakdown of fibrin in the blood, thus reducing its level in the blood.
2. Reduced blood fibrin may diminish the chances of development of fibrin atherosclerosis.
3. Reduced blood fibrin as a result of exercise may reduce the chance of a clot forming in the blood vessel.

THE CORONARY COLLATERAL CIRCULATION THEORY

There is evidence that regular exercise can improve coronary collateral circulation and thus reduce the risk of heart disease.

Within the heart, there are many tiny branches of the coronary arteries that supply blood to the heart muscle, as can be seen in Figure 3.2. These interconnecting arteries can supply blood to any region of the heart as it is needed. If a person is relatively inactive, these interconnecting arteries are functionally closed. During regular exercise, these extra blood vessels are opened up to provide the heart muscle with the necessary blood and oxygen. For a person with atherosclerosis (and evidence suggests most of us have some atherosclerosis beginning early in life) or a person who has suffered a heart attack, coronary collateral circulation may be very important. There is also evidence that the size of the coronary arteries increase as a result of exercise.

Improved coronary circulation may provide protection against a heart attack because a larger artery would require more atherosclerosis to occlude it. In addition, the development of collateral blood vessels supplying the heart may diminish the effects of an attack if one does occur. These "extra" (or collateral) blood vessels may take over the function of regular blood vessels during a heart attack.

THE LOAFER'S HEART THEORY

The heart of the inactive person is less able to resist stress and is more susceptible to "an emotional storm" that may precipitate a heart attack.

The heart is rendered inefficient by the following circumstances: high heart rate, high blood pressure, and excessive stimulation. Any of the above conditions requires the heart to use more oxygen than is normally necessary and decreases the heart's ability to adapt to stressful situations.

The "loafer's heart" is one that beats rapidly because it is dominated by the sympathetic nervous system, which speeds up the heart rate. Thus, the heart continually beats rapidly, even in resting situations, and never has a true rest period. Further, high blood pressure makes the heart work harder and contributes to its inefficiency.

Research indicates the following concerning exercise and the "loafer's heart."

1. Regular exercise leads to parasympathetic dominance rather than sympathetic dominance; thus heart rate is reduced and the heart works efficiently.
2. Regular exercise helps the heart rate return to normal faster after emotional stress.
3. Regular exercise strengthens the "loafer's heart," making the heart better able to weather "emotional storms."
4. Regular exercise may be one effective method of reducing high blood pressure.
5. Regular exercise decreases sympathetic dominance and its associated hormonal effects on the heart, thus lessening the chances of altered heart contractibility and the likelihood of the circulatory problems that accompany this state.

The theories of heart disease are compatible and it is likely that most cases of coronary heart disease are related in some way to more than one theory.

It is likely that any or all of the listed theories are correct and that exercise may help reduce the incidence of coronary heart disease in several ways. Since recent evidence indicates a decreased age for the onset of coronary heart disease, it seems especially important that any factor that might reduce heart attacks is considered.

There is no single cause or prevention of coronary heart disease. However, exercise is one of several factors that significantly relates to the incidence of coronary heart disease. There are benefits to the circulatory system, other than those already described, that may result from regular exercise.

1. Regular exercise may be *one* effective method of reducing high blood pressure (hypertension).
2. Regular exercise is necessary for the efficient return of venous blood to the heart after it is pumped to the body parts. People in standing occupations, such as barbers, dentists, etc., can improve venous return by regular exercise, especially exercise of the leg muscles. Excessive pooling of the blood in the legs resulting from inactivity may result in varicose veins.
3. There is some evidence that regular exercise may improve peripheral circulation (circulation to the arms, legs, and body parts other than the heart).
4. There is evidence that regular exercise may result in greater blood volume and a greater number of red blood cells, thus making the delivery of oxygen to the body more efficient.

THE FACTS ABOUT EXERCISE, MUSCLE FITNESS, AND BACK PAIN

Active people, who possess good flexibility, strength, and muscular endurance, are less likely to have back problems than inactive and unfit people.

Because few people die from it, back pain does not receive the attention that is heaped on such medical problems as heart disease and cancer. But back pain is considered to be the number one medical complaint in the United States, resulting in millions of hours of lost work annually, not to mention the hours of discomfort for those who are afflicted.

Over twenty-five years ago, medical doctors began to associate back problems with the lack of physical fitness. It is said that at least 85 percent of the common complaints are a result of poor muscle fitness, including poor flexibility, strength, and muscular endurance. Early tests done on patients complaining of back problems showed that they were exceptionally low in fitness. Results of similar tests of schoolchildren showed a failure rate of nearly 60 percent for American children as compared to less than 10 percent for children in four other countries. Current evidence indicates that as many as 50 percent of American children are still lacking in muscle fitness.

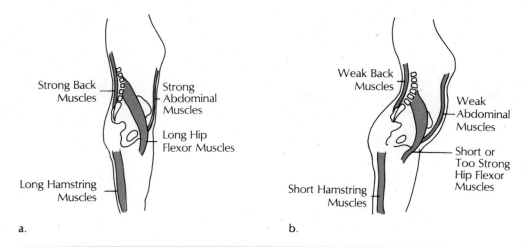

a.   b.

FIGURE 3.3 *(a)* Healthy and *(b)* Unhealthy Back

Inactivity statistics among adults in North America suggest that back problems will continue to be a problem until good muscle fitness becomes the rule rather than the exception. People who exercise in the target zones for building flexibility, strength, and muscular endurance can reduce the risk of musculoskeletal problems.

Regular exercise and good muscle fitness are not the only factors associated with risk of back pain.

Though lack of fitness is probably the leading reason for back pain in western society, there are many other factors that increase the risk of this ailment including poor posture, improper lifting and work habits, heredity, and other disease states, such as scoliosis and arthritis. Some of these will be discussed in greater detail in Concept 21.

There are many reasons why exercise can be effective in reducing the risk of back pain.

Proper exercise helps to prevent lordosis (excessive low back curve), muscle fatigue, referred pain, and muscle injury, all major factors in back pain.

Lordosis usually results from weak abdominals and short hip flexor muscles.

As can be seen in Figure 3.3, the lower part of the back normally has a slight inward curvature. If the lower back curve is too great, the muscles of the low back are more easily fatigued, are more likely to suffer muscle spasms, and are more likely to be injured.

The best way to prevent lordosis is to have strong abdominal muscles and long, but not too strong, hip flexor muscles. The strong abdominal muscles pull the bottom of the pelvis upward and help keep the top of the pelvis tipped backward, eliminating excessive back curve.

If the hip flexor muscles are too strong, or not long enough, they have the opposite effect of strong abdominal muscles; that is, they tip the top of the pelvis

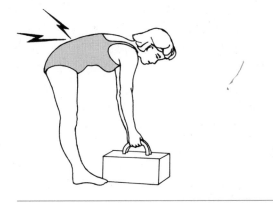

FIGURE 3.4 Muscle Spasms Result in Back Pain

forward causing excessive low back curve (lordosis). This is why it is important to have long, but not too strong, hip flexor muscles. As a general rule, flexibility exercises to lengthen the hip flexor muscles, as well as strength and endurance exercises for the abdominal muscles, are recommended. For obvious reasons, exercises to increase the strength of the hip flexor muscles are not recommended for those with back pain.

People who sit most of the day are especially likely to have short, weak back muscles, especially if they do no special exercises to lengthen and strengthen them. Through disuse, the muscles become short and weak so that even the slightest strain, as from improper lifting or sudden vigorous exercise, could result in muscle injury.

Hours of standing, on the other hand, as is done by a dentist or a store clerk, can result in muscle fatigue. Muscle fatigue and muscle injury can each result in muscle spasms evidenced in back pain. Regular, well-planned exercise to strengthen and lengthen the back muscles is important in the prevention of such pain. (See Figure 3.4.)

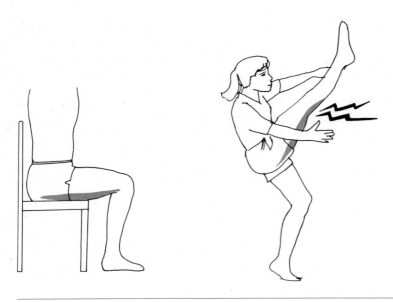

FIGURE 3.5   Referred Pain

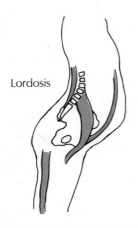

Lordosis

FIGURE 3.6   Back Pain Caused by Protruding Abdomen

Referred pain from short leg muscles can result in back pain.

Inactive people, especially those who sit a lot, are likely to have short muscles in the back of the upper leg or hamstring muscles (see Fig. 3.5). When short hamstring muscles are overstretched, spasms or injury may occur. Often the pain from hamstring muscle soreness can be referred to the low back and result in low back pain. Referred pain, or pain felt in an area other than where the pain originates, can be reduced by doing regular exercise to lengthen the short muscles.

Protruding abdomen can increase the risk of back pain.

If the abdomen or "gut" sticks out too far over the belt line, problems with the back muscles can result. The extra weight of the protruding "gut" can cause lordosis by pulling the top of the pelvis forward. This can result in extra strain on the low back muscles and can precipitate muscle fatigue, soreness, or injury. Strengthening of the abdominal muscles and a loss of body fat are advised for those with this problem (Fig. 3.6).

Back pain caused by muscle spasms can usually be reduced or relieved with static stretching of back and leg muscles.

A stretch held for twenty to sixty seconds can break what is known as the "spasm cycle," helping to relieve the muscle pain. (See Concept 16, exercises 9–14.)

THE FACTS ABOUT EXERCISE, HEALTH-RELATED FITNESS, AND OTHER HYPOKINETIC CONDITIONS

Many musculoskeletal problems, including poor posture, neck, leg, and foot pain are associated with inactivity and poor health-related physical fitness.

Regular exercise, particularly exercise designed to increase strength, muscular endurance, and flexibility, can help alleviate neck, leg, and foot pain and can help improve posture. Slow stretching and tension reduction exercises, such as those described in Concept 19, can help relieve the symptoms of muscle tension.

Obesity, as well as lesser degrees of overfatness, is not a disease state in itself, but is a hypokinetic condition that is associated with a multitude of far-reaching complications.

Obesity is associated with serious organic impairments, shortened life, psychological maladjustments, poor relationships with peers (especially among children), awkward physical movement, and a lack of achievement in athletic activities. Obesity can be both a cause and an effect of physical unfitness. Those who are overfat have a higher risk of respiratory infections, a prevalence of high blood pressure and atherosclerosis, and are prone to disorders of the circulatory, respiratory, and kidney systems. The symptoms of adult-onset diabetes are associated with excessive fatness. (Fortunately, fat loss to normal levels is usually followed by remission of diabetic symptoms.) Because exercise, together with sound nutritional management, is an effective means of lowering body fat, it can be helpful in reducing the risks of those conditions associated with overfatness and obesity.

Bone degeneration due to atrophy (osteoporosis) can be considered a hypokinetic condition.

Studies indicate that excessive bed rest can result in deterioration of the bones. When the long bones do not bear weight, they lose calcium and become porous and fragile. Even excessive sitting can result in bone deterioration, regardless of age. Bones are strengthened, not only by bearing weight, but by the pull of active muscles. Regular exercise is as necessary for healthy bone development as it is for healthy muscle development. The osteoporosis commonly seen in older adults (especially women) is caused by a loss of hormone, as well as this lack of activity.

Common stress-related disorders can be considered hypokinetic conditions.

Some of the stress-related conditions prevalent in modern society are discussed in Concept 19. However, a few that are associated with inactive lifestyles are discussed here.

Insomnia is a condition that afflicts many people in our culture and one that is often stress-related. Results of a survey of American adults indicates that 52 percent feel that one of the benefits of regular exercise is that it helps them to sleep better.

Depression is another stress-related condition that is experienced by many adults. In fact, one study found that 33 percent of inactive adults claimed that they often felt depressed. For some, depression is a serious psychosis and exercise alone will not cure it; however, recent research does indicate that exercise, combined with other forms of therapy, can be effective in its treatment. For those with minor depression, exercise may also be helpful. Studies show 34 percent of those considered to be very active, feel that regular exercise helps them to better cope with life's pressures. deVries found exercise was as effective as an antidepressant drug in relieving depression.

Even more common than depression and insomnia is the condition called *Type A behavior.* "Type A personalities" are stress-prone individuals with a greater than normal incidence of diseases. A "Type A" person is tense, overly competitive, and worried about meeting time schedules. Regular exercise can be of special benefit to the "Type A" person, though non-competitive exercise would probably be best.

In many cases, gastric ulcers may be considered a hypokinetic condition.

In their classic work, *Hypokinetic Disease,* Kraus and Raab theorized that gastric ulcers could be considered a hypokinetic condition because inactive individuals have a higher mortality rate from the condition than active people. Their conclusion must be considered tentative at best; however, the lesser incidence of ulcer disease among active people, plus the fact that exercise can be effective in helping to manage stress and tension levels often associated with ulcer disease, suggest that regular exercise may be useful for some people in the prevention or management of symptoms of the disease.

Hypokinetic diseases and conditions have many different causes.

Regular exercise is only one of the factors associated with reduced risk of hypokinetic diseases and conditions. Whereas exercise is the focus of this concept, nutrition (see Concept 18), smoking, lifestyles, heredity, stress (see Concept 19), age (see Concept 22), and environment cannot be overlooked as important risk factors. Many of these important hypokinetic disease risk factors are discussed in Concept 21.

CHART 3.1 Incidence of Hypokinetic Diseases and Conditions

Listed here are various hypokinetic diseases and conditions. In the column beside each condition or disease, place a check (✔) if you possess it, if one of your close relatives possesses it, or if one of your close friends possesses it. Close relatives are the four or five people you consider to be closest to you, whether parents, brothers, sisters, grandparents, spouse, or children. Close friends are the four or five nonrelatives you care about most. You need not live close to the individual to classify him or her as a close friend or relative.

The Hypokinetic Disease or Condition	Self	Close Relative	Close Friend
1. Heart disease	☐	☐	☐
2. High blood pressure	☐	☐	☐
3. Back pain or problems	☐	☐	☐
4. Overfat or obese	☐	☐	☐
5. Ulcer	☐	☐	☐
6. Diabetes	☐	☐	☐
7. Insomnia	☐	☐	☐
8. Depression	☐	☐	☐
9. Type A personality	☐	☐	☐
Column Totals	————	————	————

REFERENCES

Boyer, J. L. "Effects of Chronic Exercise on Cardiovascular Function." *Physical Fitness Research Digest* 2(1972):1.

Brownell, K. D., et al. "Changes in Plasma Lipid and Lipoprotein Levels in Men and Women after a Moderate Exercise Program." *Circulation* 65(1982):477.

Clarke, H. H., ed. "Exercise and Fat Reduction." *Physical Fitness Research Digest* 5(1975):1.

Clarke, H. H., ed. "Update: Exercise and Some Coronary Risk Factors." *Physical Fitness Research Digest* 9(1979):1.

Connor, J. F., et al. "Effects of Exercise on Coronary Collateralization: Angiographic Analysis of Six Patients in a Supervised Exercise Program." *Medicine and Science in Exercise and Sports* 8(1976):145.

Corbin, C. B., and M. L. Noble. "Flexibility." *Journal of Physical Education, Recreation and Dance* 51(1980):23.

Corbin, C. B., ed. *A Textbook of Motor Development*. Dubuque, IA: Wm. C. Brown Publishers, 1980.

Corbin, C. B. "Flexibility." In *Clinics in Sportsmedicine: Profiling*, edited by J. Nicholas and E. Hershman. Philadelphia: W. B. Saunders Co., 1984.

Cunningham, D. A., et al. "The Effects of Training: Physiological Responses." *Medicine and Science in Sports and Exercise* 11(1979):379.

de Vries, H. A. "Physiological Effects of an Exercise Training Regimen upon Men Aged 52–88." *Journal of Gerontology* 25(1970):325.

Durrah, M. I., and R. L. Engen. "Beneficial Effects of Exercise on 1–Isoproterenol-Induced Myocardial Infarction in Male Rats." *Medicine and Science in Sports and Exercise* 14(1982):76.

Felig, P., and J. Wahren. "Fuel Homeostasis in Exercise." *New England Journal of Medicine* 293(1975):559.

Felig, P., et al. "Hypoglycemia during Prolonged Exercise in Normal Men." *New England Journal of Medicine* 306(1982):895.

Frey, M. A., et al. "Exercise Training, Sex Hormones, and Lipoprotein Relationships in Men." *Journal of Applied Physiology* 55(1983):757.

*Friedman, M., and K. H. Rosenman. *Type A Behavior and Your Heart*. New York: A. A. Knopf, 1974.

Gibbons, L. W., et al. "The Acute Risk of Strenuous Exercise." *Journal of the American Medical Association* 244 (1980):1979.

Griest, J. H., et al. "Running Through Your Mind." In *Psychology of Running*, edited by M. H. Sacks and M. L. Sachs. Champaign, IL: Human Kinetics, 1981.

Hall, J. A. "Effects of Diet and Exercise on Peripheral Vascular Disease." *Physician and Sportsmedicine* 10(1982):90.

Harris, L., and Associates. *The Perrier Study: Fitness in America.* New York: Great Waters of France, 1979.

Hartung, G. H., and W. G. Squires. "Exercise and HDL Cholesterol in Middle-Aged Men." *Physician and Sportsmedicine* 8(1980):74.

Hartung, G. H., et al. "Relation of Diet to High Density-Lipoprotein Cholesterol in Middle-Aged Marathon Runners, Joggers, and Inactive Men." *New England Journal of Medicine* 302(1980):357.

Heaton, W. H., et al. "Beneficial Effect of Physical Training on Blood Flow to the Myocardium Perfused by Chronic Collaterals in the Exercising Dog." *Circulation* 57(1978):575.

Kannel, W. B., and P. Sorlie. "Some Health Benefits of Physical Activity: The Framingham Study." *Archives of Internal Medicine* 139(1979):857.

Keim, H. A., and W. H. Kirkaldy-Willis. "Low Back Pain." *Clinical Symposia* 32(1980):6.

Knight, D. R., and H. L. Stone. "Alteration of Ischemic Cardiac Function in the Normal Heart by Daily Exercise." *Journal of Applied Physiology* 55(1983):52.

Kornitzer, M. "Belgian Heart Disease Prevention Project: Incidence and Mortality Results." *Lancet* 8333(1983):1066.

Kransch, D. M., et al. "Reduction of Coronary Atherosclerosis by Moderate Conditioning Exercise in Monkeys on an Atherogenic Diet." *New England Journal of Medicine* 305(1981):1983.

*Kraus, H., and W. Raab. *Hypokinetic Disease.* Springfield, IL: Charles C. Thomas, 1961.

Lamb, D. R. *Physiology of Exercise.* New York: MacMillan Publishers, 1978.

Lehtonin, A., and J. Viikari. "Serum Lipids in Soccer and Ice Hockey Players." *Metabolism* 29(1980):36.

Levy, R. "Declining Mortality in Cardiovascular Disease." *Atherosclerosis* 5(1981):312.

Lindsey, R., et al. *Fitness for Health, Figure/Physique and Posture.* 5th ed. Dubuque, IA: Wm. C. Brown Publishers, 1983.

Maciejko, J., et al. "Apolipoprotein A-I as a Marker of Angiographically Assessed Coronary-Artery Disease." *New England Journal of Medicine* 309(1983):385.

Mann, G. V. "The Influence of Obesity on Health." *New England Journal of Medicine* 291(1974):178.

Mayer, J. *Overweight Causes, Costs and Control.* Englewood Cliffs, NJ: Prentice-Hall, 1968.

Montoye, H. J., et al. "Bone Mineralization in Tennis Players." *Scandinavian Journal of Sport Science* 2(1980):26.

Multiple Risk Factor Intervention Trial Research Group. "Multiple Risk Factor Intervention Trial." *Journal of the American Medical Association* 248(1982):1465.

Nabisco/AAU. *Toasted Wheat and Raisins/AAU Fitness Profile of American Youth.* Chicago: Golin-Harris, 1983.

Paffenbarger, R. S., et al. "Current Exercise and Heart Attack Risk." *Cardiac Rehabilitation* 10(1979):1.

*Paffenbarger, R. S., and R. T. Hyde. "Exercise as Protection Against Heart Attack." *New England Journal of Medicine* 302(1980):1026.

Research and Forecasts, Inc. *The Miller Lite Report on American Attitudes toward Sports.* Milwaukee: Miller Brewing Co., 1983.

Rose, G., et al. "The United Kingdom Heart Disease Prevention Project: Incidence and Mortality Results." *Lancet* 8333(1983):1062.

Ryan, A. "Heart Size and Sports." *Physician and Sportsmedicine* 8(1980):30.

*Sherin, K. "Aerobic Exercise: Can You Answer Questions Patients Ask?" *Postgraduate Medicine* 73(1983):157.

Simons, D. G., and J. G. Travell. "Myofascial Origins of Low Back Pain." *Postgraduate Medicine* 73(1983):157.

Skinner, J. "Longevity, General Health, and Exercise." In *Exercise Physiology,* edited by H. B. Falls. New York: Academic Press, 1968.

Smith, M. P., et al. "Exercise Intensity, Dietary Intake and High-Density Lipoprotein Cholesterol in Young Female Competitive Swimmers." *American Journal of Clinical Nutrition* 36(1983):251.

Storer, T. W., and R. O. Ruhling. "Essential Hypertension and Exercise." *Physician and Sportsmedicine* 9(1981):58.

Thompson, P. D., et al. "Incidence of Death during Jogging in Rhode Island from 1975 through 1980." *Journal of the American Medical Association* 247 (1982):2535.

Travell, J. G., and D. G. Simons. *Myofascial Pain and Dysfunction.* Baltimore: Williams and Williams, 1983.

Williams, R. S., et al. "Physical Conditioning Augments the Fibrinolytic Response to Venous Occlusion in Healthy Adults." *New England Journal of Medicine* 302(1980):987.

World Health Organization European Collaborative Group. "Multifactorial Trial in the Prevention of CHD." *European Heart Journal* 3(1982):184.

World Health Organization European Collaborative Group. "Changes in Risk Factors with Intervention." *European Heart Journal* 4(1983):141.

Zung, V. T., et al. "The Effects of Exercise on Blood Lipids and Lipoproteins: A Metaanalysis of Studies." *Medicine and Science in Sports and Exercise* 15(1983):393.

4
PREPARING FOR EXERCISE

CONCEPT 4

Proper preparation can help make exercise enjoyable, effective, and safe.

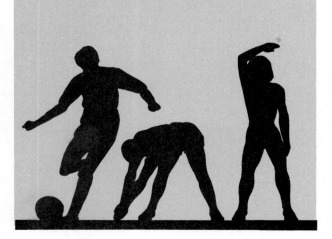

INTRODUCTION

More than at any other time in recent history, adults are engaging in some form of regular exercise during their free time. Unfortunately, all too often those who start an exercise program with good intentions "drop out" after a few days, weeks, or months. As noted in Concept 1, a part of the problem is that people lack information concerning the correct way to exercise.

For those just beginning an exercise program, adequate preparation may be the key to persistence. It is hoped that a person armed with good information about preparing for exercise will become involved and stay involved with that exercise for a lifetime. To be effective, exercise must be something that is a part of a person's normal lifestyle. Some facts that will help you to prepare for exercise and help you to make it part of your normal routine are presented in this concept.

TERMS

PAR-Q—A questionnaire designed to help you determine if you are medically suited to begin an exercise program; the Physical Activity Readiness Questionnaire.

PAR-X—A form used by physicians to determine a person's readiness for a program of regular physical activity; the Physical Activity Readiness Examination.

Achilles Tendon—The long tendon that attaches the calf muscles (the back of the lower leg) to the heel bone (on the back of the foot).

Warm-Up Exercise—Light to moderate activity, including stretching, done prior to serious exercise. Its purpose is to reduce the risk of injury and soreness and possibly to improve performance in a physical activity.

Cool-Down Exercise—Light to moderate tapering-off activity after vigorous exercise; often consisting of the same exercises used in the warm-up.

THE FACTS

Before beginning a regular exercise program, it is important to establish that you are medically ready to participate.

There is no way to be absolutely sure that you are medically sound to begin an exercise program. Even a thorough exam by a physician cannot guarantee that a person does not have some limitations that may cause a problem during exercise. However, an exam is the surest way to make certain that you are ready to participate.

The American College of Sports Medicine, in its guidelines for evaluating health status for exercise participation, suggests that people who are physically active and who have no symptoms of heart disease do not need special medical consultation except after an illness or injury, or when planning to make major modifications in their current exercise programs. The College advises medical consultation especially for those thirty-five years of age or older. For those less than thirty-five who are inactive, but who have no symptoms of heart disease, medical consultation is not necessary unless there is a question about the person's health status or if the person is at high risk for heart disease (high blood pressure, smoker, abnormal ECG, etc.). If an individual is at high risk (see Lab 21 to check your own risk) of heart disease, and even if he or she has no disease symptoms, a medical exam is recommended. For those thirty-five or older who are inactive, the College recommends a medical exam even for those without a high risk of heart disease.

Recently the British Columbia (Canada) Ministry of Health conducted extensive research to devise a procedure that would help people know when it was advisable to seek medical consultation prior to beginning or altering an exercise program. The goal was to prevent unnecessary medical examinations, while at the same time giving a reasonable assurance that regular exercise was appropriate for a given individual. The research resulted in the development of two questionnaires, both now used nationally in Canada. The first, the PAR-Q, consists of seven simple questions you can ask yourself to determine if medical consultation is necessary prior to exercise involvement. The second, the PAR-X, is a special form developed for use by physicians. It aids the physician in knowing what to include in a pre-exercise exam and in giving advice to prospective exercisers after an exam.

To help you decide whether to have a complete medical exam before you begin or modify your exercise program, or whether to adopt the American College of Sports Medicine Guidelines, complete the PAR-Q, provided in the Lab Resource Materials on page 31. Those who choose to seek medical consultation, including an examination, may wish to make the PAR-X form available to the examining physician (see Appendix A).

It is important to dress properly for exercise.

The clothing you wear for exercise should be specifically for that exercise. It should be comfortable and not too tight or binding at the joints. Though appearance is important to everyone, comfort in exercise is more important than looks. Clothing should not restrict movement in any way, and it is preferable that the clothing that comes in direct contact with the body be porous to allow for sweat absorption. Some women, especially those who need extra support, should consider using an exercise bra, and men will need an athletic supporter. Warm-up suits rather than other exercise apparel are recommended because they can be removed during exercise if desired. Many exercise suits are nonporous and so, by themselves, are not desirable for exercise.

Proper exercise footwear is important.

There are many types of exercise footwear. Jogging/running shoes and multipurpose shoes are the most common, although some sports participants, such as basketball players, prefer a high top shoe. Jogging/running shoes are specialty shoes designed specifically for jogging and running, although they are suitable for walking. These shoes should have a high back to support the Achilles tendon, a wide, cushioned, and elevated heel, good arch support, and adequate room for the toes. The exterior of the heel should be rounded and the exterior sole should be flexible with a rippled or dimpled tread.

A multipurpose shoe is not recommended for jogging and running, but is well suited for most court sports. It should have a cushioned heel, a good arch support, and adequate toe room. But unlike the running shoe, the multipurpose shoe should have a smooth or court sole tread and a narrower, nonelevated heel.

Regardless of the type of shoe worn, exercise shoes should generally be one-half size larger than your regular shoes, and if you wear two pairs of socks while exercising, you should wear two pairs when trying on the shoes. It is important to try on the shoes and move around in them before making a purchase. Make sure they feel good to you. Quality should not be sacrificed for appearance or to save a few dollars. Good quality shoes can help prevent foot and leg problems that make exercise ineffective and unenjoyable.

Probably the biggest "shoe" mistake is failure to replace them when they are worn-out. The condition of the sole of the shoe is far less important than the breakdown of the heel (rundown to the inside or outside), or disproportionate wear that results in unusual movement patterns. It is better to replace shoes too soon than to risk injury from worn-out shoes.

It takes time for exercise to benefit health-related physical fitness.

Sometimes people just beginning an exercise program expect immediate results. They expect to see large losses in body fat in short periods of time, or great increases in muscle strength in just a few days. Evidence tells us, however, that improvements in health-related physical fitness and the associated health benefits take several weeks to become apparent. Though some people report psychological benefits, such as "feeling better" and a "sense of personal accomplishment," almost immediately after beginning regular exercise, the physiological changes will take considerably longer to be realized. Proper preparation for exercise includes learning not to expect too much too soon, nor to do too much too soon. Attempts to "overdo it" and to try to "get fit fast" will probably be counterproductive, resulting in soreness and even injury. The key is to start slowly, stay with it, and enjoy the exercise. Benefits will come to those who persist.

A warm-up prior to exercise is important.

There are two good reasons for warming up prior to exercise. The first is to stretch the skeletal muscles to help prevent muscle soreness and injury. The second is to prepare the heart muscle for exercise.

The skeletal muscle warm-up should include static stretching of the major muscle groups involved in the exercise that is to follow (see Concepts 9 and 14). It should be emphasized that even though warming up prior to an activity may help reduce the chance of muscle injury, it is not a substitute for a regular program of exercise designed to improve flexibility.

A warm-up designed to prepare the heart muscle for moderate to vigorous exercise should include approximately two minutes of walking, jogging, or mild exercise. Research shows that for some people, starting vigorous exercise abruptly is not wise. Apparently in some exercises, the increased blood flow to the heart and other muscles does not immediately increase when the exercise begins, at least not for all people. Adults who do this type of warm-up do not experience electrocardiogram abnormalities that are apparent in some people who do not warm up.

We have included a warm-up that is suitable for walking, jogging, running, cycling, and even basketball. This warm-up can be used for other activities if stretching exercises for the major muscle groups involved in various activities are added. (Some good stretching exercises are described in Concept 14.) The cardiovascular warm-up is suitable for most activities, but other mild exercise, such as a slow, two-minute swim for swimmers, or a slow, two-minute ride on a bicycle for cyclists, can be substituted.

There is a minimal and an optimal amount of exercise for producing improvements in health-related physical fitness.

Each component of health-related physical fitness has a "threshold of training" (minimal amount of exercise) necessary for improvement. Each component also has a "target zone;" that is, an optimal frequency, intensity, and time (duration) of exercise necessary to produce fitness gains. A properly prepared program includes exercise *above* the threshold level and *in* the target zone for *each part of health-related fitness.* (The general concepts of threshold of training and exercise target zones are covered in greater depth in Concept 5. Specific threshold and target zone recommendations for each of the five components of health-related fitness are included in Concepts 6–10.)

A cool down after exercise is important.

Proper exercise planning is very important. One part of this planning is the organization of each exercise session. Each session should include a **warm-up,** a **workout,** and a **cool down.** The warm-up has already been discussed. The workout, or actual exercise, is discussed in greater detail in later concepts. The cool down is done immediately after the workout.

Like the warm-up, there are two principal components of a cool down: static muscle stretching and an activity for the cardiovascular system. Some experts believe that static muscle stretching *after* the workout is more important than stretching before because it can help reduce delayed localized soreness, or muscle pain, felt the day after exercise, as well as help to prevent shortening of the muscles in general. There is still some controversy about the best time to stretch and about the benefits of warming up and cooling down. However, given current evidence, both a warm-up and cool down seem wise.

The exercises shown here can be used before an aerobic workout as a warm-up, or after workout as a cool down. This sample program would be good before jogging, walking, or cycling. It includes slow cardiovascular exercise, as well as stretching for the lower and upper legs, the hip and back, and the trunk. If the activity you plan to do requires considerable use of different areas of the body, you should add stretching and circulatory exercises for those areas of the body (see Concept 14). Perform the exercises slowly. Do not bounce or jerk against the muscle. Hold each stretch for at least ten seconds. Perform each exercise at least once and up to three times. You may wish to have someone passively assist you in doing the exercise but, if so, you should read Concept 9 first.

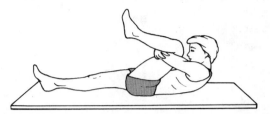

Leg Hug (For the Hip and Back)

Lie on your back. Bend one leg and grasp the thigh under the knee. Hug it to your chest. Keep the other leg straight and on the floor. Curl your head, then your shoulders, forward and upward. Hold. Repeat with the opposite leg.

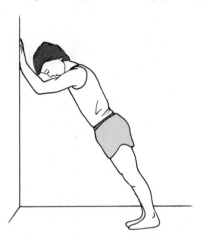

Calf Stretcher (For Back of Lower Leg)

Face a wall with your feet two to three feet away. Lean forward to allow both hands to touch the wall. Turn the toes inward slightly, keeping your heels on the ground, the knees straight, and the buttocks tucked in. Lean forward by bending the arms and allowing the head to move nearer the wall. Hold.

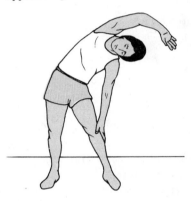

Side Stretch

With the feet apart approximately shoulder width, lean to one side. Reach down with the arm on that side and reach up over your head with the opposite arm. Let your body weight stretch the muscles as you lean downward. Do not twist. Hold. Repeat to the other side.

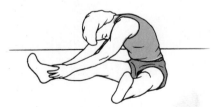

Toe Touch (For Back of Upper Leg)

Sit on the floor. Spread your feet two to three feet apart. Bend at the hip and reach forward with both hands. Grasp one foot, ankle, or calf, depending upon how far you can reach. Pull forward with your arms trying to touch your head to your knee. Keep your knee relatively straight. Hold. Repeat with the opposite leg.

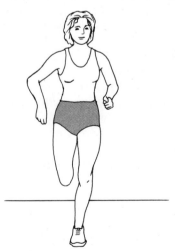

The Cardiovascular Warm-up

Before you perform a vigorous workout, walk or jog slowly for two minutes. After exercise, do the same.

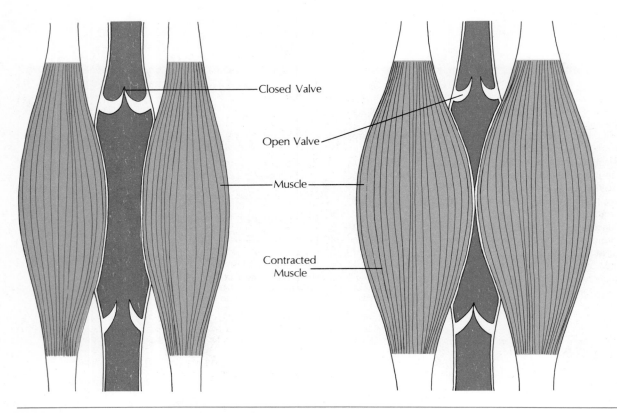

Closed Valve

Open Valve

Muscle

Contracted Muscle

FIGURE 4.1 The Pumping Action of the Muscles

A cardiovascular cool down is also important. During exercise, the heart pumps a large amount of blood to the working muscles to supply the oxygen necessary to keep moving. The muscles squeeze the veins (Fig. 4.1), which forces the blood back to the heart. Valves in the veins prevent the blood from flowing backward. As long as exercise continues, the blood is moved by the muscles back to the heart, where it is once again pumped to the body. If exercise is stopped abruptly, the blood is left in the area of the working muscles and has no way to get back to the heart. In the case of the runner, the blood pools in the legs. Because the heart has less blood to pump, blood pressure may drop. This can result in dizziness, and can even cause a person to pass out. The best way to prevent this problem is to taper off or slow down gradually after exercise. A cardiovascular cool down should include approximately two minutes of walking or slow jogging, or any nonvigorous activity that uses the muscles that were involved in the workout.

The same program used for the warm-up (see page 29) may be used to cool down after exercise. For variety, you can choose some of the stretching exercises included in Concept 14.

It may be necessary to alter exercise programs or adjust exercise schedules to accommodate the weather and environmental conditions.

Good preparation for exercise includes making adjustments in the content and the time of the exercise workout to account for cold, heat, humidity, and other environmental factors that might make exercise less enjoyable, less effective, or unsafe. For more information on appropriate dress and guidelines for working out in different climatic conditions, refer to Concept 17.

PHYSICAL ACTIVITY READINESS QUESTIONNAIRE (PAR-Q)*
A Self-administered Questionnaire for Adults

PAR Q & YOU

PAR-Q is designed to help you help yourself. Many health benefits are associated with regular exercise, and the completion of PAR-Q is a sensible first step to take if you are planning to increase the amount of physical activity in your life.

For most people physical activity should not pose any problem or hazard. PAR-Q has been designed to identify the small number of adults for whom physical activity might be inappropriate or those who should have medical advice concerning the type of activity most suitable for them.

Common sense is your best guide in answering these few questions. Please read them carefully and check the ☑ YES or NO opposite the question if it applies to you.

YES NO

☐ ☐ 1. Has your doctor ever said you have heart trouble?

☐ ☐ 2. Do you frequently have pains in your heart and chest?

☐ ☐ 3. Do you often feel faint or have spells of severe dizziness?

☐ ☐ 4. Has a doctor ever said your blood pressure was too high?

☐ ☐ 5. Has your doctor ever told you that you have a bone or joint problem such as arthritis that has been aggravated by exercise, or might be made worse with exercise?

☐ ☐ 6. Is there a good physical reason not mentioned here why you should not follow an activity program even if you wanted to?

☐ ☐ 7. Are you over age 65 and not accustomed to vigorous exercise?

If You Answered

YES to one or more questions

If you have not recently done so, consult with your personal physician by telephone or in person BEFORE increasing your physical activity and/or taking a fitness test. Tell him what questions you answered YES on PAR-Q, or show him your copy.

programs

After medical evaluation, seek advice from your physician as to your suitability for:
- unrestricted physical activity, probably on a gradually increasing basis.
- restricted or supervised activity to meet your specific needs, at least on an initial basis. Check in your community for special programs or services.

NO to all questions

If you answered PAR-Q accurately, you have reasonable assurance of your present suitability for:
- A GRADUATED EXERCISE PROGRAM - A gradual increase in proper exercise promotes good fitness development while minimizing or eliminating discomfort.
- AN EXERCISE TEST - Simple tests of fitness (such as the Canadian Home Fitness Test) or more complex types may be undertaken if you so desire.

postpone

If you have a temporary minor illness, such as a common cold.

---

* Developed by the British Columbia Ministry of Health. Conceptualized and critiqued by the Multidisciplinary Advisory Board on Exercise (MABE).
Reference: PAR-Q Validation Report, British Columbia Ministry of Health, May, 1978.
* Produced by the British Columbia Ministry of Health and the Department of National Health & Welfare.

REFERENCES

*American College of Sports Medicine. *Guidelines for Graded Exercise Testing and Exercise Prescription.* 2d ed. Philadelphia: Lea and Febiger, 1980.

*Barnard, R. J. "The Heart Needs a Warm-Up Time." *Physician and Sportsmedicine* 4 (1976):40.

*Chisholm, D. M., et al. "Physical Activity Readiness." *British Columbia Medical Journal* 17 (1975):375.

Chisholm, D. M., et al. *Par-Q Validation Report.* Victoria, British Columbia: British Columbia Ministry of Health, 1978.

Corbin, C. B. "Flexibility." *Clinics in Sports Medicine: Profiting,* edited by J. Nicholas and E. Hershman. Philadelphia: W. B. Saunders Co., 1984.

de Vries, H. A. *Physiology of Exercise.* 3d ed. Dubuque, IA: Wm. C. Brown Publishers, 1980.

Mead, W. F. and R. Hartwig. "Fitness Evaluation and Exercise Prescription." *Journal of Family Practice* 13 (1981):1039.

*Shellock, F. G. "Physiological Benefits of Warm-Up." *Physician and Sportsmedicine* 11 (1983):134.

5

Threshold of Training and Target Zones for Health-Related Physical Fitness

CONCEPT 5

There is a minimal
and an optimal amount of exercise necessary
for developing each of
the health-related aspects of physical fitness.

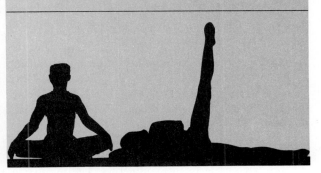

INTRODUCTION

Just as there is a correct dosage of medicine for treating an illness, there is a correct dosage of exercise for developing physical fitness. The minimum amount (dose) of exercise is called the *threshold of training*. The fitness *target zone* is the optimal amount of physical activity for developing physical fitness.

TERMS

Fitness Target Zone—A range of exercise from the minimum necessary to improve fitness, to the maximum amount, beyond which exercise may be counterproductive. If you exercise above the minimum and below the maximum, you are exercising in the fitness target zone.

The Overload Principle—A basic principle of physical fitness that specifies that for a component of fitness to improve, you must "overload" by putting more stress on the muscle than it normally encounters in daily use.

Threshold of Training—The minimum amount of exercise that will improve physical fitness.

THE FACTS

The overload principle is the basis for improving physical fitness.

In order for a muscle (including the heart muscle) to get stronger, it must be "overloaded," or worked against a load greater than normal. To increase flexibility, a muscle must be stretched longer than is normal. To increase muscular endurance, muscles must be exposed to sustained exercise for a longer than normal period. If overload is less than normal for a specific component of fitness, the result will be a decrease in that particular component of fitness. A normal amount of exercise will maintain the current fitness level.

There is no substitute for overload in developing physical fitness.

Many people do not overload enough to develop good fitness. Often the programs found in health clubs and in exercises described in popular books and magazines do not provide for adequate overload. Some people try exercise machines, special foods or medicines, or quack devices that violate the overload principle and are therefore ineffective.

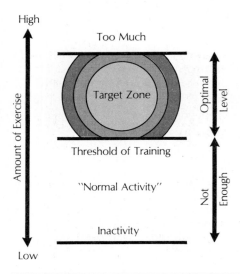

High

Amount of Exercise

Low

Too Much

Target Zone

Threshold of Training

"Normal Activity"

Inactivity

Optimal Level

Not Enough

FIGURE 5.1 Exercise Target Zones *Adapted from Laurie, D. R., and Corbin, C. B.* How Much Exercise Is Enough? *Manhattan, KS: Master Teacher, 1980. An audiovisual program.*

To get fit, you must overload above the threshold of training.

The threshold of training is the minimum amount of exercise necessary to produce gains in fitness. What you normally do, or just a little more than your normal exercise, is not enough to cause improvements in fitness. Figure 5.1 shows the threshold of training and target zones for physical fitness improvement.

To get optimal benefits of regular exercise, you should exercise in the fitness target zone.

The fitness target zone begins at the threshold of training and stops at the point where the benefits of exercise become counterproductive, as shown in Figure 5.1. This is the optimal level of exercise.

The principle of specificity is an important law of exercise that should be observed if optimal fitness is to be obtained.

The principle of specificity simply states that to develop a certain characteristic of fitness, you must overload specifically for that particular fitness component. For example, exercises that build strength may do little for developing cardiovascular fitness, and exercises for flexibility may do little for altering body composition.

Just as overload is specific to each component of fitness, it is also specific to each body part. If you exercise the legs, you build fitness of the legs. If you exercise the arms, you build fitness of the arms. For this reason, it is not unusual to see some people with disproportionate fitness development. Some gymnasts, for example, have good upper body development but poor leg development, whereas some soccer players have well-developed legs but lack upper body development.

Specificity is important in designing your warm-up, cool down, and training program for specific activities. Training is most effective when it closely resembles the activity for which you are training. For example, if your goal is to improve your skill in putting the shot, it is not enough to overload the arm muscles. You should perform a training activity that requires overload while doing a putting motion that closely resembles that used in the actual sport.

There is a threshold of training and a fitness target zone for each component of fitness.

Some people incorrectly associate the concepts of threshold of training and fitness target zones with only cardiovascular fitness. As the principle of specificity suggests, each component of fitness has its own threshold and target zone. Details for each of the health-related aspects of fitness are presented in Concepts 6–10.

The principle of progression is an important corollary of the overload principle.

The progression concept indicates that overload should not be increased too slowly nor too rapidly if fitness is to result. Obviously, the concepts of threshold of training and fitness target zones are based on the progression principle. Beginners can exercise progressively by starting near threshold levels and gradually increasing in frequency, intensity, and time (duration) within the target zone. Exercise above the target zone is counterproductive and can be dangerous. For example the "weekend" athlete who exercises vigorously only on weekends, does not exercise often enough, and so violates the principle of progression. Approximately 30 percent of all Americans, or 50 percent of those who consider themselves to be regular exercisers, violate the principle of progression by failing to exercise above threshold levels and in the exercise target zone. Clearly, it is possible to do too little and too much exercise to develop optimal fitness.

The word FIT can be used to remember the three important variables for determining threshold of training and fitness target zone levels.

For exercise to be effective, it must be done with enough *F*requency, and *I*ntensity, and for a long enough *T*ime. The first letter of these three words spells FIT. The acronym FIT can help you remember these important factors.

1. *Frequency* (how often)—Exercise must be performed regularly to be effective. The number of days a person exercises per week is used to determine frequency. Exercise frequency depends on the specific component to be developed. However, most fitness components require at least three days and up to six days of activity per week.

2. *Intensity* (how hard)—Exercise must be hard enough to require more exertion than normal to produce gains in health-related fitness. The method for determining appropriate intensity varies with each aspect of fitness. For example, flexibility requires stretching muscles beyond normal length, cardiovascular fitness requires elevating the heart rate above normal, and strength requires increasing the resistance more than normal.

3. *Time* (how long)—Exercise must be done for a significant length of time to be effective. Generally, an exercise period must be at least fifteen minutes in length to be effective, while longer times are recommended for optimal fitness gains. As the length of time increases, intensities of exercise may be decreased. This time of exercise involvement is also referred to as exercise duration.

Threshold levels and target zones change as your fitness level changes.

As you become more fit by doing correct exercises, your threshold of training and fitness target zones may change. Likewise, if you stop exercising for a period of time they will also change. Your threshold of training and fitness target zones are based on your current physical fitness levels and your current exercise patterns.

REFERENCES

American College of Sports Medicine. "Position Statement on the Recommended Quantity and Quality of Exercise for Developing and Maintaining Fitness in Healthy Adults." *Medicine and Science in Sports and Exercise* 10 (1978):vii.

*American College of Sports Medicine. *Guidelines for Graded Exercise Testing and Exercise Prescription.* 2d. ed. Philadelphia: Lea and Febiger, 1980.

Gilliam, T. B., et al. "Physical Activity Patterns Determined by Heart Rate Monitoring in 6-7-Year-Old Children." *Medicine and Science in Sports and Exercise* 13 (1981):65

Harris, L., and Associates. *The Perrier Study: Fitness in America.* New York: Great Waters of France, 1979.

Hickson, R. C., and M. A. Rosenkoetter. "Reduced Training Frequencies and Maintenance of Increased Aerobic Power." *Medicine and Science in Sports and Exercise* 13 (1981):13.

Laurie, D. R., and C. B. Corbin. "How Much Exercise Is Enough?" Manhattan, KS: Master Teacher, 1980.

*Pollock, M. L. "How Much Exercise Is Enough?" *Physician and Sportsmedicine* 6(1978):50.

*Pollock, M. L., and S. N. Blair. "Exercise Prescription." Journal of Physical Education and Recreation 52 (1981):30.

Research and Forecasts, Inc. *The Miller Lite Report on American Attitudes toward Sports.* Milwaukee: Miller Brewing Co., 1983.

Van Camp, S. P. "The Fixx Tragedy: A Cardiologist's Perspective." *Physician and Sportsmedicine* 12 (1984):153.

6
CARDIOVASCULAR FITNESS

CONCEPT 6

Cardiovascular fitness,
the ability of the blood, heart, lungs,
and other systems of the body
to effectively persist in effort,
is probably the most important aspect
of physical fitness and can be developed and
assessed in a number of ways.

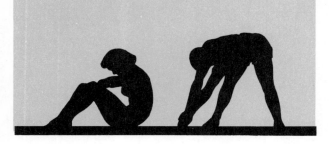

INTRODUCTION

Cardiovascular fitness is frequently considered the most important aspect of physical fitness because those who possess it are likely to have a lessened risk of coronary heart disease. Cardiovascular fitness is also referred to as cardiovascular endurance, cardiorespiratory capacity, and circulatory fitness. Regardless of the word used to describe it, cardiovascular fitness is complex because it requires fitness of several body systems.

TERMS

Aerobic Exercise—Exercise for which the body is able to supply adequate oxygen to sustain performance for long periods of time.

Anaerobic Exercise—Exercise that requires the use of the body's high-energy fuel. This type of exercise is of short duration and does not depend on the body's ability to supply oxygen.

Hemoglobin—Oxygen-carrying pigment of the red blood cells.

Liter—A metric measure of volume slightly larger than one quart.

Maximal Oxygen Uptake—A laboratory measure of fitness commonly held to be the best measure of cardiovascular fitness.

THE FACTS

Because of its importance to a healthy life, cardiovascular fitness is one of the most important aspects of physical fitness.

A considerable amount of evidence indicates that people who exercise regularly have a lower incidence of heart disease, and that exercise is an effective prescription for those who have already suffered a heart attack.

Good cardiovascular fitness requires a fit heart muscle.

The heart is a muscle; to become stronger it must be exercised like any other muscle in the body. If the heart is exercised regularly, its strength increases; if not, it becomes weaker. Contrary to the belief that strenuous work harms the heart, research has found no evidence that regular, progressive exercise is bad for the normal heart. In fact, the heart muscle will increase in size and power when called upon to extend itself. The increase in size and power allows the heart to pump a greater volume of blood with fewer strokes per minute. For example, the average individual has a resting heart rate of between seventy and eighty beats per minute, while it is not uncommon for a trained athlete's pulse to be in the low fifties or even in the forties.

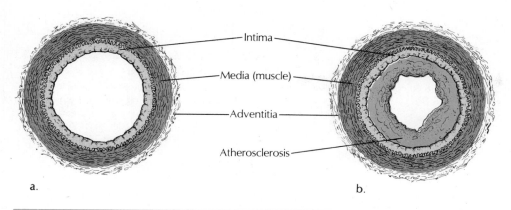

FIGURE 6.1 *(a)* Healthy, Elastic Artery and *(b)* Unhealthy Artery

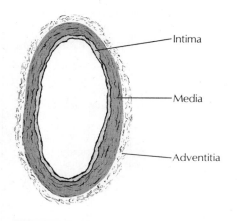

FIGURE 6.2 Healthy, Nonelastic Vein

The healthy heart is efficient in the work that it does.

The fit heart can convert about half of its fuel into energy. An automobile engine in good running condition converts about one-fourth of its fuel into energy. By comparison, the heart is an efficient engine.

The heart of a normal individual beats reflexively about 40 million times a year. During this time, over 4,000 gallons or 10 tons of blood are circulated each day, and every night the heart accomplishes a work load equivalent to carrying a thirty-pound pack to the top of the 102–story Empire State Building.

Good cardiovascular fitness requires a fit vascular system.

Blood flows in a sequence of arteries to capillaries, to veins, and back to the heart. Arteries always carry blood away from the heart. Healthy arteries are elastic, free of obstruction, and expand to permit the flow of blood. Muscle layers line the arteries and on impulse from nerve fibers, control the size of the arterial opening. Unfit arteries may have a reduced internal diameter (atherosclerosis) because of deposits on the interior of their walls, or they may have hardened, nonelastic walls (arteriosclerosis).

Fit coronary arteries are especially important to good health. The blood in the four chambers of the heart does not directly nourish the heart. Rather, numerous small arteries within the heart muscle provide for coronary circulation. Poor coronary circulation precipitated by unhealthy arteries can be the cause of a heart attack (see Fig. 6.1).

Veins have thinner, less elastic walls than arteries and contain small valves to prevent the backward flow of blood as shown in Figure 6.2. Skeletal muscles assist the return of blood to the heart. The veins are intertwined in the muscle, and when the muscle is contracted, the vein is squeezed, pushing the blood on its way back to the heart. A malfunction of the valves results in a failure to remove used blood at the proper rate. As a result, venous blood pools in the legs causing a condition known as varicose veins.

Capillaries are the transfer stations where oxygen and fuel are released to and waste products removed from the tissues. The veins receive the blood from the capillaries for the return trip to the heart.

Good cardiovascular fitness requires a fit respiratory system, fit blood, and fit muscles capable of using oxygen.

In order for a healthy heart to transmit oxygen through a healthy artery, the blood must also be healthy. It must contain adequate hemoglobin in the red blood cells (erythrocytes). Insufficient oxygen-carrying capacity of the blood is called anemia.

As fit blood travels through the lungs, adequate oxygen must be transmitted from the lungs to the blood. A limited respiratory system will limit cardiovascular fitness.

TABLE 6.1 Cardiovascular Fitness Threshold of Training and Target Zones for Aerobic Exercise*

	Threshold of Training	Target Zone
Frequency	• 3 days a week	• At least 3 and no more than 6 days a week.
Intensity	• Elevate the heart rate to 60 percent of its working range.	• Elevate the heart rate to at least 60 percent and up to 80 percent of its working range. For most young adults, the average target zone is between 135 and 170 beats per minute. For older adults, the zone for most people is between 120 and 140 beats per minute.
Time	• Exercise at the proper intensity for *a minimum of 15–30 minutes.* Another way to determine the minimal length of time for exercise is counting the calories you expend. Exercise of the proper intensity and frequency that causes a calorie expenditure of 1,500–2,000 per week is enough to improve cardiovascular fitness. As the intensity of exercise increases, the length of exercise sessions can be decreased.	• Exercise at the proper intensity for *15–60 minutes or expend from 1,500–3,000 calories* per week at the correct intensity and frequency.

*The threshold of training and target zone values depicted in this table are for healthy young adults. Older people or those who have not been active recently should begin exercising below threshold values and increase exercise gradually. Those with known medical problems should consult a physician to determine appropriate exercise amounts.

If cardiovascular fitness is to be developed, you must regularly exercise above the cardiovascular threshold of training and in the cardiovascular fitness target zone.

Three factors must be considered in designing exercise programs for developing cardiovascular fitness: frequency, intensity, and time (see Table 6.1).

Cardiovascular fitness can be achieved by doing either aerobic or anaerobic exercise.

Aerobic means "with oxygen." During aerobic exercise, the body can supply the oxygen it needs to function effectively; thus the name aerobic. Examples of aerobic exercise are walking, jogging, and swimming at moderate speeds. If exercise becomes more intense, it is likely to be at least partially anaerobic in nature. Anaerobic means "without oxygen." During anaerobic exercise, the body cannot supply adequate oxygen to meet the body's needs. For this reason, true anaerobic exercise can only be continued for less than a minute at a time. Examples of pure anaerobic exercises are all-out sprints in running or swimming.

Many activities, such as the mile run for time or a three-mile bicycle race, are part aerobic and part anaerobic. However, activities continuously performed for fifteen to sixty minutes without regular intervals of rest are primarily aerobic and are often referred to as aerobic exercise. Cooper and others advocate exercise that is principally aerobic, while Astrand and others recommend exercise that is principally anaerobic. Both can be effective in building cardiovascular fitness. Some advantages and disadvantages of each are presented in Table 6.2.

TABLE 6.2 Advantages of Aerobic and Anaerobic Exercise

Aerobic	Anaerobic
• Because it is often done slowly and continuously, rather than in short vigorous bursts, many people consider aerobic exercise to be less demanding and more enjoyable.	• Anaerobic exercise is often done using short bursts of exercise alternated with rest periods. Some people find such varied schedules of exercise interesting.
• Aerobic exercise is less intense and may be best for beginners, especially those who are older and those who are just starting an exercise program after a long layoff.	• May be the best approach for those preparing for competition in events that require bursts of speed, such as track and swimming.
• Produces aerobic fitness, or the ability to do sustained exercise.	• Produces anaerobic fitness, or the ability to do short explosive bursts of exercise.
• Less risk to older people or those with less than very good levels of fitness.	• Saves time—allows a person to do more work in a given period of time.

There is a threshold of training and a target zone for building cardiovascular fitness using aerobic exercise. Specific amounts of exercise necessary to achieve increases in cardiovascular fitness using aerobic exercise are outlined in Table 6.1.

To determine the intensity of exercise for building cardiovascular fitness, it is important to know how to count your pulse. Each time the heart beats it pumps blood into the arteries. The surge of blood causes a pulse that can be felt by holding a finger against an artery.

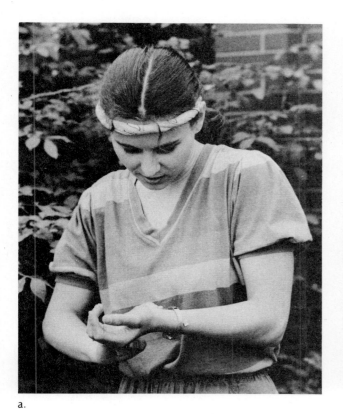

a.

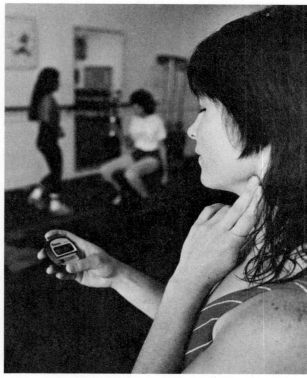

b.

FIGURE 6.3 Counting Your Own Pulse: *(a)* Wrist (Radial) and *(b)* Neck (Carotid)

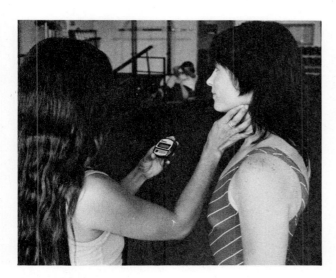

FIGURE 6.4 Counting Someone Else's Pulse: Neck (Carotid)

Major arteries that are easy to locate and are frequently used for pulse counts are the carotid (on either side of the Adam's apple), and the radial (just above the base of the thumb on the wrist). (See Figures 6.3 and 6.4.) Heart rate (pulse) is important for determining the correct intensity of exercise for building cardiovascular fitness.

To count the pulse, simply place the finger tips (index and middle finger) over the artery at one of the previously mentioned locations. Move the fingers around until a strong pulse can be felt. Press gently so as not to cut off the blood flow through the artery. Counting the pulse with the thumb is not recommended since the thumb has a relatively strong pulse of its own. This could be especially confusing when taking a pulse count for another person.

Counting the pulse at the carotid artery is the most popular procedure probably because the carotid pulse is easy to locate. Some researchers suggest that caution should be used when taking carotid pulse counts because pressing on this artery can cause a reflex that slows the heart rate. This could result in incorrect heart rate counts. More recent research indicates that when done properly, carotid palpations can be used safely to count heart rate for most people.

The radial pulse is a bit harder to find than the carotid pulse because of the many tendons near the wrist. Moving the fingers around to several locations just above the thumb on the wrist will help you to locate this pulse. For older adults or those with known medical problems, this procedure is recommended.

Though less popular, the pulse can also be counted at the brachial artery. This is located on the inside of the upper arm just below the armpit.

Once the pulse is located, the heart rate can be determined in beats per minute. At rest, this is done simply by counting the number of beats in one minute. To determine exercise heart rate it would be best to count heart beats or pulses during exercise. However, it is difficult to count the pulse during most activities. Machines do exist that can count heart beats during exercise but they are not available to most people. The most practical method is to count the pulse immediately after exercise. During exercise, the heart rate increases and immediately after exercise, it begins to slow down or return to normal. In fact, the heart rate has already slowed considerably within one minute after exercise ceases. The key is to locate the pulse quickly and to count the pulse for a short period of time. Even if the pulse is located quickly, a full one-minute pulse count after exercise does not give a good estimate of exercise heart rate because the heart rate during the end of the count is much slower than it was during exercise. Keep moving while quickly locating the pulse, then stop and take a fifteen-second count. The number of pulses counted in a fifteen-second period is multiplied by four to convert heart rate to beats per minute.

The pulse rate should be counted after regular exercise, not after a sudden burst of activity. Some runners sprint the last few yards of their daily run and then count their pulse. Such a burst of exercise will elevate the heart rate considerably. This gives a false picture of the actual exercise heart rate. It would be wise for every person to learn to accurately determine resting heart rate and to estimate exercise heart rate by quickly and accurately making pulse counts after exercise.

In order to plan aerobic exercise for building cardiovascular fitness, it is important to know how to calculate heart rate threshold levels and target zones.

In Table 6.1, it was noted that the threshold, or minimal heart rate intensity for building cardiovascular fitness, is based on a percentage of your working heart rate range. To calculate your working heart rate range, you must know your resting and your maximal heart rate.

The resting heart rate is easily determined by counting the pulse for one minute while sitting or lying down. Ideally, this should be done early in the morning when you are rested, rather than late in the day when you have been involved in many activities.

Maximal heart rate is harder to determine. It could be measured by an electrocardiogram while exercising to exhaustion; however, for most people it is safer and better to estimate *maximal heart* rate by

TABLE 6.3 Formula and Example for Calculating Target Heart Rates (Example is for a twenty-two-year-old person with a resting heart rate of 68 bpm.)

Formula for Calculating Maximal Heart Rate	Example
220 — Age (in years) = Maximal Heart Rate	220 — 22 = 198 beats per minute

Formula For Calculating Working Heart Rate	Example
Maximal Heart Rate — Resting Heart Rate = Working Heart Rate	198 — 68 = 130

Formula for Calculating Threshold of Training Heart Rate	Example
Working Heart Rate	130
× .60	× .60
+ Resting Heart Rate	= 78 + 68
Threshold of Training Heart Rate	= 146

Formula for Calculating the Upper Limit of the Target Heart Rate Zone	Example
Working Heart Rate	130
× .80	× .80
+ Resting Heart Rate	= 104 + 68
= Upper Limit for Target Heart Rate Zone	= 172

The target zone for this twenty-two-year-old is 146–172 bpm.

using a formula. This is done by subtracting your age from 220. Maximal heart rates are near 200 in young people but decrease with age. The formula for calculating your maximal heart rate and an example of the calculations for a twenty-two-year-old individual are shown in Table 6.3.

The *working heart rate* range is determined by subtracting the resting heart rate from the maximal heart rate. The heart always works in this range because the resting is the lowest and the maximal is the highest rate for your pulse. The formula for calculating the working heart rate range and an example for the twenty-two-year-old with a resting heart rate of sixty-eight are also shown in Table 6.3.

TABLE 6.4 Cardiovascular Fitness Threshold of Training and Target Zones for Anaerobic Exercise*

	Threshold of Training	Target Zone
Frequency	• Three days a week.	• Three to four days a week.
Intensity	• Short Intervals — 100% of maximum speed running, swimming, or other exercise of short duration (10–30 seconds).	• Short Intervals — 100% of maximum speed running, swimming, or other exercise of short duration (10–30 seconds).
	• Long Intervals — 90% of maximum speed running, swimming, or other exercise (30 seconds–2 minutes).	• Long Intervals — 90%–100% of maximum speed running, swimming, or other exercise (30 seconds–2 minutes).
Time	• Short Intervals — Exercise 10 seconds, rest 10 seconds. Repeat 20 times.	• Short Intervals — Same as threshold but repeat up to 30 times.
	or	
	• Exercise 20 seconds, rest 15 seconds. Repeat 10 times.	• Same as threshold but repeat up to 20 times.
	or	
	• Exercise 30 seconds, rest 1–2 minutes. Repeat 8 times.	• Same as threshold but repeat up to 18 times.
	• Long Intervals — Exercise one minute, rest 3–5 minutes. Repeat 5 times.	• Long Intervals — Same as threshold but repeat up to 15 times.
	or	
	• Exercise two minutes, rest 5–15 minutes. Repeat 4 times.	• Same as threshold but repeat up to 10 times.

*The threshold of training and target zone values depicted in this table are for healthy, young adults. For older people, or those who have not been active recently, aerobic training is recommended. Those with known medical problems should consult a physician to determine appropriate exercise amounts.

The *threshold of training, or minimum heart rate* for building cardiovascular fitness, is determined by calculating 60 percent of the working heart rate range and then adding it to the resting heart rate. The upper limit of the target zone is 80 percent of the working heart rate range added to the resting heart rate. The formula for determining threshold and the upper limit of the target heart rate zone and examples for the hypothetical exerciser are shown in Table 6.3.

You should learn to calculate your own threshold and target heart rate values. However, for convenient reference and so that you can check your calculations, Chart 6B.1 in the Lab Resource Materials on page 42 includes threshold and target heart rates for people of all ages. Once you have determined your threshold and target heart rates, you should exercise vigorously enough to bring your heart rate above threshold and into the target zone. Count your fifteen-second heart rate immediately after exercise (and multiply by four) to see if your heart rate is in the proper range. You may have to adjust the intensity of your exercise if your heart rate is not in the target zone. The heart rate of the *hypothetical* twenty-two-year-old used in the previous example should be elevated to no less than 146 and up to 172 beats per minute for optimal cardiovascular fitness benefits.

There is a threshold of training and a target zone for developing cardiovascular fitness using anaerobic exercise.

Specific amounts of exercise necessary to increase cardiovascular fitness using anaerobic exercise are outlined in Table 6.4.

Though cardiovascular fitness can be measured in many ways, maximal oxygen uptake is the best method of evaluation.

A person's maximal oxygen uptake is determined in a laboratory by measuring how much oxygen can be used in one minute of maximal work. Great endurance athletes can extract five or six liters of oxygen per minute from the environment during an all-out treadmill run or bicycle ride, as opposed to the average person, who can extract only two or three liters. In order to extract a large amount of oxygen during maximal work, a person must have a fit heart muscle, capable of pumping large amounts of blood; fit blood, capable of carrying adequate amounts of oxygen; fit arteries, free from congestion and capable of carrying large amounts of blood; and fit muscles, capable of using the oxygen supplied to the muscle. Less sophisticated tests such as the twelve-minute run, the step test, or the Astrand-Ryhming bicycle test can also be used to measure cardiovascular endurance (see the Lab Resource Materials that follow).

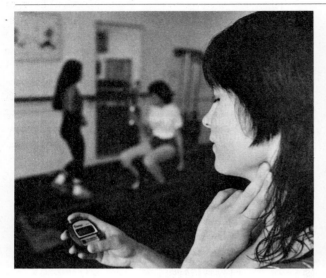 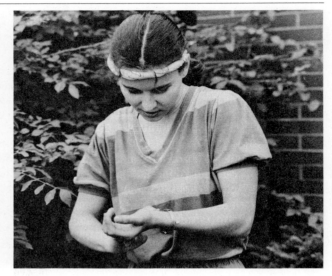

Counting the Pulse

1. *Locating the Carotid Pulse*
   Place the index and middle fingers of one hand on one side of your throat about an inch to the side of your Adam's apple. Pressing lightly, you should feel the pulse with your fingers. If not, move the fingers to another spot in the area (but do not move the fingers about the level of the Adam's apple) until a strong pulse is felt. Do not press hard as this may restrict the movement of the blood through the carotid artery.

2. *Locating the Radial Pulse*
   Place the index and middle fingers of one hand on the palm-side of the other wrist just above the base of the thumb. Pressing lightly, you should feel the pulse with your fingers. You may need to move the fingers to several spots in the area until a strong pulse is felt. Do not press hard since this may restrict the movement of the blood through the radial artery.

CHART 6B.1 Threshold of Training and Target Zone Heart Rates
(Heart rates necessary to produce improved cardiovascular fitness)*

Resting Heart Rate		Age									
		Less than 25	25–29	30–34	35–39	40–44	45–49	50–54	55–59	60–64	Over 65
below 50	Threshold	136	133	130	127	124	121	118	115	112	109
	Target zone	136–156	133–164	130–160	127–156	124–152	121–148	118–144	115–140	112–136	109–134
50–54	Threshold	138	135	132	129	126	123	120	117	114	111
	Target zone	138–167	135–165	132–161	129–157	126–153	123–149	120–145	117–141	114–137	111–135
55–59	Threshold	140	137	134	131	128	125	122	119	116	113
	Target zone	140–168	137–166	134–162	131–158	128–154	125–150	122–146	119–142	116–138	113–136
60–64	Threshold	142	139	136	133	130	127	124	121	118	115
	Target zone	142–169	139–167	136–163	133–159	130–155	127–151	124–147	121–143	118–139	115–137
65–69	Threshold	144	141	138	135	132	129	126	123	120	117
	Target zone	144–170	141–168	138–164	135–160	132–156	129–152	126–148	123–144	120–140	117–138
70–74	Threshold	146	143	140	137	134	131	128	125	122	119
	Target zone	146–171	143–169	140–165	137–161	134–157	131–153	128–149	125–145	122–141	119–139
75–79	Threshold	148	145	142	139	136	133	130	127	124	121
	Target zone	148–172	145–170	142–166	139–162	136–158	133–154	130–150	127–146	124–142	121–140
80–85	Threshold	150	147	144	141	138	135	132	129	126	123
	Target zone	150–173	147–171	144–167	141–163	138–159	135–155	132–151	129–147	126–143	123–141
85 and over	Threshold	152	149	146	143	140	137	134	131	128	125
	Target zone	152–174	149–172	146–168	143–164	140–160	137–156	134–152	131–148	128–144	125–142

*Computed using 60%–80% of the working heart rate.

Evaluating Cardiovascular Fitness

For an exercise program to be most effective, it should be based on personal needs. Some sort of testing is necessary to determine your personal need for cardiovascular fitness. A treadmill test that includes continuous EKG monitoring or assessment of Maximal Oxygen Uptake is the best test of cardiovascular fitness (see American College of Sports Medicine reference in Concept 6). However, there are some tests that do not require as much time and equipment and that can be done to give you a good estimate of cardiovascular fitness. Some of these tests are the twelve-minute run, the step test, and the Astrand-Ryhming bicycle test, all of which are described here. Prior to performing any of these tests, it is important to be sure that you are physically and medically ready (Concept 4). Prepare yourself by doing some regular exercise for three to six weeks before actually taking the tests.

The Twelve-Minute Run Test

1. Locate an area where a specific distance is already marked, such as a school track or football field; or measure a specific distance using a bicycle or automobile odometer.
2. Use a stopwatch or wristwatch to accurately time a twelve-minute period.
3. For best results, warm up prior to the test, then run at a steady pace for the entire twelve minutes (cool down after the tests).
4. Determine the distance you can run in twelve minutes in fractions of a mile. Depending upon your age, locate your score and rating on the appropriate chart here.

CHART 6C.1* Twelve-Minute Test for Ages 17–25

Classification	Men	Women
Excellent	1.9 miles	1.5 miles
Very good	1.8–1.89 miles	1.4–1.49 miles
Fair	1.6–1.79 miles	1.1–1.39 miles
Poor	1.5–1.59 miles	1.0–1.09 miles
Very poor	1.4–1.49 miles	below .9 miles

Twelve-Minute Test for Adult Men (26+)

Classification	Age 26–39	40–49	50+
Very poor	<.95 miles	<.85 miles	<.80 miles
Poor	.95–1.14 miles	.85–1.04 miles	.80–.99 miles
Fair	1.15–1.39 miles	1.05–1.29 miles	1.0–1.24 miles
Good	1.40–1.64 miles	1.30–1.54 miles	1.25–1.49 miles
Excellent	1.65+ miles	1.55+ miles	1.50+ miles

Twelve-Minute Test for Adult Women (26+)

Classification	Age 26–39	40–49	50+
Very poor	<.85 miles	<.75 miles	<.65 miles
Poor	.85–1.04 miles	.75–.94 miles	.65–.84 miles
Fair	1.05–1.24 miles	.95–1.14 miles	.85–1.04 miles
Good	1.25–1.54 miles	1.15–1.44 miles	1.05–1.34 miles
Excellent	1.55+ miles	1.45+ miles	1.35+ miles

*Adapted from K. H. Cooper, The New Aerobics. New York: M. Evans & Co., 1972.

The Step Test*

1. Prior to exercise, warm up, and after finishing, be sure to cool down.
2. Step up and down on a twelve-inch bench for three minutes at a rate of twenty-four steps per minute. One step consists of four beats, that is, "up with the left foot, up with the right foot, down with the left foot, down with the right foot."
3. Immediately after the exercise, sit down on the bench and relax. Don't talk.
4. Locate your pulse or have another person locate it for you.
5. Five seconds after the exercise ended, begin counting your pulse. Count the pulse for sixty seconds.
6. Your score is your sixty-second heart rate. Locate your score and your rating on the following chart.

CHART 6C.2 Step Test Rating Chart

Classification	Sixty-Second Heart Rate
Excellent	84 or less
Very good	85–94
Fair	95–114
Poor	115–124
Very poor	125 and above

As you grow older you would want to continue to score well on this rating chart. Because your maximal heart rate decreases as you age you should be able to score well if you exercise regularly.
Adapted from Kasch, F. W., and Boyer, J. L. Adult Fitness: Principles and Practices. Palo Alto, Calif.: Mayfield Publishers, 1968.

The Astrand-Ryhming Bicycle Test*

1. Ride a stationary bicycle ergometer for six minutes at a rate of fifty pedal cycles per minute (one push with each foot per cycle). Prior to beginning, a stretching warm-up is recommended. The test itself will serve as a cardiovascular warm-up. Cool down after the test.
2. Set the bicycle at a work load between 300 and 1,200 kpm. For less fit or smaller people, a setting in the range of 300 to 600 is appropriate. Larger or fitter people will need to use a setting of 750 to 1,200. The work load should be enough to elevate the heart rate to at least 125 bpm but no more than 170 bpm during the ride.
3. During the sixth minute of the ride (if the heart rate is in the correct range—see step 2), count the heart rate for the entire sixth minute. The carotid or radial pulse may be used.
4. Use the nomogram to determine your predicted oxygen uptake score. Connect the point that represents your heart rate with the point on the right-hand scale that represents the work load you used in riding the bike (use the ♂ scale for men and the ♀ scale for women). Read your score at the point where a straight line connecting the two points crosses the Max VO₂ line. For example, the sample score for the woman represented by the dotted line is 2.55, or nearly 2.6. She had a heart rate of 150 and worked at a load of 600 kpm.
5. Determine your score in terms of VO_2 per kilogram of body weight by dividing your weight in kilograms into the score obtained from the nomogram. To compute your weight in kilograms, divide your weight in pounds by 2.2.
6. To determine your cardiovascular fitness rating on the bicycle test, look up your VO_2 per kilogram of body weight score on the following chart.

Nomogram

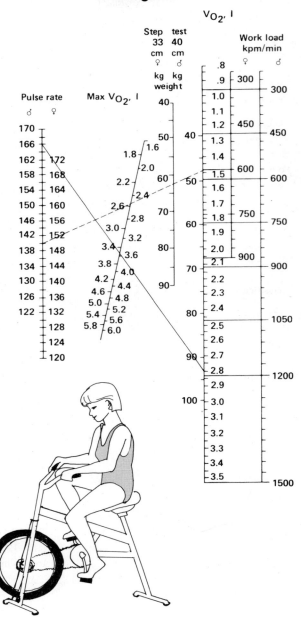

CHART 6C.3 Bicycle Test Rating Chart (ml/O$_2$ /kg)**

	Women				
Age	17–29	30–39	40–49	50–59	60–69
Excellent	49+	45+	42+	38+	35+
Very good	38–48	34–44	31–41	28–37	24–34
Fair	31–37	28–33	24–30	21–27	18–23
Poor	24–30	20–27	17–23	15–20	13–17
Very poor	23–	19–	16–	14–	12–

	Men				
Age	17–29	30–39	40–49	50–59	60–69
Excellent	53+	49+	45+	43+	41+
Very good	43–52	39–48	36–44	34–42	31–40
Fair	34–42	31–38	27–35	25–33	23–30
Poor	25–33	23–30	20–26	18–24	16–22
Very poor	24–	22–	19–	17–	15–

*Test adapted from P. O. Astrand, and K. Rodahl. Textbook of Work Physiology. *New York: McGraw-Hill, 1977.*
**Rating charts adapted from M. L. Pollock, D. H. Schmidt, and A. S. Jackson. "Measurement of Cardiorespiratory Fitness and Body Composition in the Clinical Setting." Comprehensive Therapy 6(1980):12.*

REFERENCES

American College of Sports Medicine. *Guidelines for Graded Exercise Testing and Exercise Prescription.* 2d ed. Philadelphia: Lea and Febiger, 1980.

Astrand, P. O., and K. Rodahl. *Textbook of Work Physiology.* 2d ed. New York: McGraw-Hill, 1977.

*Cantwell, J. D., et al. "Fitness, Aerobic Points, and Coronary Risk." *Physician and Sportsmedicine* 7(1979):79.

*Cooper, K. H. *The Aerobics Program for Total Well-Being.* New York: M. Evans, 1982.

Corbin, C. B., ed. *A Textbook of Motor Development.* 2d ed. Dubuque, IA: Wm. C. Brown Publishers, 1980.

*Couldry, W., C. B. Corbin, and A. Wilcox. "Carotid vs. Radial Pulse Counts." *Physician and Sportsmedicine* 10(1982):67.

deVries, H. A. *Physiology of Exercise.* 3d ed. Dubuque, IA: Wm. C. Brown Publishers, 1980.

Lamb, D. R. *Physiology of Exercise.* New York: Macmillan Publishers, 1978.

*Mahurin, J., and T. P. Martin. "Anaerobic Threshold: A Trainable Component of Cardiovascular Fitness." *Motor Skills: Theory into Practice* 6(1982):41.

Olderidge, N. B., et al. "Carotid Palpation, Coronary Heart Disease, and Exercise Rehabilitation." *Medicine and Science in Sports and Exercise* 13(1981):6.

Paffenbarger, R. S., et al. "Current Exercise and Heart Attack Risk." *Cardiac Rehabilitation* 10(1979):1.

Paffenbarger, R. S., and R. T. Hyde. "Exercise as Protection Against Heart Disease." *New England Journal of Medicine* 302(1980):1026.

Paffenbarger, R. S., et al. "A Natural History of Athleticism and Cardiovascular Health." *Journal of the American Medical Association* 252 (1984):496.

*Pollock, M. L., and S. N. Blair. "Exercise Prescription." *Journal of Physical Education and Recreation* 52(1981):30.

Sedlock, D. A., et al. "Accuracy of Subject-Palpated Carotid Pulse after Exercise." *Physician and Sportsmedicine* 11 (1983):106.

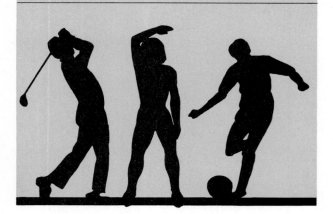

7
STRENGTH

CONCEPT 7

Strength is an important health-related component of physical fitness.

INTRODUCTION

Strength is measured by the amount of force you can produce with a single maximal effort. You need strength to increase work capacity; to decrease the chance of injury; to prevent low back pain, poor posture, and other hypokinetic diseases; to improve athletic performance; and perhaps to save life or property in an emergency situation.

TERMS

Anabolic Steroid—A synthetic hormone similar to the male sex hormone testosterone.

Antagonistic Muscles—The muscles that have the opposite action as those that are contracting (agonists); normally, antagonists reflexly relax when agonists contract.

Concentric Contraction—An isotonic muscle contraction in which the muscle gets shorter as it contracts, such as when a joint is "bent" and two body parts move closer together. An example is the biceps muscle contraction that occurs when pulling up on a chinning bar.

"Definition" of Muscle—The detailed external appearance of a muscle.

Eccentric Contraction—"Negative exercise." An isotonic muscle contraction in which the muscle gets longer as it contracts, as when a weight is gradually lowered and the contracting muscle gets longer as it gives up tension. Lowering the body from a pull-up on a chinning bar is an example of eccentric contraction.

Hypertrophy—Increase in the size of muscles as the result of strength training; increase in bulk.

Isotonic Contraction—Type of muscle contraction in which the muscle changes length, either shortening (concentrically) or lengthening (eccentrically). Isotonic exercises are those in which a resistance is raised and then lowered, as in weight training and calisthenics.

PRE—Progressive resistance exercise.

THE FACTS

There are three types of muscle tissue.

The three types of muscle tissue—smooth, cardiac, and skeletal—have different structures and functions. Smooth muscle tissue consists of long spindle-shaped fibers; each fiber usually contains only one nucleus. The fibers function as the movers of internal organs since they are located in the walls of these body parts. Cardiac muscle tissue, as the name implies, is found only in the heart and its fibers are interwoven. Smooth muscles and cardiac muscles operate involuntarily. Skeletal muscle tissues consist of long, cylindrical, multinucleated fibers. They provide for force for the movement of the skeletal system and may be controlled voluntarily.

There are several different types of skeletal muscle fibers.

The skeletal muscles are the muscles that do the work when a person runs, does calisthenics, dances, or participates in a sport. Skeletal muscles are made up of two different types of fibers, slow twitch and fast twitch. There are at least two different kinds of fast twitch fibers. While slow twitch fibers are used for prolonged or aerobic work, fast twitch fibers are used in strength and power activities.

Studies indicate that distance runners have a high number of slow twitch fibers in their muscles, and sprinters have a high number of fast twitch fibers. As a muscle is overloaded, the muscle fibers grow larger and circulation to the fibers increases. Apparently, strength training using high resistance exercises tends to selectively build fast twitch fibers. Muscular endurance training seems to promote increased functioning of the slow twitch fibers. While some people have tried to use muscle biopsies (a method of counting fast twitch and slow twitch fibers) to determine their potential for success in various sports, there is good evidence that counting the numbers of different kinds of muscle fibers is *not* an effective way to predict athletic success.

Strength is best developed by exercising against a near maximum resistance with only a few repetitions.

Strength training requires an overload in the amount of the resistance, while muscular endurance training (see Concept 8) requires an overload in the number of repetitions. Therefore, according to the law of specificity, when designing a program for strength development, high resistance and low repetitions should be used for maximum effectiveness.

There is a threshold of training and a target zone for muscular development.

Experts generally agree that in progressive resistance exercise (PRE), using a maximum load (resistance) for one to ten repetitions in two to three sets three or four times per week will develop strength. Experts do *not* agree, however, on the ideal combination of reps and sets. Table 7.1 compares the thresholds and target zones of isotonic exercise, isometric exercise, and isokinetic exercise using generally accepted practices.

TABLE 7.1 Strength Threshold of Training and Fitness Target Zones

	Threshold of Training			Target Zone		
	Isometrics	Isotonics	Isokinetics	Isometrics	Isotonics	Isokinetics
Frequency	• 3 days a week.	• 3 days a week.	• 3 days a week.	• Daily.	• Every other day.	• 4–5 times a week.
Intensity	• Use two-thirds maximum contractions.	• During the first set, lift one-half of maximum; during the second set, lift three-fourths maximum; and during the third set, lift maximum weight.	• Two-thirds of maximum contractions.	• Use maximal contractions.	• Maximum contraction.	• Maximum contraction.
Time	• Hold for 2–5 seconds. • Repeat once a day.	• Perform 2 sets of each exercise. • Do 5 repetitions of each exercise.	• 3 repetitions lasting 1–3 seconds.	• Hold for 6–8 seconds. • Repeat 5–10 times a day.	• Perform 3 sets of each exercise. • Do 10 repetitions.	• 5 repetitions lasting 1–3 seconds.

TABLE 7.2 Advantages and Disadvantages of Isometric, Isotonic, and Isokinetic Exercises

Isometrics	Isotonics	Isokinetics
1. Can be done in small area.	1. Develops more strength than isometrics.	1. Good to train for athletic skill.
2. No equipment needed.	2. May aid coordination.	2. Equal to isotonics for strength development.
3. No feedback, so lack of motivation is a problem.	3. Faster recovery from fatigue.	3. Provides maximum resistance at all angles in the range of motion.
4. Good in rehabilitation where no joint movement is desired.	4. Strengthens throughout range of motion.	4. Less injury and soreness than isotonics.
5. Builds strength only at the joint angle practiced.	5. Produces greater hypertrophy.	5. Machines very expensive; devices less expensive.
6. Causes very little soreness.	6. Progress easy to follow.	6. Good for rehabilitation.
7. Easy to maintain strength.	7. More soreness and injury.	
8. Lacks movement so does not train coordination.	8. If equipment is used, it is more expensive than isometrics.	
9. May be hazardous for those with high blood pressure.	9. Strength occurs at weakest point in range of motion, so entire range not trained equally.	

Strength training should closely resemble the activity for which the strength is needed.

Specificity of training will enhance performance. If you want your arms to be stronger so you can carry heavy loads, or if you want finger strength to grip a heavy bowling ball, much of your strength exercise should be done isometrically, using the arm muscles the way you would use them to carry loads or using the fingers the same way you hold a bowling ball. On the other hand, if the task for which you are training is performed isotonically, your strength program should be primarily isotonic use of the muscles involved in that skill.

If you are not training for a specific skill, but merely wish to develop overall strength, then consider the advantages and disadvantages listed in Table 7.2. You may wish to use a variety of methods to avoid boredom.

Progressive resistance exercise (PRE) is the most effective type of strength training program.

Muscles adapt only to the load placed upon them. So in order to continue increasing strength, you must progressively increase the stress on the muscle as it adapts to each new load. Muscle groups differ in their strength potential, so each muscle group must have an individualized program. For example, the legs and trunk can usually lift greater loads than the arms.

There are several good PRE programs for strength development, each having advantages and disadvantages.

Progressive resistance exercise can be performed in properly designed programs of weight training using free weights, constant resistance weight machines, or variable resistance isokinetic weight machines; pulley devices; isometric exercises and calisthenics. (See Figure 7.1.) Concept 13 describes some sample exercises and compares some of these programs. Weight training is considered the fastest and best method of improving strength. However, properly designed calisthenics are adequate for developing strength in most people.

The most popular form of strength exercise utilizes isotonic contractions of the muscles.

As used in Table 7.2, isotonic exercise refers to such activities as weight lifting, calisthenics, and pulley weights, in which the muscles alternately shorten and lengthen. Typically, the stress on the muscle in these types of exercises varies with the joint position and the muscle length. Thus, the muscle may work harder at the beginning of a lift than it does near the end of the range of motion, or than it does as the weight is lowered.

Isokinetics, plyometrics, and "negative" exercises are special forms of isotonic exercise. These are discussed later in this concept.

Isometric strength exercises have advantages and disadvantages.

Isometric exercises are effective for developing strength and require no equipment and only minimal space. But these exercises do not develop as much strength as isotonic and isokinetic exercises, nor do muscles hypertrophy as much. They work the muscle only at the angle of joint used in the exercise. Isometrics can be dangerous for those with high blood pressure or cardiovascular disease. (See Table 7.2 for a comparison with other types of exercise.)

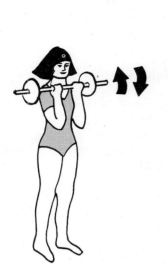

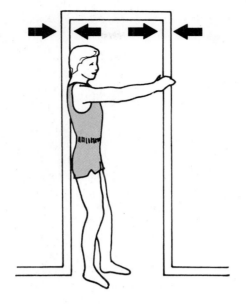

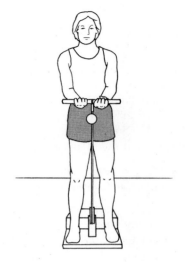

Isotonic Exercise: Raising and Lowering a Barbell

Isometric Exercise: Against an Immovable Object

Isokinetic Exercise: With an Isokinetic Device

FIGURE 7.1 Examples of Three Strength Exercises

Isokinetic exercises are effective for developing strength.

Isokinetic exercises are isotonic exercises performed with a device or machine that provides "accommodating resistance" or "variable resistance." This resistance is equal to the force applied throughout the range of motion, so it automatically compensates for changes in the torque of the body segments at different joint angles. There is no evidence that it develops more strength, but it has the advantage of being safer because resistance is constantly controlled. Examples of these devices include Exer-Genie, Apollo, Mini-Gym, and Nautilus machines. (See Table 7.2 for comparison with other exercise types.)

"Negative" exercise has no advantage over other types of exercise for strength development.

Contrary to the claims of some enthusiasts, there does not seem to be any difference between eccentric (negative) exercise, and concentric (positive) exercise (see definitions) in terms of their effectiveness in developing strength. Eccentric exercise is performed more comfortably even though more weight can be handled. It is particularly useful in rehabilitation settings, but has a tendency to cause more muscle soreness. This type of exercise also requires the assistance of another person or the use of a very large, expensive machine.

Plyometrics may be useful in athletic training for certain sports events.

A quick prestretch, or eccentric contraction of a muscle, immediately followed by an isometric or concentric contraction can produce more power. This has been called "preexertion countermovement" or "wind up" or "plyometrics." Russian Olympic coaches have pioneered in this area, developing drills for their athletes. Track and field athletes may, for example, perform a hopping drill for thirty to sixty seconds or for thirty to one hundred meters.

The "double progressive system" is an effective variation of the PRE system.

The "double progressive system" of progression periodically adjusts both the resistance and the number of repetitions. For example, you may begin with three reps for the arms. Once a week, you add one rep. When you have progressed to ten reps, increase the arm weight by five pounds. Decrease the reps to three and begin the progression again.

Strength capacity differs with sex and age.

Because of differences in hormones and muscle mass, women have only about two-thirds of the strength of men. Women are as strong as men, however, when strength is expressed per unit of cross section of the muscles. Maximum strength is usually reached in the twenties and then declines with age. But regardless of age, strength can be improved.

Training for "bulk" (hypertrophy) and "definition" may differ from strength training.

Most body builders use three to seven sets of ten to fifteen reps, rather than the three sets of five or six reps recommended for most weight trainers. Sometimes, definition is difficult to obtain because it is obscured by fat. It should be noted that those with the largest-looking muscles are not always the strongest.

Strength developed in one limb can be transferred to another unexercised limb.

When the right arm is trained with biceps curls until its strength increases, the unexercised left arm will also increase in strength though not as much as the exercised arm. This phenomenon is called "transfer of training," "bilateral transfer," or "cross-education." The reason for this is not fully understood, but the phenomenon is sometimes applied to rehabilitation to prevent a limb from atrophying.

The amount of force you can exert during a strength test depends upon the speed of contraction, muscle length, warm-up, and other muscle-related factors.

If you want to score high on a strength test, consider some of the "secrets of success" used by experienced lifters and proven by research. Generally, a muscle exerts the least force as it becomes shorter (toward the end of a movement), and can exert more force during an isometric contraction than when it is shortening. The muscle can exert the most force when it is lengthening (lowering a weight). If a muscle is placed on a slight stretch immediately before it contracts, it can exert more force than it could if it started from a resting length.

Speed of contraction affects the amount of force that can be exerted. A slow contraction can lift a heavier weight than a fast contraction. If muscles are warmed up before lifting, more force can be exerted and heavier loads lifted.

There is a proper way to perform strength exercises.

The following are some guidelines for safe and effective strength training:

1. Make sure you are well prepared to begin. (See Concept 4 for details).
2. To ensure overall development, include all body parts and balance the strength of antagonists. For example, the ratio of quadriceps strength to hamstring strength should be 60:40. Exercise large muscles before small muscles.
3. When beginning a weight program, start with weights that are too light so you can learn proper technique and avoid soreness and injury. Novices might, for example, start with one-fourth of their body weight for the military press; ten pounds less than the press for the curl; ten pounds more than the press for the bench press; and half of the body weight for back and leg exercises.
4. Progress gradually. For example, use two sets of four reps with a light weight to begin; add two reps when it gets easy, then another, until you reach two sets of ten reps; then drop back to four reps and add a third set. After this, the "double progressive system" (previously described) can be used, increasing the weight and the reps.
5. Athletes should train muscles the way they will be used in their skill, using similar patterns, range of motion, and speed (the principle of specificity). This applies to anyone who knows the precise skill for which he or she is training.
6. Sports participants should include some eccentric training, such as plyometrics, to prevent injury to decelerating muscles during sports events and to develop power in accelerating muscles.
7. Choose an exercise sequence that alternates muscle groups so muscles have a rest period before being used in another exercise.
8. Beginning weight trainers should probably train for endurance initially (see Concept 8). For example, ten to fifteen reps at fifty to seventy percent of the maximum amount of weight they can lift for one repetition might be a reasonable goal.

9. Move from one station to another with no waste of time, allowing about forty-five seconds of rest between stations when circuit training.
10. Isometric training should be done at several joint angles.
11. To avoid boredom, especially when you reach a plateau or "sticking point," use such motivating techniques as music, record keeping, partners, competition, and variation in routine.
12. To prevent injury:
    a. warm up ten minutes before the workout and stay warm during the workout (see Concept 4).
    b. do not hold your breath while lifting. This may cause blackout or hernia.
    c. avoid hyperventilation before lifting a weight.
    d. avoid dangerous or high-risk exercises.
    e. progress slowly.
    f. use good shoes with good traction.
    g. avoid arching your back. Keep the pelvis tipped backward.
    h. keep the weight close to the body.
    i. do not lift from a stoop.
    j. do not let the hips come up before your upper body when lifting from the floor.
    k. for bent-over rowing, put the head on a table and bend the knees.
    l. stay in a squat as short a time as possible and do not do a full squat.
    m. be sure collars are on free weights tightly.
    n. use a moderately fast, continuous, controlled movement and hold the final position a few seconds.
    o. do not pause between reps.
    p. try to keep a definite rhythm.
    q. do not allow the weights to drop or bang.
    r. do not train if you have a hernia, high blood pressure, fever, infection, recent surgery, or heart disease.
    s. use chalk or a towel to keep hands dry when handling weights.

There are many fallacies, myths, and superstitions associated with strength training.

Some of these misconceptions have been refuted.

1. It is *not* true that you will become "muscle-bound" and lose flexibility just because you do strength training. This could happen only if you train improperly.
2. It is *not* true that women will become masculine-looking if they develop strength. Contrary to popular belief, most women will not be able to develop large and bulky muscles as a result of strength training. As a group, females lack muscle mass and testosterone, the hormone necessary for developing muscle bulk. Those females who have a relatively large muscle mass without training will most likely be able to further develop bulk through training.
3. Strength training does *not* make you move more slowly or make you more uncoordinated. Up to a point, an increase in strength may help to increase speed.
4. The expression "no pain, no gain" is a fallacy. It may be helpful to strive for a burning sensation in the muscle, but this is not painful. If it hurts, you are probably harming yourself.
5. Supplements of wheat germ, liver, brewer's yeast, yogurt, blackstrap molasses, protein, and vitamins do *not* benefit muscle mass or strength building. You do need a balanced diet.
6. Anabolic steroids should *not* be used. They produce such side effects as liver damage or liver cancer, endocrine disturbance, testicular atrophy, impotency, and in women, masculinity and changes in the reproductive system.
7. Strength training is *not* effective for cardiovascular fitness, nor flexibility or weight loss. Muscles will get firmer, and desirable changes may occur in girth, but other aspects of fitness are specific and so require specific training.
8. It does *not* require two hours to complete a workout in weight training—unless you are a competitive lifter or body builder. If you are training for athletics, you will need forty-five to ninety minutes; the beginner or the person training for fitness or recreation can complete a circuit in thirty to forty-five minutes.

Evaluating Isotonic Strength

Tests		Point Value
I.	1. One bent knee push-up, keeping your body straight and rigid.	1

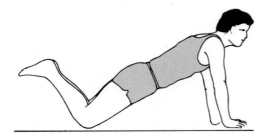

	2. One straight-leg push-up, keeping your body rigid.	3

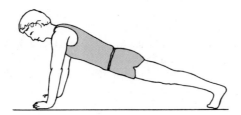

	3. One straight-leg push-up, keeping your body rigid and your feet on bench.	5

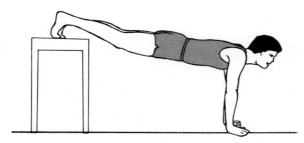

	4. Same as no. 2, except have partner do a push-up on back of your shoulders at the same time.	7

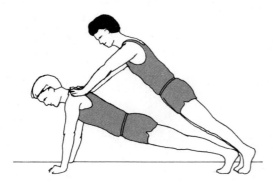

Tests		Point Value
	5. Same as no. 2, except use only one arm.	10

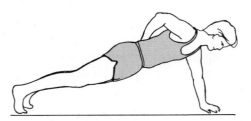

II.	1. a. Hang from a bar placed at the height of the lower end of your sternum. b. Body should be inclined at a forty-five degree angle. c. Have partner brace your feet. d. Pull up until your chin or chest touches the bar.	1

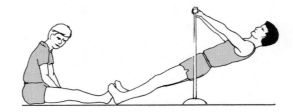

	2. a. Stand on a chair and assume a position with palms facing body, elbows bent, and chin over bar. b. Remove chair. c. Hang in this position for ten seconds.	3

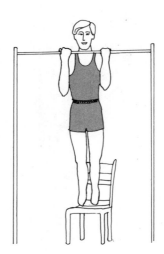

Evaluating Isotonic Strength *continued*

Tests	Point Value
3. Perform one regulation chin-up (pull-up) from a hanging position with palms facing your body.	5

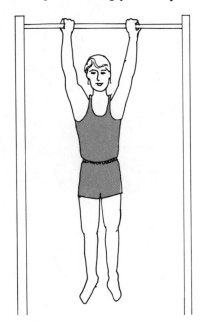

4. Same as no. 3, except pull up while two bleach bottles filled with water are suspended on the ends of a short rope across the back of your neck.   7

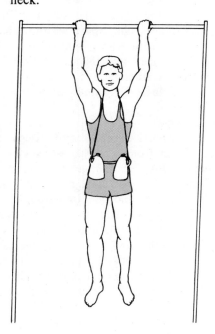

Tests	Point Value
5. Climb a rope to a height of ten feet above your head, using arms only (no leg use).	10

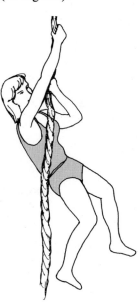

III. Squat on one leg and pick up a paper cup with one hand; return to a stand. Keep the back erect and maintain balance.
    1. Use one leg only.   3
    2. Use right leg only, then use left only.   5

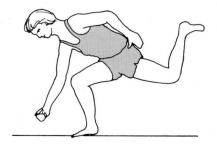

Tests	Point Value
IV. Lie prone, hands clasped behind your neck. Lift your upper trunk as high as possible from the floor; keep your feet on the floor. Measure height of your chin.	
4–5 inches	1
6–7 inches	3
8–9 inches	5
10–11 inches	7
12+ inches	10

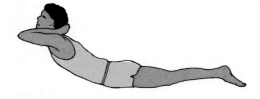

Tests	Point Value
V. Lie on a mat and have your partner mark your body length (height) from head to toe on the mat. Perform a standing long jump the distance of your body height if possible. Measure the jump.	
Half your height	1
Three-quarters your height	3
Full body height, third try	5
Full body height, second try	7
Full body height, first try	10

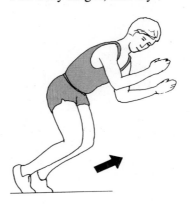

CHART 7A.1 Isotonic Strength Rating Chart

Classification	Total Score
Excellent	40–45
Good	33–40
Fair	25–32
Poor	15–24
Very poor	0–14

Evaluating Isometric Strength

1. *Grip Strength*
   Adjust a hand dynamometer to fit your hand size. Squeeze it as hard as possible. You may bend or straighten the arm, but do not touch the body with your hand, elbow, or arm. Perform with both right and left hands.

2. *Leg Strength*
   Use the belt provided and place it low over the hips; attach the belt to the handle. Hold the bar with both hands in the center of the handle, palms down, so it rests at the level of the hip joint. Place the feet parallel, six inches apart, with the chain centered between them. Knees should be bent 115–124 degrees. The arms and the back should be kept straight, the head erect, and the chest up. Pull as hard as possible on the chain by trying to straighten the legs.

3. *Back Strength*
   Stand as in no. 2 except keep the legs straight. Place hands on front of thighs. Adjust chain length so handle is just below finger tips. Bend at hips, keep head up and eyes straight ahead; grasp bars at ends of handles, one palm forward and one palm backward. Lift steadily, pulling as hard as possible on the chain as you roll your shoulders back.

4. When not being tested, perform the isometric strength exercises in Concept 13, or try to crush an aluminum can with two hands or with one hand; or try to squeeze and indent a new tennis ball.

CHART 7B.1 Isometric Strength Rating Scales

Strength Rating Scale for Women (pounds)

Classification	Left Grip	Right Grip	Back Strength	Leg Strength	Total Score	Strength per/lb/wt
Excellent	77+	86+	241+	261+	665+	5.30+
Very good	71–76	76–85	215–240	226–260	588–664	4.60–5.29
Fair	48–70	56–75	125–214	145–225	370–587	2.90–4.59
Poor	40–47	49–55	95–124	105–144	280–369	2.20–2.89
Very poor	below 39	below 48	below 94	below 104	below 279	below 2.19

Strength Rating Scale for Men (pounds)

Classification	Left Grip	Right Grip	Back Strength	Leg Strength	Total Score	Strength per/lb/wt
Excellent	131+	141+	460	476+	1200	7.26+
Very good	111–130	126–140	390–459	421–475	1050–1201	6.96–7.25
Fair	95–110	105–125	277–389	352–420	826–1049	4.82–6.95
Poor	86–94	91–104	201–276	301–351	676–825	4.81–5.20
Very poor	below 85	below 90	below 200	below 300	below 675	below 4.80

Because there is typically some loss of muscle tissue as you grow older, persons older than age 50 may wish to make an approximately 10 percent adjustment in the scores presented above.

REFERENCES

Basmajian, J. V. *Therapeutic Exercise.* Baltimore: Williams and Wilkins, 1984.

Buck, J. A., L. R. Amundsen, and D. H. Nielsen. "Systolic Blood Pressure Response during Isometric Contractions of Large and Small Muscle Groups." *Medicine and Science in Sports and Exercise* 12 (1980):145.

Chaffin, D. B., F. Lee, and A. Friewalds. "Muscle Strength Assessment from E.M.G. Analysis." *Medicine and Science in Sports and Exercise* 12 (1980):205.

*Cook, Brian, and G. W. Stewart. *Get Strong.* Ganges, B. C., Canada: 3S Fitness Group, 1981.

DeVries, H. A. *Physiology of Exercise.* 3d. ed. Dubuque, IA: Wm. C. Brown Publishers, 1980.

Fardy, P. S. "Isometric Exercise and the Cardiovascular System." *Physician and Sportsmedicine* 9 (September 1981):42.

*Gettman, L. R., and M. L. Pollock. "Circuit Weight Training: A Critical Review of its Physiological Benefits." *Physician and Sportsmedicine* 9 (June 1981):44.

Hage, P. "Prescribing Exercises: More Than Just a Running Program." *Physician and Sportsmedicine* 11 (May 1983):123.

Hay, J. G., J. G. Andrews, and C. L. Vaugh. "The Effect of Lifting Rate on Elbow Torques during Arm Curl Exercises." *Medicine and Science in Sports and Exercises* 15 (1983):63.

Hickson, R. S., M. A. Rosen Roetter, and M. M. Brown. "Strength Training Effects on Aerobic Power and Short-Term Endurance." *Medicine and Science in Sports and Exercise* 12 (1980):336.

Katch, V., et al. "Muscular Development and Lean Body Weight in Body Builders and Weight Lifters." *Medicine and Science in Sports and Exercise* 12 (1980):340.

Kottke, F. J., G. K. Stillwell, and J. F. Lehmann. *Krusen's Handbook of Physical Medicine and Rehabilitation.* 3d ed. Philadelphia: W. B. Saunders Co., 1982.

Kreighbaum, E., and K. M. Barthels. *Biomechanics.* Minneapolis: Burgess Publishing Co., 1981.

Kuntzleman, C. T., and Editors of Consumer Guide. *Rating the Exercises.* New York: William Morrow and Co., Inc., 1978.

Kusinitz, I., M. Fine, and Editors of Consumer Reports Books. *Physical Fitness for Practically Everybody.* Mount Vernon, NY: Consumers Union, 1983.

Lamb, D. R. *Physiology of Exercise.* New York: Macmillan Publishers, 1978.

Pollock, M., J. Willmore, and S. Fox. *Health and Fitness through Physical Activity.* New York: John Wiley and Sons, 1978.

*Rasch, P. J. *Weight Training.* 4th ed. Dubuque, IA: Wm. C. Brown Publishers, 1982.

Salle, A., et al. "New Muscle Fiber Production During Compensatory Hypertrophy." *Medicine and Science in Sports and Exercise* 12 (1980):268.

Schwane, J. A., et al. "Is Lactic Acid Related to Delayed-Onset Muscle Soreness?" *Physician and Sportsmedicine* 11 (March 1983):124.

Sports Medicine Technology 1 (June 1983):1.

Wilt, F., "Plyometrics: What It Is—How It Works." *The Athletic Journal* 55 (1975):76.

8
MUSCULAR ENDURANCE

CONCEPT 8

Muscular endurance
is an important health-related component
of physical fitness.

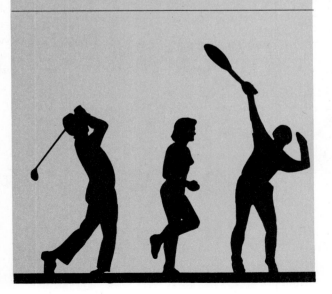

INTRODUCTION

Muscular endurance is the capacity of a muscle or group of muscles to continue contracting over a long period of time against a light-to-moderate resistance. This is your ability to resist fatigue when you hold a position or carry things for an extended period of time. And this is your ability to repeat a movement over and over without getting tired. You need muscular endurance to prevent undue fatigue from your daily activities and for greater success and enjoyment in athletic and recreational endeavors.

TERMS (Also see Concept 7 terms)

Dynamic Endurance—A muscle's ability to contract and relax repeatedly. This is usually measured by the number of times (repetitions) you can make a body movement in a given period of time.

Static Endurance—A muscle's ability to remain contracted for a long period of time. This is usually measured by the length of time you can hold a body position.

THE FACTS

Dynamic muscular endurance is developed with progressive resistance exercises using light-to-moderate resistance and a moderate-to-high number of repetitions.

While strength is developed by high resistance and low rep exercises, muscular endurance requires just the opposite—high reps and low resistance. Because of the principle of specificity, training for each should be designed differently.

There is a threshold of training and a target zone for muscular endurance exercises.

There is a level of frequency, intensity, and time at which a training effect will begin to take place (threshold). There is also an optimal range, or target zone, where the most effective and efficient improvement will occur (see Table 8.1). We do not know the optimum range, but studies suggest that it has wide limits. The intensity, or resistance (load), is less important than the number of reps or the length of time a muscle contracts.

Muscular endurance is slightly related to cardiovascular endurance, but it is not the same thing.

Cardiovascular endurance depends primarily upon the efficiency of the heart muscle, circulatory system, and the respiratory system. It is developed with activities that stress these systems, such as running, cycling, and swimming. Muscular endurance depends upon the efficiency of the local skeletal muscles and the nerves that

TABLE 8.1 Muscular Endurance Threshold of Training and Fitness Target Zone

	Threshold of Training	Target Zone
Dynamic Endurance		
Frequency	• 3 days per week.	• Every other day.
Intensity	• Lift resistance 20%–30% of the maximum you can lift.	• Lift resistance 40%–70% of the maximum you can lift.
Time	• One set of 8 repetitions of each exercise.	• 2–5 sets of 9–25 repetitions.
Static Endurance		
Frequency	• 3 days per week.	• Every other day.
Intensity	• Hold a weight 50%–100% of the weight you ultimately will need to hold in your work or leisure activity.	• Hold a weight equal to and up to 50% greater than the amount you will need to hold in your work or leisure activity.
Time	• Hold for lengths of time 10%–50% shorter than the time you plan to do the activity. Repeat 10–20 times.	• Hold for lengths of time equal to and up to 20% greater than the time you plan to do the activity. For longer times, use fewer repetitions (5–10).

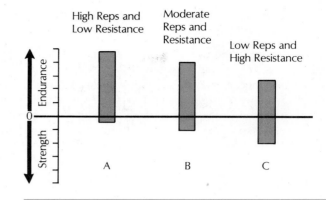

FIGURE 8.1 A Comparison of Absolute Endurance and Strength Developed by Different Exercise Regimes *Adapted from Anderson and Kearney, 1982.*

control them. You might train for cardiovascular endurance by running, but if the leg muscles lack the muscular endurance to continue contracting for more than five minutes, the cardiovascular system will not be stressed, even if it is in good condition.

Muscular endurance is related to strength, but is different.

Studies show that the person who is strength-trained will fatigue as much as four times faster than the person who is endurance-trained. However, there is a slight correlation between strength and endurance because the person who trains for strength will develop some endurance, and the person who trains for muscular endurance will develop some strength (Fig. 8.1).

Look at the graph in Figure 8.1, an illustration of the relationship between strength and muscular endurance. In *A,* the training program calls for a high number of repetitions and light resistance. This results in a small gain in strength (the area of the bar below the line), and a large increase in endurance (the area of the bar above the line). In *B,* the training program calls for a moderate number of reps (less than in *A*), and a moderate resistance (more than in *A*). This results in slightly less endurance and slightly more strength than in program *A.* Program *C* results in the least gain in endurance and the most gain in strength because it uses high resistance and low reps. Thus, if

you are primarily interested in muscular endurance, program *A* is your optimal choice.

Some endurance tests penalize the weaker person.

If you are tested on the number of times you can move a designated number of pounds, a stronger person has an advantage. However, if you are tested on the number of times you can move a designated percentage of the maximum load you can lift (1RM), the stronger person does not have the advantage and men and women can compete more evenly.

There are a variety of effective programs for developing muscular endurance.

All of the methods used in strength development are applicable to endurance development. Weight training, calisthenics, isometrics, isokinetics, and such activities as running, swimming, and aerobic dance can all be designed to increase muscular endurance. Even games, such as rope climbing, tug-o-war, Indian wrestling, and hopping races, can contribute to muscular endurance. It is well to keep in mind, however, that the endurance is specific to the muscles being used and that training should be specific to the type of activity for which you are training.

Guidelines for muscular endurance training programs are the same as those for strength development.

Performance guidelines for safety and effectiveness presented in Concept 7 should be reviewed before starting a program of exercise. It is particularly important that all muscle groups are exercised. For example, if your program for cardiovascular fitness stresses the muscles of the legs (front and back), then these might be omitted from your muscular endurance program and special attention given to the muscles on the inside and the outside of the legs and the muscles of the trunk and upper extremities.

Some training methods can interfere with athletic performance.

Some research studies have shown that certain techniques used in training may actually cause a decrease in performance. For example, when distance runners were trained with weighted wristlets, anklets, and belts, they performed worse than runners who did not wear the weights in training. In another study, when running and bicycling for aerobic endurance six days per week were combined with strength training five days per week, there was a decrease in strength development near the upper limits.

For optimal benefits, the exercise should resemble the actual activity for which you are training.

Studies show that you do better if your training closely resembles (mimics) the activity for which you are training. This is another example of specificity of training. If you are trying to develop endurance for a dynamic task, you should do isotonic exercises. If you need endurance in muscles that hold you in a static position, do isometric exercises. If the activity requires a rapid movement, it is better to train with fast movements. There may be transfer from fast practice to slow movement in a skill, but the reverse is not true.

Exercises to "slim" the figure/physique should be of the muscular endurance type.

Women in particular seem interested in exercises designed to decrease girth measurements. The high rep, low resistance exercise is suitable for this because it usually brings about some strengthening and, therefore, some "firming" of flabby muscles, which in turn, changes body contour. Exercises do *not* "spot reduce" fat (see Concept 25). Endurance exercises do speed up the metabolism so more calories are burned, but if weight or fat reduction is desired, aerobic (cardiovascular) exercises are best. To increase girth, strength exercises such as those power lifters use for hypertrophy are best (see Concept 7).

LAB RESOURCE MATERIALS (FOR USE WITH LAB 8, PAGE 207)

Evaluating Muscular Endurance

1. *Sitting Tucks*
   Sit on the floor so that your back and feet are off the floor. Interlock your fingers on top of your head. Alternately draw your legs to your chest and extend them away from your body. Keep your feet and back off the floor. Repeat as many times as possible up to thirty-five.

2. *Chins or Bent Arm Hang*
   a. *Chins*—Pull your body weight above the horizontal bar, gripping the bar with palms facing the bar. Repeat as many times as possible.
   b. *Bent Arm Hang*—(For men and women who cannot perform one chin.) Hang from a horizontal bar with palms facing the bar. Count the number of seconds that your chin can be held above the bar. *This test is only for people who cannot do one chin.* A separate rating chart is provided for this measure of muscular endurance.

CHART 8.1 Rating Scale for Muscular Endurance

Classification	Men		Women	
	Sitting Tuck	**Chins**	**Sitting Tuck**	**Chins**
Excellent	35+	15+	22	2
Very good	25–34	11–14	16–21	1
Fair	12–24	7–10	8–15	—
Poor	7–11	4–6	5–7	—
Very poor	6 or less	3 or less	4 or less	—

Adjust scores downward by 10 percent after age 50.

CHART 8.2 Rating Scale for Flexed Arm Hang (For people who cannot do one chin)

Classification	Score in Seconds
Making progress toward chin-up	25
Poor	12
Very poor	8 or less

REFERENCES

Anderson, T., and J. T. Kearney. "Effects of Three Resistance Training Programs on Muscular Strength and Absolute and Relative Endurance." *Research Quarterly for Exercise and Sport* 53 (1982):1.

Basmajian, J. V. *Therapeutic Exercise.* Baltimore: Williams and Wilkins, 1984.

Cook, B., and G. W. Stewart. *Get Strong.* Ganges, B. C., Canada: 3S Fitness Group, 1981.

Kottke, F. J., G. K. Stillwell, and J. F. Lehmann. *Krusen's Handbook of Physical Medicine and Rehabilitation.* 3d ed. Philadelphia: W. B. Saunders Co., 1982.

Kreighbaum, E., and K. M. Barthels. *Biomechanics.* Minneapolis: Burgess Publishing Co., 1981.

Kroll, W., P. M. Clarkson, G. Kamen, and J. Lambert. "Muscle Fiber Type Composition and Knee Extension Isometric Strength Fatigue Patterns in Power and Endurance Trained Males." *Research Quarterly for Exercise and Sport* 51 (1980):323.

Kusinitz, I., M. Fine and Editors of Consumer Reports Books. *Physical Fitness for Practically Everybody.* Mount Vernon, NY: Consumers Union, 1983.

Lamb, D. R. *Physiology of Exercise.* New York: Macmillan Publishers, 1978.

*Lindsey, R., B. Jones, and A. V. Whitley. *Fitness.* 5th ed. Dubuque, IA: Wm. C. Brown Publishers, 1983.

*Rasch, P. J. *Weight Training* 4th ed. Dubuque, IA: Wm. C. Brown Publishers, 1982.

9
FLEXIBILITY

CONCEPT 9

Adequate flexibility permits
freedom of movement and may contribute
to ease and economy of muscular effort,
success in certain activities,
and less susceptibility to some types of injuries
or musculoskeletal problems.

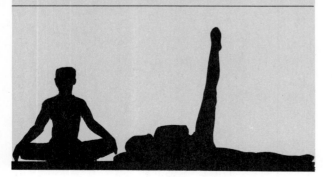

INTRODUCTION

Flexibility is a measure of the range of motion available at a joint or group of joints. It is determined by the shape of the bones and cartilage in the joint, and by the length of muscles and ligaments that cross the joint. Traditionally, it has been the most neglected of the five health-related components of physical fitness. However, there has been a recent surge of interest in "stretching exercises" by athletes, fitness buffs, and researchers.

The range of movement at a joint may vary. It may be restricted so that it will not bend or straighten, and is said to be "tight" or "stiff" or have "contractures." The deformed hand of an arthritic is an example of this extreme. At the other end of the spectrum is a high degree of flexibility referred to as "loose jointed," "hypermobility," or erroneously, "double-jointedness." An example of this extreme is the contortionist seen at the circus. Each person, depending upon his or her individual needs, must have a reasonable amount of flexibility to perform efficiently and effectively in daily life.

TERMS

Antagonist-Stretch—Muscles are stretched by the force of the contraction of the opposing, or antagonist, muscle. For example, when doing a toe-touch exercise, the muscles on the front of the thigh (quadriceps) contract to cause a stretch of the muscles on the back of the thigh (hamstrings). (See Figure 9.1a.)

Assisted-Stretch—Stretch imposed on a muscle by someone or something other than the opposing muscle. For example, when doing the toe-touch exercise, the force causing the stretch is provided by an assist from another person pushing gently on your back (Fig. 9.1b); or you may grasp your ankles and pull with your arms (Fig. 9.1c); or you could use gravity; or might also use an extra weight to provide the assist.

Ballistic-Stretch—Muscles are stretched by the force of momentum of a body part that is bounced, swung, or jerked, as in, for example, the toe-touch exercise shown in Figure 9.1d and e. The trunk is bounced forward either by antagonist muscle force or by an assist from another person.

Dysmenorrhea—Painful menstruation.

Flexibility—Range of motion (ROM) in a joint or group of joints. Because muscle length is a major factor limiting the range of motion, those having long muscles that allow for good joint mobility are considered to have good flexibility.

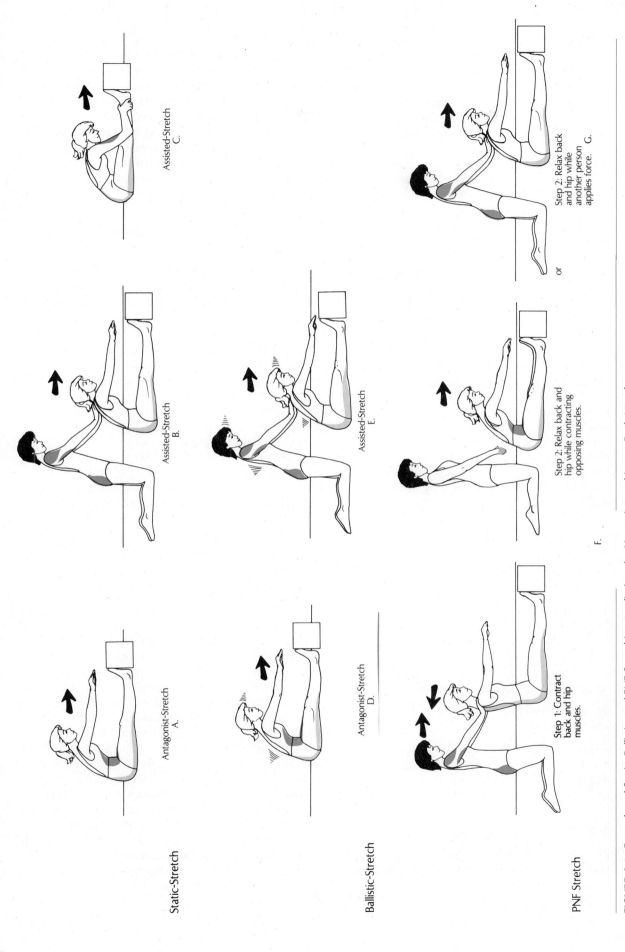

Static-Stretch

Antagonist-Stretch
A.

Assisted-Stretch
B.

Assisted-Stretch
C.

Ballistic-Stretch

Antagonist-Stretch
D.

Assisted-Stretch
E.

PNF Stretch

Step 1: Contract back and hip muscles.

Step 2: Relax back and hip while contracting opposing muscles.
F.

or

Step 2: Relax back and hip while another person applies force.   G.

FIGURE 9.1 Examples of Static, Ballistic, and PNF Stretching Applied to the Hamstring and Lower Back Muscles

Note: Muscles shown in dark color are the muscle groups that are contracting. Those shown in light color are those being stretched.

Hamstrings—Muscles that cross the back of the hip joint and the back of the knee joint causing hip extension and knee flexion. They make up the bulk on the back of the thigh.

Laxity—Looseness or slackness of the muscles and ligaments (soft tissue) surrounding a joint.

Ligaments—Bands of tissue that connect bones.

Lumbar Muscles—Erector spinae and other muscles of the lower back (lumbar region of the spine); the muscles in the "small of the back." These muscles are used to arch (hyperextend) the lower back.

PNF Exercise—(Proprioceptive Neuromuscular Facilitation) Special exercise techniques to increase the contraction or the relaxation of muscles through reflex mechanisms (Fig. 9.1f and g).

Reciprocal Innervation—When a muscle (agonist) contracts, its opposing muscle (antagonist) will reflexly relax.

Static-Stretch—A muscle is slowly stretched and then held in that stretched position for several seconds. For example, if you lie on your back and pull one knee to your chest and hold it there with your arms for a count of ten, you are placing a static stretch on your back muscles.

Trigger Point—An especially irritable spot, usually a tight band or "knot" in a muscle or fascia. This often refers pain to another area of the body. For example, a trigger point in the shoulder might cause a headache. This condition is referred to as "myofascial pain syndrome" and is often caused by muscle tension, fatigue, or strain.

THE FACTS

To increase the length of a muscle, you must stretch it more than its normal length.

There is much that is not known about flexibility, but the best evidence suggests that muscles should be stretched to about 10 percent beyond their normal length to bring about an improvement in flexibility. Exercises that do not cause an "overload" by stretching beyond normal will not increase flexibility.

There are several effective methods of exercising to develop flexibility.

There are three commonly used types of stretching exercises. These are static, ballistic, and PNF. Each of these can be performed as an antagonist-stretch or as an assisted-stretch. All are effective in developing flexibility.

Static stretching is widely recommended because it is less apt to cause injury and soreness.

Because static stretching is done slowly and held for a period of time, there is less probability of tearing the soft tissue, particularly if the force comes from your own muscles. When antagonist-stretch is used, the opposing muscles contract. This makes the muscles you are trying to stretch relax (reflexly) so that they can be stretched farther. When stretching is done with an assist by something other than the antagonist muscle, the reflex relaxation does not occur, so there is more potential for injury. For this reason, assisted stretching is not as effective as the antagonist-static stretch. Because the antagonist-stretch is safest, it is particularly suitable for beginners, for older adults, and for the early stages of warm-up. (See Figure 9.1, exercises a, b, and c, for further clarification.)

Ballistic stretching may be an important technique for active people.

A ballistic-stretch uses momentum to produce the stretch. Momentum is produced by vigorous motion, such as flinging a body part, or rocking it back and forth to create a bouncing or jerking movement. Because this produces a sudden stretch on the muscle, and may stretch it farther than other methods, there is the potential for injury. Most people avoid this type of stretching, but everyone does not agree that its disadvantages outweigh its advantages.

Since so many athletic activities are ballistic in nature, many experts recommend the use of predominantly static stretching in early training, but with an increasing amount of ballistic exercise as flexibility improves. The principle of specificity of training implies that one should use the type of stretching movements that are most apt to occur in the activity for which one is training. Ballistic exercises are illustrated in Figure 9.1d and e.

Some PNF (Proprioceptive Neuromuscular Facilitation) techniques have proven to be effective methods of improving flexibility.

PNF has been popular for rehabilitation since the 1960s. It consists of dozens of techniques to stimulate muscles to contract more strongly or to relax more fully so that they can be stretched. Two of those techniques have become popular in fitness programs to improve the flexibility of healthy people: "Contract-Relax-Contract," and "Contract-Relax."

The "Contract-Relax-Contract" technique involves three steps: (1) move the limb so the muscle to be stretched is elongated initially, then contract it isometrically for five to ten seconds; (2) relax the muscle; (3) stretch the muscle immediately by contracting the antagonist for twenty to sixty seconds. Recent research suggests that this type of PNF stretch is more effective than a simple static-stretch without the preceding isometric contraction. An example of the "Contract-Relax-Contract" PNF exercise is shown in Figure 9.1f.

A variation of this PNF procedure is "Contract-Relax." This is the same procedure as the "Contract-Relax-Contract" technique except that the static-stretch is done with an assist. Following the isometric

TABLE 9.1 Flexibility Threshold of Training and Fitness Target Zones

	Threshold of Training			Target Zones		
	Static	Ballistic	PNF	Static	Ballistic	PNF
Frequency	• 3 days per week for all methods.			• 3 to 7 days per week for all methods.		
Intensity	• Stretch as far as you can go without pain with slow movement, hold at the end of the range of motion.	• Stretch muscle beyond normal length with gentle bounce or swing, but do not exceed 10% of antagonist-static range of motion.	• Same as static except use a maximum isometric contraction of the muscle prior to stretch.	• When *antagonist-stretch* is used, the muscle should be stretched as far as possible using only the antagonist muscles. • When *assisted-stretch* is used, the muscle should not be stretched more than 10% beyond its normal range of motion, and it should not reach the point of pain. Care should be taken to avoid overstretch.		
Time (Duration)	• Hold the stretch for 10 seconds.	• 3 sets of 5 repetitions; 10-second rest between sets.	• Hold isometric contraction 6 seconds; hold stretch 10 seconds. Repeat 3 times.	• Hold 20–60 seconds for 1–3 sets.	• 5 sets of 5–10 reps.	• Hold isometric contraction 6 seconds. • Hold stretch 20–60 seconds for 1–3 sets.

contraction, another person applies force to stretch the muscles. There is no contraction of the opposing muscles during the stretch.

It is possible to combine these two techniques so that the opposing muscles contract while another person assists in applying the stretch. Theoretically, the muscle would be elongated more by this procedure, but any time assistance is provided by another person or a machine, there is danger of overstretching the muscle. This modification is shown in Figure 9.1g.

There is a minimum amount of exercise (threshold of training) and an optimal amount of exercise (target zone) necessary for developing flexibility.

The threshold of training and target zones for static, ballistic, and PNF stretching are presented in Table 9.1. The time required to stretch tissue varies inversely with the force used. Low force requires more time, whereas high force requires less time.

Each form of flexibility exercise has its advantages and disadvantages.

The advantages and disadvantages of ballistic, static, and PNF exercises using both antagonist-stretch and assisted-stretch methods are summarized in Table 9.2. The best method or methods for you may depend upon your physical condition, and whether or not you wish to increase or maintain your range of motion.

For maximal effectiveness and minimal harm, there are guidelines that should be followed in performing flexibility exercises.

There is a correct and an incorrect way to exercise, and some exercises can even be harmful. Concept 14 presents guidelines for flexibility exercises and some samples of the exercises defined in this concept.

Lack of use, injury, or disease can decrease joint mobility.

Arthritis and calcium deposits can damage a joint, and inflammation can cause pain that prevents movement. Failure to regularly move a joint through its full range of motion can lead to a shortening of muscles and ligaments. Static positions held for longer periods of time, such as in poor posture, working postures, and when a body part is immobilized by a cast, lead to shortened tissue and loss of mobility. Improper exercise that over-develops one muscle group while neglecting the opposing group results in an imbalance that restricts flexibility.

Flexibility is specific to each joint of the body.

No one flexibility test will give an indication of your overall flexibility. For example, "tight" hamstrings or back muscles might be revealed by a toe-touch test, but the range of motion in other joints may be quite different.

TABLE 9.2 Comparison of Advantages and Disadvantages of Six Types of Flexibility Exercises

A. Antagonist-Stretch

Static-Antagonist-Stretch	Ballistic-Antagonist-Stretch	PNF-Antagonist-Stretch ("Contract-Relax-Contract")
1. Will not overstretch tissue.	1. If done vigorously, can overstretch tissue, especially in presence of scar tissue or pathology.	1. Will not overstretch tissue; therapists use PNF in treatment of arthritics.
2. May be ineffective in producing enough stretch to increase muscle length. It can be used to maintain current flexibility levels or in combination with *assisted-stretch* to improve flexibility.	2. Is effective for increasing flexibility because momentum produces overload.	2. More effective than static and ballistic for increasing flexibility, especially if combined with *assisted-stretch.*
3. Useful if combined with *assisted-stretch* to relieve muscle cramps.	3. Not recommended for cramps.	3. Useful if combined with *assisted-stretch* to relieve muscle cramps.
4. Useful if combined with *assisted-stretch* for some types of muscle soreness.	4. If done vigorously, may cause soreness.	4. Useful if combined with *assisted-stretch* for some types of muscle soreness.
5. Does not develop strength.	5. Does not develop strength.	5. Strength is developed in muscle being stretched.
6. Stretched muscle relaxes through reciprocal innervation with contracting agonist.	6. Stretched muscle relaxes through reciprocal innervation with contracting agonist.	6. Stretched muscle relaxes because of reciprocal innervation and because of previous isometric contraction.
7. Stretch will elicit mild reflex contraction that will gradually subside as stretch is held.	7. Stretch reflex will be elicited more strongly, but muscle will not strengthen because it is not overloaded during contraction.	7. Stretch will elicit mild reflex contraction that will gradually subside as stretch is held.
8. May become boring.	8. More nearly resembles movements needed in some athletics and daily activities.	8. Easier to do if another person applies resistance.

B. Assisted-Stretch

Static-Assisted-Stretch	Ballistic-Assisted-Stretch	PNF with Assisted-Stretch ("Contract-Relax")
1. May overstretch tissue.	1. Most apt to overstretch tissue.	1. May overstretch tissue.
2. Effective for increasing flexibility, but better if combined with *antagonist-stretch* or if muscle is consciously relaxed.	2. Effective for increasing flexibility, but better if combined with *antagonist-stretch,* or if muscle is consciously relaxed.	2. Not as effective as *antagonist-static* or PNF with *antagonist-stretch,* but would be better if combined with *antagonist-stretch* or if muscle was consciously relaxed.
3. Can aid in relief of soreness, but more effective if combined with *antagonist-stretch* or if the muscle is consciously relaxed.	3. More apt to cause soreness.	3. Can aid in relief of soreness, but more effective if combined with *antagonist-stretch* or if the muscle is consciously relaxed.
4. Can aid in relief of muscle cramps, but more effective if combined with *antagonist-stretch* or if the muscle is consciously relaxed.	4. Not recommended for muscle cramps.	4. Can aid in muscle cramps, but more effective if combined with *antagonist-stretch* or if the muscle is consciously relaxed.
5. Does not develop strength.	5. Does not develop strength.	5. Develops strength in muscle being stretched.
6. Muscle being stretched does not relax unless combined with *antagonist-stretch* or with conscious relaxation.	6. Muscle being stretched does not relax unless combined with *antagonist-stretch* or with conscious relaxation.	6. Muscle being stretched will relax because of previous isometric contraction, especially if conscious relaxation is used.
7. Will elicit mild myotatic reflex that is lessened if combined with *antagonist-stretch* or with conscious relaxation.	7. Will elicit mild myotatic reflex that is lessened if combined with *antagonist-stretch* or with conscious relaxation.	7. Will elicit mild myotatic reflex that is lessened if combined with *antagonist-stretch* or with conscious relaxation.
8. Requires outside force: another person, other body parts, or gravity.	8. Requires outside force: another person, other body parts, or gravity.	8. Easier to do if another person applies stretch, but any outside force may be used.

Flexibility is influenced by age and sex.

As children grow older, their flexibility increases until adolescence when they become progressively less flexible. As a general rule, girls tend to be more flexible than boys. This is probably due to anatomical differences in the joints, as well as differences in the type and extent of activities the two sexes tend to choose. In adults, there is less difference between the sexes.

Scores on flexibility tests may be influenced by several factors.

Range of motion may be influenced by your motivation to exert maximum effort, warm-up preparation, the presence of muscular soreness, tolerance for pain, room temperature, and your ability to relax. Contrary to popular opinion, there is very little relationship between leg or trunk length and the scores made on flexibility tests.

Stretching exercises are useful in preventing and remediating some cases of dysmenorrhea.

Painful menstruation of some types can be prevented or reduced by stretching the pelvic and hip joint fascia.

Static muscle stretching appears to be effective in relieving muscle soreness and "shin splints."

One theory suggests that local muscle soreness may be caused by slight reflex contractions. There is the belief that a static-stretch of the affected muscle may relieve these slight contractions and thus relieve the pain. Even some cases of nonpathological shin splints may be relieved by such exercise.

Adequate flexibility may help prevent muscle strain and such orthopedic problems as backache.

Short, tight muscles are more apt to be injured by overstretching than are long muscles. One common cause of backache is shortened lumbar and hip flexor muscles. (See Concept 20 for more discussion on back problems.) Stretching exercises may help prevent or alleviate some backaches, muscle cramps, and muscle strains.

Trigger points may sometimes be prevented or inactivated by static, or PNF stretching, of the muscles involved.

When body parts are held in static positions for long periods of time, or when muscles are chronically overloaded, fatigued or chilled, myofascial trigger points may cause stiffness and local or referred pain. Often the trigger point can be deactivated and the pain relieved by gentle but persistent stretching of the muscle, especially if accompanied by or followed by the application of heat.

Assisted stretching may exceed the limits of extensibility of the muscles, tendons, and ligaments and cause injury.

When force that is not under the control of the exerciser is applied to stretch the soft tissue around a joint, it may result in torn tissue. A partner, therapist, or machine can not "feel" how much stretch is being applied and so may cause injury.

Too much flexibility in certain joints may make a person more susceptible to injury or hamper performance.

Muscles and tendons have both extensibility and elasticity. Ligaments are extensible but lack elasticity. When stretched, ligaments remain in the lengthened state. When this occurs, the joint may lack stability and so is susceptible to chronic dislocation or movement in an undesirable plane. This is particularly true of weight-bearing joints, such as the hip, knee, and ankle. Loose ligaments may allow the joint to twist abnormally, tearing the cartilage and other soft tissue.

On the other hand, joint laxity does not necessarily mean instability. While most studies show no relationship between laxity and subsequent injury, there is some evidence that loose knees are detrimental in football and in ballet. Dancers seem to have a decreased ability to judge how much movement has taken place in the knee and, therefore, may be more susceptible to injury.

In the fifth century, Hippocrates noted the disadvantage of hyperextension of the elbow in archery. The hyperextended position for elbows and knees is not an efficient position from which to move because of a poor angle of muscle pull. For example, it is difficult to perform push-ups when the elbows lock into hyperextension because extra effort is required to "unlock" the joint.

Good flexibility may bring about improved athletic performance.

A hurdler must have good hip joint mobility to clear the hurdle. A swimmer requires shoulder and ankle flexibility for powerful strokes. A diver must be able to reach his or her toes in order to perform a good jackknife. Low back flexibility allows a runner to lengthen the stride. The fencer needs long hamstrings and hip adductors in order to lunge a long distance.

It is not necessary to sacrifice flexibility in order to develop strength.

A person with bulging muscles may become muscle-bound, or have a restricted range of motion, if strength training is done improperly. In any progressive resistance program, both agonists and antagonists should receive equal training and all movements should be carried through the full range of motion. Properly conducted strength training does not cause a person to be muscle-bound. Furthermore, there is no evidence that a flexible muscle is any less strong than an inflexible one.

There is no ideal standard for flexibility.

It is not known how much flexibility any one person should have in a joint. There are test "norms" available that list how hundreds of subjects of various ages, of both sexes, and from many walks of life have performed. But there is little scientific evidence to indicate that a person who can reach two inches past his or her toes on a sit-and-reach test is any less fit than a person who can reach eight inches past the toes. Too much flexibility could be as detrimental as too little.

LAB RESOURCE MATERIALS (FOR USE WITH LAB 9, PAGE 209)

Flexibility Tests

Since it is impractical to test the flexibility of all joints, perform these tests for the joints used most frequently in movement performance.

1. *Flexibility Test of Lower Back and Hamstrings*
   a. Sit on the floor with your knees together and your feet flat against a bench turned on its side.
   b. With a partner holding your knees straight, reach forward with your arms fully extended.
   c. Measure the distance your fingertips reach on the yardstick fixed on the bench. (The six-inch mark of the yardstick should be flush with the end of the bench.)

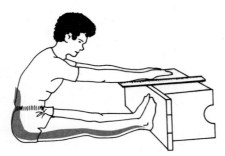

Note: Ruler extends six inches over the end of the bench

2. *Shoulder Flexibility*
   a. Raise your right arm, bend your elbow, and reach down across your back as far as possible.
   b. At the same time, extend your left arm down and behind your back, bend your elbow up across your back, and try to cross your fingers over those of your right hand as shown in the accompanying illustration.
   c. Measure the distance to the nearest half-inch. If your fingers overlap, score as a plus; if they fail to meet, score as a minus; use a zero if your fingertips just touch.
   d. Repeat with your arms crossed in the opposite direction (left arm up). Most people will find that they are more flexible on one side than the other.

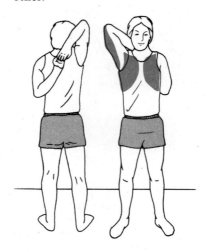

3. *Flexibility Stunt (Multiple Joint Flexibility)*
   a. Grasp a wand or broom stick with palms down and about shoulder width apart.
   b. Reach the end of the wand and your left hand between the legs.
   c. Step with your left leg around the outside of your arm and into the "hole" between the stick and your body.
   d. Slide the stick over your left knee, left hip, and back (see accompanying picture).
   e. Step your right foot over the stick and stand erect, holding the stick in front of your body, palms up (without ever having released grip on stick).
   f. Score yourself on the basis of the number of attempts needed to succeed. You may find that you perform better when you start with the right leg. This is permissible. If you succeed up to the point of stepping out of the "hole," (step d) or to step e before dropping the wand, you still rate.

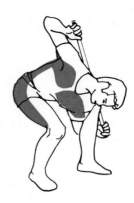

CHART 9.1 Flexibility Rating Scale

Classification	Men				Women			
	Test 1	**Test 2**		**Test 3**	**Test 1**	**Test 2**		**Test 3**
		R up	L up			R up	L up	
Excellent	14+	7+	7+	1 trial	15+	8+	8+	1 trial
Very good	11–13	6	3–6	2–3 trials	12–14	7	6–7	2–3 trials
Fair	7–10	4–5	0–2	step d	7–11	5–6	0–5	step d
Poor	4–6	1–3	−2–1	step e	4–6	1–4	−2–1	step e
Very poor	3 or less	less than 0	−3 or less	fail	3 or less	less than 0	−3 or less	fail

Though many people become less flexible as they grow older, for optimal health, it is recommended that you attempt to maintain adequate levels of flexibility on the above chart throughout life.

REFERENCES

Barrack, R. L., H. B. Skinner, M. E. Brunet, and S. D. Cook. "Joint Laxity and Proprioception in the Knee." *Physician and Sportsmedicine* 11 (1983):130.

Beaulieu, J. E. "Developing a Stretching Program." *Physician and Sportsmedicine* 9 (1981):59.

Brodie, D. A., H. A. Bird, and V. Wright. "Joint Laxity in Selected Athletic Populations." *Medicine and Science in Sports and Exercise* 14 (1980):190.

Corbin, C. B., and L. Noble. "Flexibility." *Journal of Physical Education, Recreation, and Dance* 51 (1980):23.

*Corbin, C. B. "Profiling for Flexibility." In Nicholas, J. A. and Herschberger, J. *Clinics in Sports Medicine: Profiling.* Philadelphia: W. B. Saunders Co., 1984.

Daniels, L., and C. Worthingham. *Therapeutic Exercise for Body Alignment and Function.* Philadelphia: W. B. Saunders Co., 1977.

De Vries, H. A. *Physiology of Exercise for Physical Education and Athletics.* Dubuque, IA: Wm. C. Brown Publishers, 1980.

*Dominguez, R. H., and R. S. Gajda. *Total Body Conditioning.* New York: Charles Scribners Sons, 1982.

Grahame, R., and J. M. Jenkins. "Joint Hypermobility—Asset or Liability." *Annals of Rheumatic Disease* 31 (1972):109.

Hartley-O'Brien, S. J. "Six Mobilization Exercises for Active Range of Hip Flexion." *Research Quarterly of Exercise and Sport* 51 (1980):625.

Holt, L. E., T. M. Travis, and T. Okita. "Comparative Study of Three Stretching Techniques." *Perceptual and Motor Skills* 31 (1970):611.

Knott, M., and D. Voss *Proprioceptive Neuromuscular Facilitation: Patterns and Techniques.* New York: Harper and Row, 1968.

Kreighbaum, E., and K. M. Barthels. *Biomechanics: A Qualitative Approach for Studying Human Movement.* Minneapolis: Burgess Publishing Co., 1981.

Lindsey, R., B. Jones, and A. Whitley. *Fitness for Health, Figure/Physique, Posture.* 5th ed. Dubuque, IA: Wm. C. Brown Publishers, 1983.

Millar, A. P. "Strains of the Posterior Calf Musculature (Tennis Leg)." *American Journal of Sports Medicine* 7 (1979):172.

Millar, A. P. "An Early Stretching for Calf Muscle Strains." *Medicine and Science in Sports* 8 (1976):39.

Montoye, H. J. *An Introduction to Measurement in Physical Education.* Boston: Allyn and Bacon, Inc., 1978.

Moore, M. A., and R. S. Hutton. "Electromyographic Investigation of Muscle Stretching Techniques." *Medicine and Science in Sports and Exercise* 12 (1980):322.

O'Neil, R. "Prevention of Hamstring and Groin Strain." *Athletic Training* 11 (1976):27.

Nicholas, J. A. "Injuries to the Knee Ligaments." *Journal of the American Medical Association* 212 (1970):2236.

Rivera, M. L. "Effects of Static, Ballistic, and Modified Proprioceptive Neuromuscular Stretching Exercises on the Flexibility and Retention of Flexibility in Selected Joints." Master's thesis, University of Kansas, 1979.

*Rogers, J. L. "PNF: A New Way to Improve Flexibility." *Track Technique* 12 (1978):2345.

Sapega, A. A., T. C. Quedenfeld, R. A. Moyer, and R. A. Butler. "Biophysical Factors in Range of Motion Exercise." *Physician and Sportsmedicine* 9 (1981):57.

*Schultz, P. "Flexibility: Day of the Static Stretch." *Physician and Sportsmedicine* 7 (1979):109.

Surburg, P. R. "Neuromuscular Facilitation Techniques in Sports Medicine." *Physician and Sportsmedicine* 9 (1981):115.

Tanigawa, M. C. "Mobilization on Increasing Muscle Length." *Physical Therapy* 52 (1972):725.

Travell, J. G., and D. G. Simons. *Myofascial Pain and Dysfunction: The Trigger Point Manual.* Baltimore: Williams and Wilkins, 1983.

10
BODY COMPOSITION/ WEIGHT CONTROL

CONCEPT 10

Obesity is a significant health problem that can be controlled, in most cases, with a proper balance between caloric consumption (diet) and caloric expenditure (physical activity).

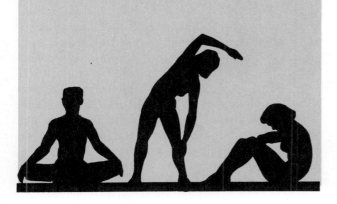

INTRODUCTION

Appearance is probably the major reason why most people are concerned about weight control. However, proper body composition is also very important to total health and fitness. The following discussion presents facts about weight control, including information about diet and physical activity. Special consideration is given to the use of exercise as an effective means of maintaining ideal body weight.

TERMS

Calorie—A unit of energy supplied by food; the quantity of heat necessary to raise the temperature of a kilogram of water one degree centigrade (actually a kilocalorie but usually called a calorie for weight control programs).

Caloric Balance—Consuming calories in amounts equal to the number of calories expended.

Diet—The usual food and drink for a person or animal.

M.E.T.—MET is an acronym for the basic amount of energy expended at rest. As you work, your metabolism increases. METs are multiples of the amount of energy expended at rest.

Obesity—Extreme weight, often considered as 20 to 35 percent above "normal;" probably best defined as an extreme overfat condition.

Overfat—Having too much body composition as fat; for men, having more than 19 percent of the total body composition as fat; and for women, 26 percent.

Overweight—Having weight in excess of normal. Not harmful unless it is accompanied by overfatness.

Somatotype—Inherent body build: ectomorph (thin); mesomorph (muscular); and endomorph (fat).

THE FACTS

Overfat rather than overweight is more important in determining health.

Individuals who are interested in controlling their weight usually consult a height-weight chart to determine "desirable" weight. Being 20 percent or more above the ideal chart weight is the commonly accepted criterion of obesity. While proper chart weights are good general guidelines, it is now clear that for most people, the height-weight chart is not as accurate an indication of health as is the percentage of body fat.

It is possible to estimate the percentage of the body that is fat. Some individuals having muscular body types have been overweight and even obese in terms of height-weight charts, yet they possess very little body fat. Since the amount of body fat, not the amount of

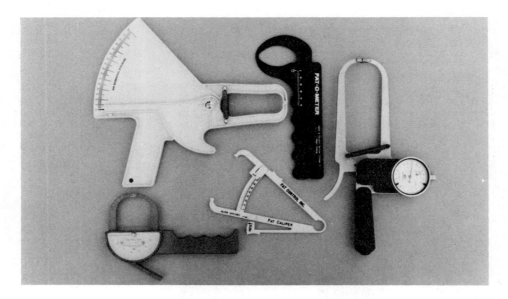

FIGURE 10.1 Skinfold Calipers

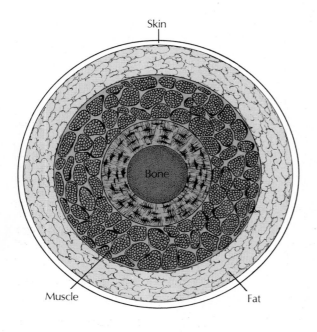

FIGURE 10.2 Location of Body Fat

weight, is the important factor in living a healthy life, it is wise to use "overfat" rather than "overweight" as the measure.

There are many ways to assess body fatness and leanness.

Underwater weighing is one of the better methods for determining the amount of your body that is composed of fat. Because this procedure takes a considerable amount of time, equipment, and specialized training, it is not practical for use except in well-equipped laboratories. Other ways of estimating body fatness are body girth measurements, X rays, and skinfold measurements. Skinfold measurements are often used because they can be taken fairly easily using a caliper (see Fig. 10.1). This is not nearly as costly as underwater weighing or X rays. The better, more accurate calipers cost several hundred dollars. However, considerably less expensive calipers are now available. When used by a trained person, these calipers give a good estimate of fatness (see the Lab Resource Materials on page 75). An expert's estimate of your body fatness determined by skinfold measurements is informative. It will also be useful for you to learn to correctly use a caliper so that you can take your own measurements throughout your life.

Body fat is distributed throughout the body. About one-half of the body's fat is located inside the body around the various body organs and in the muscles. The other half of the body's fat is located just under the skin, or in skinfolds (Fig. 10.2). A skinfold is two thicknesses of skin and the amount of fat that lies just under the skin. At certain locations in the body, the thickness of the skinfolds can be used to obtain a good estimate of the fatness of the total body (Fig. 10.3).

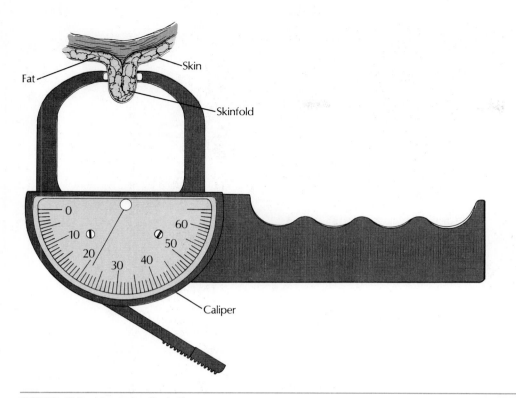

Fat

Skin

Skinfold

0
10
20
30
40
50
60

Caliper

FIGURE 10.3 Measuring Body Fat

Obesity is a problem experienced by too many Americans.

Some experts indicate that as many as 60 million people or half of all the adults, in the United States are overweight. Others suggest that at least one-third of adult Americans are overfat. In addition to the problem of adult obesity, statistics indicate that as many as 10 million schoolchildren can be classified as overfat or obese.

In some cases, glandular problems cause an obese condition. However, these conditions are quite rare. Obesity is usually a result of an imbalance between caloric intake and output. Crash diets, spot reducing, and passive exercise "gimmick" machines are *not* effective in producing lasting fat loss.

Overfatness or obesity can contribute to degenerative diseases, health problems, and even shortened life.

Some diseases and health problems associated with overfatness and obesity were presented in Concept 4. In addition to the higher incidence of certain diseases and health problems, there is evidence that people who are moderately overfat have a 40 percent higher than normal risk of shortened life. More severe obesity results in a 70 percent higher than normal death rate.

This is evidenced by the exorbitant life insurance premiums paid by obese individuals.

Recent statistics indicating that underweight people had a higher than normal risk of premature death are very deceptive. Many people included in the data were underweight because of terminal illnesses. The truth is, most experts agree those people who are free from disease and who have lower than average amounts of body fat have a lower than average risk of premature death.

Excessive concern for being thin or low in body fat can result in health problems.

More and more Americans are becoming aware of the dangers of obesity. While this awareness is good, excessive concern for thinness can also become a problem. For example, several medical conditions that are particularly prevalent among children and teenagers are anorexia nervosa, bulemia, and "fear of obesity." All conditions are, to a large extent, modern-day and western-world disorders. Anorexia, which means "loss of appetite," is a condition associated with an extreme desire to be lean and thin. It can result in dramatic and dangerous losses in body weight from failure to eat, regurgitating food to prevent digestion, and compulsive

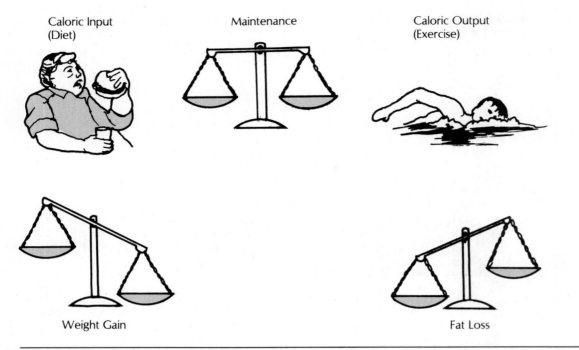

Caloric Input
(Diet)

Maintenance

Caloric Output
(Exercise)

Weight Gain

Fat Loss

FIGURE 10.4 Weight Loss and Gain

exercise to prevent weight gain. This is a serious medical-psychological disorder that can be fatal. Those suffering from bulimia are also overly conscious of gaining weight, and so eat erratically and regurgitate to prevent digestion.

"Fear of obesity" is a newly discovered condition that is not as severe as anorexia nervosa, but that can still have negative health consequences. This condition is most common among achievement-oriented teenagers who impose a self-restriction on caloric intake as a result of the fear of obesity. Consequences include stunting of growth, delayed puberty including delayed sexual development, and decreased physical attractiveness. It is important to avoid excessive eating and inactivity to prevent the problems associated with overfatness and obesity. However, it is also important to realize that overconcern for leanness can result in serious health problems, too.

To lose body fat, decreased caloric intake, increased caloric expenditure, or a combination of the two is necessary.

The threshold of training and a target zone for exercise are not the only determinants of minimal and optimal body fatness. Exercise is one effective way to reduce body fat levels. Decreasing caloric intake (dieting) is another. Of course, a combination of the two is preferable (Fig. 10.4). Threshold of training and target zones for body fat reduction, including information for both exercise and diet, are presented in Table 10.1.

Exercise is one effective means of controlling body fat.

Though physical activity or exercise will not result in immediate and large decreases in body fat levels, there is increasing evidence that fat loss resulting from exercise may be more lasting than fat loss from dieting. Vigorous exercise can increase the resting energy expenditure up to thirteen times (13 METs).

TABLE 10.1 Threshold of Training and Target Zones for Body Fat Reduction

	Threshold of Training*		Target Zones*	
	Exercise	Diet	Exercise	Diet
Frequency	• To be effective, exercise must be regular, preferably daily, though fat can be lost over the long haul with almost any frequency that results in increased caloric expenditure.	• It is best to reduce caloric intake consistently and daily. To restrict calories only on certain days is *not* best, though fat can be lost over a period of time by reducing caloric intake at any time.	• Daily moderate exercise is recommended. For those who do regular vigorous activity, 5 or 6 days per week may be best.	• It is best to diet consistently and daily.
Intensity	• To lose 1 pound of fat, you must expend 3,500 calories more than you normally expend.	• To lose 1 pound of fat, you must eat 3,500 calories fewer than you normally eat.	• Slow, low-intensity aerobic exercise that results in no more than 1–2 pounds of fat loss per week is best.	• Modest caloric restriction resulting in no more than 1–2 pounds of fat loss per week is best.
Time	• To be effective, exercise must be sustained long enough to expend a considerable number of calories. At least 15 minutes per exercise bout is necessary to result in consistent fat loss.	• Eating moderate meals is best. Skipping meals is *not* most effective.	• Exercise durations similar to those for achieving aerobic cardiovascular fitness seem best. An exercise duration of 30–60 minutes is recommended.	• Eating moderate meals is best. Skipping meals or fasting is *not* most effective.

Note: It is best to combine exercise and diet to achieve the 3,500 caloric imbalance necessary to lose a pound of fat. Using both exercise and diet in the target zone is most effective.

If a person exercises moderately for fifteen minutes a day (all other things being equal), a loss of more than ten pounds in a year's time may be seen. Regular walking, jogging, swimming, or any type of sustained exercise can be effective in producing losses in body fat.

Exercise that can be sustained for relatively long periods of time is probably the most effective for losing body fat.

Table 10.2 shows the caloric expenditures for one hour of involvement in various recreational physical activities. The heavier the person, the more calories expended because more work is required to move larger bodies. Activities that are extremely vigorous can help in losing body fatness if done regularly. But for many people, these may not be as effective as some less vigorous activities. For example, running at ten miles per hour (a six-minute mile) will cause a 150-pound person to expend 900 calories in one hour. Jogging about one-half as fast, or at five and one-half miles per hour (approximately an eleven-minute mile), will result in an expenditure of about 650 calories in the same amount of time. At first glance, the more vigorous exercise seems to be a better choice. But how many people can continue to run at a ten-mile-per-hour pace for a full hour? Each mile run at ten miles per hour results in an expenditure of 90 calories, while each mile run at five and one-half miles per hour results in an expenditure of 118 calories. Per mile, you expend more calories in slow running. It takes longer to run a mile, but by the same token, you can also persist longer. The key is to expend as many calories as possible during each regular exercise period. Doing less vigorous activity for longer periods of time is better for fat control than doing very vigorous activities that can be done only for short periods of time.

TABLE 10.2   Calories Expended Per Hour in Various Physical Activities

| Activity | Calories Used per Hour | | | | |
	100 lbs.	120 lbs.	150 lbs.	180 lbs.	200 lbs.
Archery	180	204	240	276	300
Backpacking (40-lb. pack)	307	348	410	472	513
Badminton	255	289	340	391	425
Baseball	210	238	280	322	350
Basketball (halfcourt)	225	255	300	345	375
Bicycling (normal speed)	157	178	210	242	263
Bowling	155	176	208	240	261
Canoeing (4 mph)	276	344	414	504	558
Circuit Training*	247	280	330	380	413
Dance, Ballet (choreographed)	240	300	360	432	480
Dance, Exercise	315	357	420	483	525
Dance, Modern (choreographed)	240	300	360	432	480
Dance, Social	174	222	264	318	348
Fencing	225	255	300	345	375
Fitness Calisthenics	232	263	310	357	388
Football	225	255	300	345	375
Golf (walking)	187	212	250	288	313
Gymnastics	232	263	310	357	388
Handball	450	510	600	690	750
Hiking	225	255	300	345	375
Horseback Riding	180	204	240	276	300
Interval Training*	487	552	650	748	833
Jogging (5½ mph)	487	552	650	748	833
Judo/Karate	232	263	310	357	388
Mountain Climbing	450	510	600	690	750
Pool; Billiards	97	110	130	150	163
Racquetball; Paddleball	450	510	600	690	750
Rope Jumping (continuous)	525	595	700	805	875
Rowing, Crew	615	697	820	943	1025
Running (10 mph)	625	765	900	1035	1125
Sailing (pleasure)	135	153	180	207	225
Skating, Ice	262	297	350	403	438
Skating, Roller	262	297	350	403	438
Skiing, Cross-Country	525	595	700	805	875
Skiing, Downhill	450	510	600	690	750
Soccer	405	459	540	621	775
Softball (fast)	210	238	280	322	350
Softball (slow)	217	246	290	334	363
Surfing	416	467	550	633	684
Swimming (slow laps)	240	272	320	368	400
Swimming (fast laps)	420	530	630	768	846
Table Tennis	180	204	240	276	300
Tennis	315	357	420	483	525
Volleyball	262	297	350	403	483
Walking	204	258	318	372	426
Waterskiing	306	390	468	564	636
Weight Training	352	399	470	541	558

Note: Locate your weight to determine the calories expended per hour in each of the activities shown in the table based on recreational involvement. More vigorous activity, as occurs in competitive athletics, may result in greater caloric expenditures.
From C. B. Corbin and R. Lindsey. *Fitness for Life,* 2d ed., Glenview, IL: Scott, Foresman, Inc., 1983, 105. Used by permission.

The only satisfactory way to control diet is to count caloric content of commonly eaten foods.

When accurate records are not kept, most people greatly underestimate the amount they eat. A calorie table (Appendix A) shows the caloric content of the most commonly eaten foods. Use this table and the diet recall procedure from Lab 18A (nutrition) to help keep accurate records of your own caloric intake.

A combination of regular exercise and dietary restriction is the most effective means of losing body fat.

Recent studies indicate that exercise combined with dietary restriction may be the *most* effective method of losing fat. One study of adult women indicated that diet alone resulted in loss of weight, but much of this lost weight was lean body tissue. Those studied who were dieting as well as exercising experienced similar weight losses, but this loss included more body fat. On the basis of this research, all weight loss programs should combine lowered caloric intake with a good physical exercise program.

Good exercise and diet habits can be useful in maintaining desirable body composition.

Table 10.1 illustrates how fat can be lost through regular exercise and proper dieting. However, not all people want to lose fat. For those who wish to maintain their current body composition, a balance between caloric intake and expenditure is effective. For those who want to increase their lean body weight, increased caloric intake with increased exercise can result in the desired changes.

Appetite is not necessarily increased through exercise.

The human animal was intended to be an active animal. For this reason, man's "appetite thermostat" (called the appestat by some) is set as if all people are active. Those who are inactive do not have a decreased appetite. Likewise, if one is sedentary and then begins regular exercise, the appetite does not necessarily increase because this "appetite thermostat" expects activity. Very vigorous activity does not necessarily cause an appetite increase that is proportional to the calories expended in the vigorous exercise.

Fat children may become fat adults.

Retention of "baby fat" is not a sign of good health. On the contrary, excess body fat in the early years is a health problem of considerable concern. As many as 25 percent of American schoolchildren are overfat. Of these children, four of five will become overfat adults. Twenty-eight of twenty-nine teenagers who are too fat will become overfat adults. There is evidence that children who are obese may actually increase the number

as well as the size of their fat cells, thus making them predisposed to obesity in later life.

Inactivity contributes to childhood obesity.

Studies of fat children show that activity restriction is more often a cause of obesity than is overeating. Many fat children eat less but are considerably less active than their nonfat peers.

"Creeping obesity" often accompanies an increase in age.

Many of the "too fat Americans" are between the ages of thirty and sixty. As you grow older, changes in metabolism cause a decrease in caloric expenditure necessary to sustain life. Unless activity is increased or diet is restricted, a gain in weight will occur. Activity usually decreases while eating habits remain fairly constant with age. Thus, obesity creeps up on an individual. To prevent "creeping obesity," it is suggested that the average person cut caloric intake 3 percent each decade after twenty-five, so that by age sixty-five, caloric intake is at least 10 percent less than it was at age twenty-five.

LAB RESOURCE MATERIALS (FOR USE WITH LABS 10A AND 10B, PAGES 211–14)

Evaluating Body Fatness

Skinfold Measurements

Skinfold measurements are made with a skinfold caliper. Some of the more accurate and expensive calipers are the Harpenden, the Lange, and the Lafayette calipers. Some of the less expensive calipers include the Slimguide, the Fat-O-Meter, and the Adipometer. Regardless of the type employed, it is important to use a consistent procedure for "drawing up" or "pinching up" a skinfold and making the measurement with the caliper. The following procedures should be used for each skinfold site.

1. Lay the caliper down on a nearby table. Use the thumbs and index fingers of both hands to "draw up" a skinfold or layer of skin and fat. The fingers and thumbs of the two hands should be about one inch apart or half an inch on either side of the location where the measurement is to be made.
2. The skinfolds are normally "drawn up" in a vertical line rather than in a horizontal line. However, if the natural tendency of the skin aligns itself less than vertical, the measurement should be done on the natural line of the skinfold, rather than vertically.
3. Do not "pinch" the skinfold too hard. Draw it up so that your thumbs and fingers are not compressing the skinfold.

CHART 10A.1* Percent Fat Estimates for Men, Sum of Chest, Abdominal, and Thigh Skin Folds**

Sum of Skin Folds (mm)	Under 22	23 to 27	28 to 32	33 to 37	38 to 42	43 to 47	48 to 52	53 to 57	Over 58
				Age to the Last Year					
8-10	1.3	1.8	2.3	2.9	3.4	3.9	4.5	5.0	5.5
11-13	2.2	2.8	3.3	3.9	4.4	4.9	5.5	6.0	6.5
14-16	3.2	3.8	4.3	4.8	5.4	5.9	6.4	7.0	7.5
17-19	4.2	4.7	5.3	5.8	6.3	6.9	7.4	8.0	8.5
20-22	5.1	5.7	6.2	6.8	7.3	7.9	8.4	8.9	9.5
23-25	6.1	6.6	7.2	7.7	8.3	8.8	9.4	9.9	10.5
26-28	7.0	7.6	8.1	8.7	9.2	9.8	10.3	10.9	11.4
29-31	8.0	8.5	9.1	9.6	10.2	10.7	11.3	11.8	12.4
32-34	8.9	9.4	10.0	10.5	11.1	11.6	12.2	12.8	13.3
35-37	9.8	10.4	10.9	11.5	12.0	12.6	13.1	13.7	14.3
38-40	10.7	11.3	11.8	12.4	12.9	13.5	14.1	14.6	15.2
41-43	11.6	12.2	12.7	13.3	13.8	14.4	15.0	15.5	16.1
44-46	12.5	13.1	13.6	14.2	14.7	15.3	15.9	16.4	17.0
47-49	13.4	13.9	14.5	15.1	15.6	16.2	16.8	17.3	17.9
50-52	14.3	14.8	15.4	15.9	16.5	17.1	17.6	18.2	18.8
53-55	15.1	15.7	16.2	16.8	17.4	17.9	18.5	18.1	19.7
56-58	16.0	16.5	17.1	17.7	18.2	18.8	19.4	20.0	20.5
59-61	16.9	17.4	17.9	18.5	19.1	19.7	20.2	20.8	21.4
62-64	17.6	18.2	18.8	19.4	19.9	20.5	21.1	21.7	22.2
65-67	18.5	19.0	19.6	20.2	20.8	21.3	21.9	22.5	23.1
68-70	19.3	19.9	20.4	21.0	21.6	22.2	22.7	23.3	23.9
71-73	20.1	20.7	21.2	21.8	22.4	23.0	23.6	24.1	24.7
74-76	20.9	21.5	22.0	22.6	23.2	23.8	24.4	25.0	25.5
77-79	21.7	22.2	22.8	23.4	24.0	24.6	25.2	25.8	26.3
80-82	22.4	23.0	23.6	24.2	24.8	25.4	25.9	26.5	27.1
83-85	23.2	23.8	24.4	25.0	25.5	26.1	26.7	27.3	27.9
86-88	24.0	24.5	25.1	25.7	26.3	26.9	27.5	28.1	28.7
89-91	24.7	25.3	25.9	25.5	27.1	27.6	28.2	28.8	29.4
92-94	25.4	26.0	26.6	27.2	27.8	28.4	29.0	29.6	30.2
92-97	26.1	16.7	27.3	27.9	28.5	29.1	29.7	30.3	30.9
98-100	26.9	27.4	28.0	28.6	29.2	29.8	30.4	31.0	31.6
101-103	27.5	28.1	28.7	29.3	29.9	30.5	31.1	31.7	32.3
104-106	28.2	28.8	29.4	30.0	30.6	31.2	31.8	32.4	33.0
107-109	28.9	29.5	30.1	30.7	31.3	31.9	32.5	33.1	33.7
110-112	29.6	30.2	30.8	31.4	32.0	32.6	33.2	33.8	34.4
113-115	30.2	30.8	31.4	32.0	32.6	33.2	33.8	34.5	35.1
116-118	30.9	31.5	32.1	32.7	33.3	33.9	34.5	35.1	35.7
119-121	31.5	32.1	32.7	33.3	33.9	34.5	35.1	35.7	36.4
122-124	32.1	32.7	33.3	33.9	34.5	35.1	35.8	36.4	37.0
125-127	32.7	33.3	33.9	34.5	35.1	35.8	36.4	37.0	37.6

Percent fat calculated by the formula by Siri. Percent fat = [4.95/BD) – 4.5] × 100, where BD = body density.

**Taken from Pollock, M. L., Schmidt, D. H., and Jackson, A. S. "Measurement of Cardiorespiration Fitness and Body Composition in the Clinical Setting." *Comprehensive Therapy*, 6 (September 1980):12–27.

CHART 10A.2* Percent Fat Estimates for Women, Sum of Triceps, Iliac Crest, and Thigh Skin Folds**

Sum of Skinfolds (mm)	Age to the Last Year								
	Under 22	23 to 27	28 to 32	33 to 37	38 to 42	43 to 47	48 to 52	53 to 57	Over 58
23-25	9.7	9.9	10.2	10.4	10.7	10.9	11.2	11.4	11.7
26-28	11.0	11.2	11.5	11.7	12.0	12.3	12.5	12.7	13.0
29-31	12.3	12.5	12.8	13.0	13.3	13.5	13.8	14.0	14.3
32-34	13.6	13.8	14.0	14.3	14.5	14.8	15.0	15.3	15.5
35-37	14.8	15.0	15.3	15.5	15.8	16.0	16.3	16.5	16.8
38-40	16.0	16.3	16.5	16.7	17.0	17.2	17.5	17.7	18.0
41-43	17.2	17.4	17.7	17.9	18.2	18.4	18.7	18.9	19.2
44-46	18.3	18.6	18.8	19.1	19.3	19.6	19.8	20.1	20.3
47-49	19.5	19.7	20.0	20.2	20.5	20.7	21.0	21.2	21.5
50-52	20.6	20.8	21.1	21.3	21.6	21.8	22.1	22.3	22.6
53-55	21.7	21.9	22.1	22.4	22.6	22.9	23.1	23.4	23.6
56-58	22.7	23.0	23.2	23.4	23.7	23.9	24.2	24.4	24.7
59-61	23.7	24.0	24.2	24.5	24.7	25.0	25.2	25.5	25.7
62-64	24.7	25.0	25.2	25.5	35.7	26.0	26.7	26.4	26.7
65-67	25.7	25.9	26.2	26.4	26.7	26.9	27.2	27.4	27.7
68-70	26.6	26.9	27.1	27.4	27.6	27.9	28.1	28.4	28.6
71-73	27.5	27.8	28.0	28.3	28.5	28.8	28.0	29.3	29.5
74-76	28.4	28.7	28.9	29.2	29.4	29.7	29.9	30.2	30.4
77-79	29.3	29.5	29.8	30.0	30.3	30.5	30.8	31.0	31.3
80-82	30.1	30.4	30.6	30.9	31.1	31.4	31.6	31.9	32.1
83-85	30.9	31.2	31.4	31.7	31.9	32.2	32.4	32.7	32.9
86-88	31.7	32.0	32.2	32.5	32.7	32.9	33.2	33.4	33.7
89-91	32.5	32.7	33.0	33.2	33.5	33.7	33.9	34.2	34.4
92-94	33.2	33.4	33.7	33.9	34.2	34.4	34.7	34.9	35.2
95-97	33.9	34.1	34.4	34.6	34.9	35.1	35.4	35.6	35.9
98-100	34.6	34.8	35.1	35.3	35.5	35.8	36.0	36.3	36.5
101-103	35.3	35.4	35.7	35.9	36.2	36.4	36.7	36.9	37.2
104-106	35.8	36.1	36.3	36.6	36.8	37.1	37.3	37.5	37.8
107-109	36.4	36.7	36.9	37.1	37.4	37.6	37.9	38.1	38.4
110-112	37.0	37.2	37.5	37.7	38.0	38.2	38.5	38.7	38.9
113-115	37.5	37.8	38.0	38.2	38.5	38.7	39.0	39.2	39.5
116-118	38.0	38.3	38.5	38.8	39.0	39.3	39.5	39.7	40.0
119-121	38.5	38.7	39.0	39.2	39.5	39.7	40.0	40.2	40.5
122-124	39.0	39.2	39.4	39.7	39.9	40.2	40.4	40.7	40.9
125-127	39.4	39.6	39.9	40.1	40.4	40.6	40.9	41.1	41.4
128-130	39.8	40.0	40.3	40.5	40.8	41.0	41.3	41.5	41.8

*Percent fat calculated by the formula of Siri.³⁹ Percent fat $= [(4.95/\text{BD}) - 4.5] \times 100$, where $\text{BD} = $ body density.

**Taken from Pollock, M. L., Schmidt, D. H., and Jackson, A. S. "Measurement of Cardiorespiration Fitness and Body Composition in the Clinical Setting." *Comprehensive Therapy*, 6 (September 1980):12–27.

4. Once the skinfold is "drawn up," let go with your right hand and pick up the caliper. Open the jaws of the caliper and place them over the location of the skinfold to be measured and one-half inch from your left index finger and thumb. Allow the tips, or jaw faces, of the calipers to close on the skinfold at a level about where the skin would be normally.

5. Let the reading on the caliper "settle" for two or three seconds, then read the thickness of the skinfold in millimeters.

6. Three measurements should be taken at each location. Use the middle of the three values to determine your measurement. For example, if you had values of 10, 11, and 9, your measurement for that location would be 10. If the three measures vary by more than three mm from the lowest to the highest, you may want to take additional measurements.

Skinfold Locations for Women

A. *Triceps Skinfold*—Make a mark on the back of the right arm one-half the distance between the tip of the shoulder and the tip of the elbow. Make the measurement at this location.

B. *Iliac Crest Skinfold*—Make a mark at the top front of the iliac crest. This skinfold is taken slightly diagonally because of the natural line of the skin.

C. *Thigh Skinfold*—Make a mark on the front of the thigh midway between the hip and the knee. Make the measurement vertically at this location.

Skinfold Locations for Men

A. *Chest Skinfold*—Make a mark above and to the right of the right nipple (one-half the distance from the midline of the side and the nipple). The measurement at this location is often done on the diagonal because of the natural line of the skin.

B. *Abdominal Skinfold*—Make a mark on the skin approximately one inch to the right of the navel. Make a vertical measurement at that location.

C. *Thigh Skinfold*—Make a mark on the front of the thigh midway between the hip and the knee. Make a vertical measurement at this location.

CHART 10A.3 Fatness Rating Scale

Classification	Men	Women
Very lean	10 or less	15 or less
Lean	11–14	16–17
Fair	15–18	18–25
Fat	19–22	26–30
Obese	28 +	31 +

CHART 10B.1 Determining Frame Size Using Wrist Size in Inches

	Men	Women
Small frame	6½″ or less	5½″ or less
Medium frame	6¼″–7¼″	5¾″
Large frame	7½″ or more	6″ or more

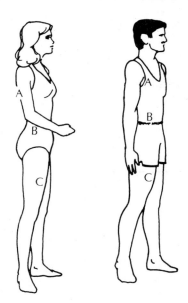

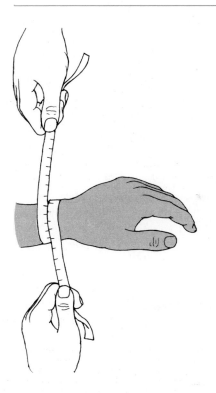

CHART 10B.2 Determination of "Desirable" Weight for Men

Height Feet	Inches	Small Frame	Medium Frame	Large Frame
5	2	128–134	131–141	138–150
5	3	130–136	133–143	140–153
5	4	132–138	135–145	142–156
5	5	134–140	137–148	144–160
5	6	136–142	139–151	146–164
5	7	138–145	142–154	149–168
5	8	140–148	145–157	152–172
5	9	142–151	148–160	155–176
5	10	144–154	151–163	158–180
5	11	146–157	154–166	161–184
6	0	149–160	157–170	164–188
6	1	152–164	160–174	168–192
6	2	155–168	164–178	172–197
6	3	158–172	167–182	176–202
6	4	162–176	171–187	181–207

Weights at ages 25–59 based on lowest mortality. Weight in pounds according to frame (in indoor clothing weighing 3 lbs., shoes with 1″ heels). Adapted from tables provided courtesy of Metropolitan Life Insurance Co.

CHART 10B.3 Determination of "Desirable" Weight for Women

Height Feet	Inches	Small Frame	Medium Frame	Large Frame
4	10	102–111	109–121	118–131
4	11	103–113	111–123	120–134
5	0	104–115	113–126	122–137
5	1	106–118	115–129	125–140
5	2	108–121	118–132	128–143
5	3	111–124	121–135	131–147
5	4	114–127	124–138	134–151
5	5	117–130	127–141	137–155
5	6	120–133	130–144	140–159
5	7	123–136	133–147	143–163
5	8	126–139	136–150	146–167
5	9	129–142	139–153	149–170
5	10	132–145	142–156	152–173
5	11	135–148	145–159	155–176
6	0	138–151	148–162	158–179

Weights at ages 25–59 based on lowest mortality. Weight in pounds according to frame (in indoor clothing weighing 3 lbs., shoes with 1″ heels). Adapted from tables provided courtesy of Metropolitan Life Insurance Co.

CHART 10B.4 Determination of Desirable Body Weight for Men

Actual Body Weight	Percent Fat 6	8	10	12	14	16	18	20	22	24	26	28	30	32	34	36	38	40
240	263	258	254	249	244	240	234	230	225	220	215	210	206	201	196	191	186	182
235	257	253	248	243	239	235	266	225	220	215	210	206	201	196	192	187	182	178
230	252	247	243	238	233	230	224	220	215	210	206	201	197	192	187	183	178	174
225	247	243	238	234	229	225	220	216	211	207	202	198	193	189	184	180	175	171
220	241	237	233	228	223	221	215	211	206	202	197	193	189	184	180	175	171	167
215	236	231	227	223	218	215	210	206	201	197	193	188	184	180	175	171	167	163
210	230	226	222	217	215	210	205	202	200	192	188	184	180	175	171	167	163	159
205	224	220	216	212	208	205	200	197	191	187	183	179	175	171	167	163	159	155
200	220	216	212	208	204	200	196	192	188	184	180	176	172	168	164	160	156	152
195	214	210	206	202	198	195	190	187	183	179	175	171	167	163	159	155	151	148
190	208	204	201	197	193	190	185	182	178	174	170	166	163	159	155	151	147	144
185	202	199	195	191	187	185	180	177	173	169	165	162	158	154	151	147	143	140
180	197	193	190	186	182	180	175	172	168	164	161	157	154	150	146	143	139	136
175	192	189	185	182	178	175	171	168	164	161	157	154	150	147	143	140	136	133
170	186	183	180	176	173	170	166	163	159	156	152	149	146	142	139	135	132	129
165	181	177	174	171	167	165	161	158	154	151	148	144	141	138	134	131	128	125
160	175	172	169	165	162	160	157	153	149	146	143	140	137	133	130	127	124	121
155	169	166	163	160	157	155	151	148	144	141	138	135	132	129	126	123	120	117
150	165	162	159	156	153	150	147	144	141	138	135	132	129	126	123	120	117	114
145	159	156	153	150	147	145	141	139	136	133	130	127	124	121	118	115	112	110
140	153	150	148	145	142	140	136	134	131	128	125	122	120	117	114	111	108	100
135	147	145	142	139	137	135	131	129	126	123	120	118	115	112	110	107	104	102
130	142	139	137	134	131	130	126	124	121	118	116	113	111	108	105	103	102	98
125	137	135	132	130	127	125	122	120	117	115	112	110	107	105	102	100	97	95
120	131	129	121	129	122	120	117	115	112	110	107	105	103	100	98	95	93	91

Along the side locate your actual body weight and across the top locate your estimated percent fat. The intersection of the two entries is your desirable weight (fat-free body weight plus 16 percent fat). Example: 175 pounds is the desirable weight for a man who weighs 195 pounds and currently has a body fat amount of 26 percent.

CHART 10B.5 Determination of Desirable Body Weight for Women

Actual Body Weight	Percent Fat 6	8	10	12	14	16	18	20	22	24	26	28	30	32	34	36	38	40
200	228	224	220	216	212	208	204	200	196	192	188	184	180	176	172	168	164	160
195	222	218	214	210	206	202	198	195	191	187	183	179	175	171	167	163	159	156
190	216	212	209	205	201	197	193	190	186	182	178	174	171	167	163	159	155	152
185	210	207	203	199	196	192	188	185	181	177	173	170	166	162	159	155	151	148
180	205	201	198	194	190	187	183	180	176	172	169	165	162	158	154	151	147	144
175	199	196	192	189	185	182	178	175	171	168	164	161	157	154	150	147	143	140
170	193	180	177	173	170	166	163	170	166	163	159	156	153	149	146	142	139	136
165	188	184	181	178	174	171	168	165	161	158	155	151	148	145	141	138	135	132
160	182	179	176	172	169	166	163	160	156	153	150	147	144	140	137	134	131	128
155	176	173	170	167	164	161	158	155	151	148	145	142	139	136	133	130	127	124
150	171	168	165	162	159	156	153	150	147	144	141	138	135	132	129	126	123	120
145	165	162	159	156	153	150	147	145	142	139	136	133	130	127	124	121	118	116
140	159	156	154	151	148	145	142	140	137	134	131	128	126	123	120	117	114	112
135	153	151	148	145	143	140	137	135	132	129	126	124	121	118	116	113	110	108
130	148	145	143	140	137	135	132	130	127	124	122	119	117	114	111	109	106	104
125	142	140	137	135	132	130	127	125	122	120	117	115	112	110	107	105	102	100
120	136	134	132	129	127	124	122	120	117	115	112	110	108	105	103	100	98	96
115	131	128	126	124	121	119	117	115	112	110	108	105	103	101	98	96	94	92
110	125	123	121	118	116	114	112	110	107	105	103	101	99	96	94	92	90	88
105	119	117	115	113	111	109	107	105	102	100	98	96	94	92	90	88	86	84
100	114	112	110	108	106	104	102	100	98	96	94	92	90	88	86	84	82	80
95	108	106	104	102	100	98	96	95	93	91	89	87	85	83	81	79	77	76
90	102	100	99	97	95	93	91	90	88	86	84	82	81	79	77	75	73	72

Along the side locate your actual body weight and across the top locate your estimated percent fat. The intersection of the two entries is your desirable weight (fat-free body weight plus 20 percent fat). Example: 150 pounds is the desirable weight for a woman who weighs 160 pounds and currently has a body fat amount of 26 percent.

REFERENCES

Blair, S. N., H. B. Falls, and R. R. Pate. "A New Physical Fitness Test." *Physician and Sportsmedicine* 11 (1983):87.

Clarke, H. H., ed. "Exercise and Fat Reduction." *Physical Fitness Research Digest* 5 (1975):1.

Corbin, C. B., ed. *A Textbook of Motor Development.* 2d ed. Dubuque, IA: Wm. C. Brown Publishers, 1980.

Corbin, C. B., and R. Pate. "The AAHPERD Health-Related Fitness Test: Implications for Physical Education Curriculum." *Journal of Physical Education and Recreation* 52 (1981):36.

Corbin, C. B., and W. B. Zuti. "Body Density and Skinfold Thickness of Children." *American Corrective Therapy Journal* 36 (1982):50.

Corbin, C. B., and R. Lindsey. *The Ultimate Fitness Book.* New York: Leisure Press, 1984.

Hafen, B. Q. *Nutrition, Food, and Weight Control.* Boston: Allyn and Bacon, 1981.

Hirsch, J., and J. L. Knittle. "Cellularity of Obese and Nonobese Adipose Tissue." *Federation Proceedings* 29 (1970):1518.

Jackson, A. S., M. L. Pollock, and A. Ward. "Generalized Equations for Predicting Body Density of Women." *Medicine and Science in Sports and Exercise* 12 (1980):175.

Katch, F. I., and W. D. McArdle. *Nutrition, Weight Control, and Exercise.* Philadelphia: Lea and Febiger, 1982.

Katch, F. I., and V. L. Katch. "Measurement and Prediction Errors in Body Composition Assessment and the Search for the Perfect Prediction Equation." *Research Quarterly of Exercise and Sport* 51 (1980):249.

Lindsey, R., B. Jones, and A. Whitley. *Fitness for Health, Figure/Physique, Posture.* 5th ed. Dubuque, IA: Wm. C. Brown Publishers, 1983.

*Lohman, T. G. "Skinfold and Body Density and Their Relation to Body Fatness: A Review." *Human Biology* 53 (1981):181.

Lohman, T. G., and M. L. Pollock. "Skinfold Measurements: Which Caliper?" *Journal of Physical Education and Recreation* 52 (1981):27.

*Lohman, T. G. "Body Composition Methodology in Sports Medicine." *Physician and Sportsmedicine* 10 (1982):46.

Oscai, L. B. "Exercise or Food Restriction: Effect of Adipose Cellularity." *American Journal of Physiology* 27 (1974):902.

Pate, R. R. "A New Definition of Youth Fitness." *Physican and Sportsmedicine* 11 (1983):77.

Pollock, M. L., D. H. Schmidt, and A. S. Jackson. "Measurement of Cardiorespiratory Fitness and Body Composition in the Clinical Setting." *Comprehensive Therapy* 6 (1980):12.

*Pugliese, M. T., et al. "Fear of Obesity: A Cause of Short Stature and Delayed Puberty." *New England Journal of Medicine* 309 (1983):513.

Sinning, W. E. "Use and Misuse of Anthropometric Estimates of Body Composition." *Journal of Physical Education and Recreation* 51 (1980):43.

Smith, N. J. "Gaining and Losing Weight in Athletics." *Journal of the American Medical Association* 236 (1976):149.

*Svoboda, M. "Addressing Weight Management in Physical Education." *Journal of Physical Education and Recreation* 51 (1980):49.

Williams, M. H. *Nutrition for Fitness and Sports.* Dubuque, IA: Wm. C. Brown Publishers, 1983.

Zuti, W. B., and L. A. Golding. "Comparing Diet and Exercise as Weight Reduction Tools." *Physician and Sportsmedicine* 4 (1976):49.

11

SKILL-RELATED PHYSICAL FITNESS

CONCEPT 11

Skill-related fitness is essential
to performance in games and sports as well as
to working efficiency.

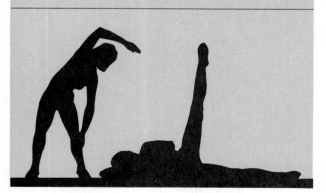

INTRODUCTION

Skill-related fitness consists of six different components: balance, agility, coordination, speed, power, and reaction time (see Concept 2 for definitions). Although these aspects of physical fitness do not necessarily make you healthier, possessing these fitness characteristics makes you better at games and sports as well as improving your work efficiency. In a society that is becoming increasingly interested in leisure and recreation, skill-related physical fitness can be important to living a meaningful and enjoyable life.

TERMS

Sports Fitness—A term commonly used for skill-related physical fitness.
Motor Fitness—Another term commonly used for skill-related physical fitness.

THE FACTS

Good skill-related fitness may help you achieve good health-related fitness.

Individuals who achieve good skill-related fitness have the potential to succeed in sports and games. Regular participation in these activities can lead to improved health-related fitness throughout life. In addition, people who make an effort to learn activities involving skill-related fitness are more likely to be active in sports and games for a lifetime.

Skill-related fitness may improve your ability to work efficiently.

In manual labor, skillful performance improves efficiency. For example, a ditchdigger with great ditch-digging skills uses less energy than one who has not mastered the skill. Seemingly simple skills are often quite complex and may require some proficiency in each of the skill-related fitness components.

Skill-related fitness may improve your ability to meet emergency situations.

Good agility would enable you to dodge an oncoming car; good balance would lessen the likelihood of a fall; and good reaction time would decrease the chances of being hit by a flying object. Each aspect of skill-related fitness contributes in its own way to your ability to avoid injury and meet emergencies.

Good skill-related fitness is beneficial to carrying out the normal daily routine and enjoying your leisure time.

Walking, sitting, climbing, pushing, pulling, and other such tasks require varying degrees of skill-related fitness. Accordingly, improved fitness resulting from regular practice may improve efficiency in performing daily activities and enjoying your leisure or recreational time.

The potential for possessing outstanding skill-related fitness is based on hereditary predispositions, but all aspects of skill-related fitness can be improved through regular practice.

In order for a skill to be improved, it must be repeated. Some skill-related fitness components, such as power, agility, balance, and coordination, can be enhanced greatly with practice. Others, such as speed and reaction time, can be improved somewhat but are determined to a greater extent by heredity.

Exceptional athletes tend to be outstanding in more than one component of skill-related fitness.

While people possess skill-related fitness in varying degrees, great athletes are likely to be above average in most, if not all, aspects. Indeed, exceptional athletes must be exceptional in many areas of skill-related fitness. Different sports require different skills, each of which requires varying degrees of the six components of skill-related fitness.

Excellence in one skill-related fitness component may compensate for lack in another.

Each individual possesses a specific level of each of the skill-related fitness aspects. The performer should learn his or her other strengths and weaknesses in order to produce optimal performances. For example, a tennis player may use coordination to compensate for lack of speed.

Excellence in skill-related fitness may compensate for lack of health-related fitness when playing sports and games.

As you grow older, health-related fitness potential declines. You may use superior skill-related fitness to compensate. For example, a baseball pitcher who lacks the strength and the power to dominate hitters may rely on a pitch such as a knuckleball, which is more dependent on coordination, than on power.

Skills are specific in nature.

An individual might possess ability in one area and not in another. For this reason, "General Motor Ability" probably does not really exist. Individuals do not have one general capacity for performing skills. Rather, the ability to play games or sports is determined by combined abilities in each of the separate motor skill components of agility, coordination, balance, reaction time, speed, and power. It is, however, possible and even likely that some performers will have above-average skill in many areas.

LAB RESOURCE MATERIALS (FOR USE WITH LAB 11, PAGE 215)

Evaluating Skill-Related Physical Fitness

Evaluating agility: The Illinois agility run*
An agility course using four chairs, ten feet apart, and a thirty-foot running area will be set up as depicted in this illustration.

    The test is performed as follows:

1. Lie prone with your hands by your shoulders and with your head at the starting line. On the signal to begin, the performer will run the course as fast as possible.
2. The performer's score is the time required to complete the course.

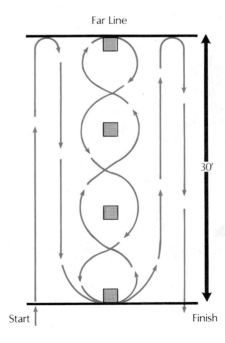

Far Line

30'

Start   Finish

CHART 11.1 Agility Rating Scale

Classification	Men	Women
Excellent	15.8 or faster	17.4 or faster
Very good	16.7–15.9	18.6–17.5
Fair	18.6–16.8	22.3–18.7
Poor	18.8–18.7	23.4–22.4
Very poor	18.9 or slower	23.5 or slower

*Adams, et al. Foundations of Physical Activity (Champaign, Ill.: Stipes and Co., 1965), p. 111.

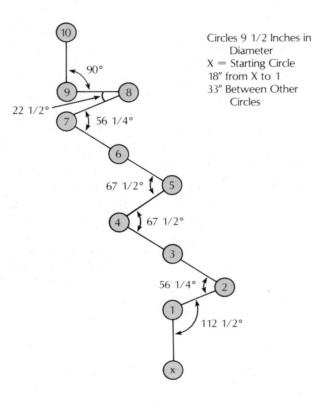

Circles 9 1/2 Inches in Diameter
X = Starting Circle
18″ from X to 1
33″ Between Other Circles

6. For every error, deduct three points each. Errors include touching the heel, moving the supporting foot, touching outside a circle, or touching any body part to the floor other than the supporting foot.
7. Scores should be plotted on the appropriate rating scales.

CHART 11.2 Bass Test Rating Scale

Rating	Score
Excellent	90–100
Very good	80–89
Fair	60–79
Poor	30–59
Very poor	0–29

*From McCloy, C. H. Tests and Measurements in Health and Physical Education. New York: Appleton-Century-Crofts, 1954, p. 106.

Evaluating coordination: The stick test of coordination
The stick test of coordination requires you to juggle three wooden wands. The wands are used to perform a one-half flip and a full flip as shown in the illustrations.

1. *One-Half Flip*—Hold two twenty-four-inch (one-half inch in diameter) dowel rods, one in each hand. Support a third rod of the same size across the other two. Toss the supported rod in the air so that it makes a half turn. Catch the thrown rod with the two held rods.
2. *Full Flip*—Perform the preceding task, letting the supported rod turn a full flip.

Evaluating balance: The Bass test of dynamic balance*
Eleven circles (9½-inch) are drawn on the floor as shown in the illustration. The test is performed as follows:

1. Stand on the right foot in circle X. *Leap* forward to circle one, then circles two through ten, alternating feet with each leap.
2. The feet must leave the floor on each leap and the heel may not touch. Only the ball of the foot may land on the floor.
3. Remain in each circle for five seconds before leaping to the next circle. (A count of five will be made for you, aloud.)
4. Practice trials are allowed.
5. The score is fifty, plus the number of seconds taken to complete the test, minus the number of errors.

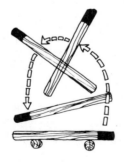

One-Half Flip

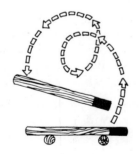

Full Flip

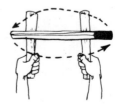

Hand Position

The test is performed as follows:

1. Practice the half-flip and the full flip several times before taking the test.
2. When you are ready, attempt a half-flip five times. Score one point for each successful attempt.
3. When you are ready, attempt the full flip five times. Score two points for each successful attempt.

CHART 11.3 Coordination Rating Scale

Classification	Men	Women
Excellent	14–15	13–15
Very good	11–13	10–12
Fair	5–10	4–9
Poor	3–4	2–3
Very poor	0–2	0–1

Evaluating power: The vertical jump test
The test is performed as follows:

1. Hold a piece of chalk so its end is even with your fingertips.
2. Stand with both feet on the floor and your side to the wall and reach and mark as high as possible.
3. Jump upward with both feet as high as possible. Swing arms upward and make a chalk mark on a $5' \times 1'$ wall chart marked off in half-inch horizontal lines placed six feet from the floor.
4. Measure the distance between the reaching height and the jumping height.
5. Your score is the best of three jumps.

CHART 11.4 Power Rating Scale

Classification	Men	Women
Excellent	25½″ or more	23½″ or more
Very good	21″–25″	19″–23″
Fair	16½″–20½″	14½″–18½″
Poor	12½″–16″	10½″–14″
Very poor	12″ or less	10″ or less

Evaluating reaction time: The stick drop test
To perform the stick drop test of reaction time, you will need a yardstick, a table, a chair, and a partner to help with the test. To perform the test, follow these procedures:

1. Sit in the chair next to the table so that your elbow and lower arm rest on the table comfortably. The heel of your hand should rest on the table so that only your fingers and thumb extend beyond the edge of the table.
2. Your partner holds a yardstick at the very top, allowing it to dangle between your thumb and fingers.
3. The yardstick should be held so that the twenty-four-inch mark is even with your thumb and index finger. No part of your hand should touch the yardstick.
4. Without warning, your partner will drop the stick and you will catch it with your thumb and index finger.
5. Your score is the number of inches read on the yardstick just above the thumb and index finger after you catch the yardstick.
6. Try the test three times. Your partner should be careful not to drop the stick at predictable time intervals so that you cannot guess when it will be dropped. It is important that you react to the dropping of the stick only.
7. Use the middle of your three scores (example: if your scores are 21, 18, and 19, your middle score is 19). The higher your score, the faster your reaction time.

CHART 11.5 Reaction Time Rating Scale

Classification	Score in Inches
Excellent	More than 21
Very good	19–21
Fair	15–18¾
Poor	13–15¾
Very poor	Below 13

Evaluating speed: Running test of speed

To perform the running test of speed, it will be necessary to have a specially marked running course, a stopwatch, a whistle, and a partner to help you with the test. To perform the test, follow this procedure:

1. Mark a running course on a hard surface so that there is a starting line and a series of nine additional lines, each two yards apart, the first marked at a distance ten yards from the starting line.

2. From a distance one or two yards behind the starting line, begin to run as fast as you can. As you cross the starting line, your partner starts a stopwatch.

3. Run as fast as you can until you hear the whistle that your partner will blow exactly three seconds after the stopwatch was started. Your partner marks your location at the time when the whistle was blown.

4. Your score is the distance you were able to cover in three seconds. You may practice the test and take more than one trial if time allows. Use the better of your distances on the last two trials as your score.

CHART 11.6 Speed Rating Chart

Classification	Men	Women
Excellent	24–26 yards	22–26 yards
Very good	22–23 yards	20–21 yards
Fair	18–21 yards	16–19 yards
Poor	16–17 yards	14–15 yards
Very poor	Less than 16 yards	Less than 16 yards

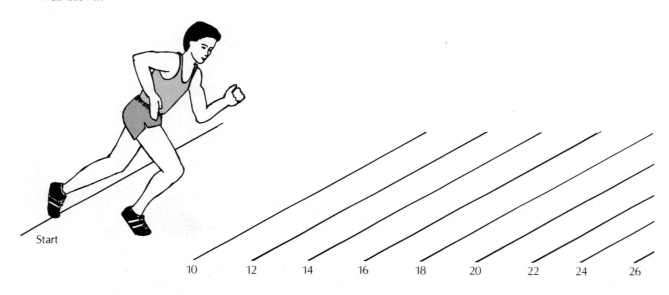

Start

10   12   14   16   18   20   22   24   26

REFERENCES

*Corbin, C. B., ed. *A Textbook of Motor Development*. 2d ed. Dubuque, IA: Wm. C. Brown Publishers, 1980.

Corbin, C. B., and R. Lindsey. *The Ultimate Fitness Book*. New York: The Leisure Press, 1984.

Csikszentmihalyi, M. *Beyond Boredom and Anxiety*. San Francisco: Jossey-Bass, 1977.

Fitness Canada, *Canada Fitness Survey—Highlights*. Ottawa, Ontario: Government of Canada, 1983.

Harris, L., and Associates. *The Perrier Study: Fitness in America*. New York: Great Waters of France, 1979.

Research and Forecasts, Inc. *The Miller Lite Report on American Attitudes toward Sports*. Milwaukee: Miller Brewing Co., 1983.

Synder, E. E., and E. Spreitzer. "Adult Perceptions of Physical Education in the Schools and Community Sports Programs for Youth." *The Physical Educator* 40 (1983):88.

Section Two
PROGRAMS OF EXERCISE

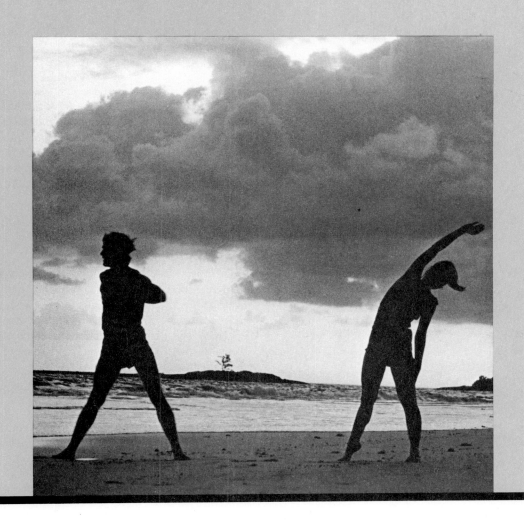

12
AEROBIC EXERCISE

CONCEPT 12

Aerobic exercise
is an excellent form of exercise for developing
health-related physical fitness,
especially cardiovascular fitness and control
of body fatness.

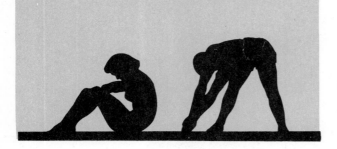

INTRODUCTION

There are many forms of aerobic exercise. In fact, almost any phyical activity that is done at a mild-to-moderate pace can be aerobic. Some of the most popular forms of aerobic exercise are described in this concept.

TERMS

Aerobic Exercise—Exercise for which the body is able to supply adequate oxygen to sustain performance for long periods of time.

Anaerobic Exercise—Exercise that requires the use of the body's high energy fuel. This type of exercise can only be sustained for short periods of time without rest and does not depend on the body's ability to supply oxygen.

Continuous Exercise—Exercise that is done for relatively long periods of time without stopping.

Intermittent Exercise—Exercise that is done in short bursts followed by rest periods.

THE FACTS

Aerobic exercise is a good way to develop several components of health-related physical fitness.

When done in the cardiovascular fitness target zone, aerobic activities are excellent for building cardiovascular fitness. Because aerobic activities can be sustained for relatively long periods of time, they can result in considerable calorie expenditure and are very good for helping to control body fatness. Aerobic activities can also be of value in developing muscular endurance (usually in the leg muscles).

Aerobic exercise can be continuous or intermittent.

Anaerobic exercise cannot be done continuously. Because it is so intense, you must alternate vigorous anaerobic exercise with frequent rest periods. Aerobic exercise, on the other hand, can be done continuously or intermittently, but for best result, it should be done continuously. For information concerning the correct frequency, intensity, and time for aerobic exercise, refer to Concepts 6 and 10.

Not all aerobic exercise is effective in building health-related physical fitness.

Bowling is aerobic exercise. So is golf. Yet these activities may do very little to contribute to the development of health-related physical fitness. Those who popularized the term "aerobics" really meant *continuous* aerobic exercise that stressed the cardiovascular system when they spoke of the health benefits of aerobic activity. As the term is commonly used now, it means activities sustained for relatively long periods of time without rest intervals.

Some activities that are at least partially anaerobic, such as basketball and racquetball, can be considered aerobic if done continuously.

Because sports, such as basketball and racquetball, involve short, vigorous bursts of exercise followed by rest or recovery periods, they are at least in part anaerobic. However, if the bursts of exercise are moderate, allowing continued participation for fifteen minutes or more without extended rest periods (i.e., the heart rate is maintained in the target zone), the activities can be considered aerobic.

Aerobic activities are exceptionally popular among adults.

Whereas activities that have a strong anaerobic component, such as sprinting, football, baseball, and sprint swimming, are very popular among youth, aerobic activities are more popular among adults. Adults report that they are most often involved in continuous swimming, jogging, cycling, walking, and calisthenics. All but vigorous calisthenics, sprint running, or sprint swimming are aerobic. When done at a slow or moderate pace, calisthenics are aerobic, and when done continuously, they can be effective in producing the same benefits as jogging, swimming, and other aerobic activities.

To be effective in building all components of health-related physical fitness, aerobic exercise should be supplemented with other forms of exercise.

As already noted, aerobic exercise can be effective in aiding cardiovascular fitness, muscular endurance, and in reducing body fat. Except for some types of continuous calisthenics, aerobic exercise must be supplemented with exercises designed to build flexibility, and strength, and, to a lesser extent, muscular endurance. If certain types of aerobic exercise are done exclusively, such as jogging, they may actually reduce flexibility.

THERE ARE MANY POPULAR FORMS OF AEROBIC EXERCISE

Some of the most popular forms of aerobic exercise are discussed briefly here.

Bicycling

Bicycling, when done continuously, is a form of aerobic exercise. This activity requires only a bicycle and some safety equipment, such as a helmet and a light and reflectors if done after dark. A tall "flag" is needed if biking in traffic. To be most effective in building physical fitness, you should pedal continuously, rather than coasting for long periods of time. Maintaining a steady pace is recommended. Riding a different course periodically can increase enjoyment of the activity.

Circuit Overload Training

Originally, circuit training was a type of physical training involving movement from one exercise station to another. A different type of exercise was performed at each station. In order to complete the circuit, you had to complete all of the exercises at the different stations. Your goal was to perform the circuit in progressively shorter periods of time.

Recently, however, circuit training has been modified by some to include several strength overload stations. These stations may involve overload exercises with free weights or exercise machines. There is some evidence that when this type of exercise is done at a moderate and continuous pace, it can be effective in building cardiovascular fitness. In these cases, circuit training can be considered an aerobic form of exercise. When repetitions of weight training exercises are followed by a relatively long rest period (longer than the exercise time) and are done very vigorously, they are primarily anaerobic. If repetitions of the exercise are done at a slow or moderate pace, and are followed by an extended rest period, they may still be aerobic, but because they are not continuous and do not elevate the heart rate for a sustained period of time, they are not effective in building cardiovascular fitness.

Cooper's Aerobics

Based on the needs of military personnel, Dr. Kenneth Cooper developed a physical fitness program that he calls aerobics. In fact, he popularized the term. His program includes a variety of aerobic activities having point values for the different types of exercises involved. To develop fitness, especially cardiovascular fitness, a person is expected to earn thirty "aerobic points" per week. Aerobic points are part of Cooper's system for helping people to know when they are exercising frequently enough, intensely enough, and long enough. Many of the activities Cooper includes in his program are described in this concept. Table 12.1 charts some of the point values for various activities. (For more complete details on the Cooper Aerobics program, refer to the reference at the end of this concept.)

TABLE 12.1 Aerobic Points Chart

Points	Walking-Running (Time for 1 Mile)	Cycling (Speed for 2 Miles)	Swimming (300 yds.)	Handball, Basketball	Stationary Running for 5 Minutes	Stationary Running for 10 Minutes	Points
0	Over 20 min.	Less than 10 mph	Over 10 min.	Less than 10 min.	Less than 60 steps/min.	Less than 50 steps/min.	0
1	20:00–14:30 min.	10–15 mph	8:00–10:00 min.	10 min.	60–70 steps/min.	50–65 steps/min.	1
2	14:29–12:00 min.	15–20 mph	7:30–8:00 min.	20 min.	80–90 steps/min.	65–70 steps/min.	2
3	11:59–10:00 min.	Over 20 mph	6:00–7:30 min.	30 min.		70–80 steps/min.	3
4	9:59–8:00 min.			40 min.		80–90 steps/min.	4
5	7:59–6:30 min.			50 min.			5
6	Less than 6:30 min.			60 min.			6

Used by permission of K. Cooper. *The New Aerobics* (New York: M. Evans and Co., 1970.)

CONTINUOUS CALISTHENICS (SAMPLE PROGRAM)

Some continuous calisthenic exercises are illustrated here.

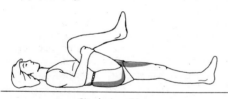

Single Leg Hug

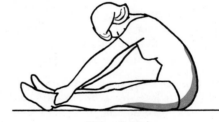

Sitting Stretches

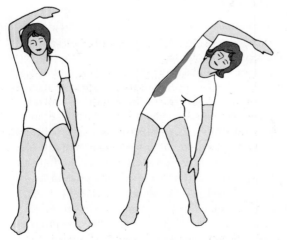

Lateral Trunk Stretchers

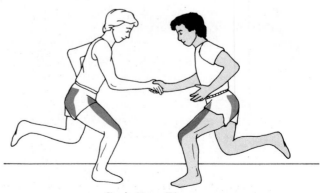

Single Knee Dips

Continuous Calisthenics

Survey results repeatedly indicate that calisthenics is one of the top two or three participant activities performed. Calisthenics, exercises such as sit-ups and push-ups, are designed to build flexibility, strength, or muscular endurance in specific muscle groups. Even though most calisthenics are aerobic, they are often done intermittently. That is, the calisthenics are done a few at a time followed by a rest period. This type of calisthenics can build flexibility, strength, and muscular endurance, but does little for cardiovascular fitness or fat control.

Continuous calisthenics, or calisthenics that are done without stopping or with walking, jogging, rope jumping, or some other aerobic activity performed during the rest period, can develop virtually all health-related aspects of physical fitness. Fitness pioneer Dr. Thomas Cureton has long advocated the use of continuous calisthenics, or what he refers to as "continuous rhythmical endurance exercise." Almost everyone can plan a continuous calisthenics program by selecting exercises for each fitness part that will elevate the heart rate to the optimal level and sustain this intensity an adequate length of time. Continuous calisthenics can be done individually, but are also excellent for group use. A sample program and some suggestions for performing them are presented in the box beginning on the preceding page.

Cross-Country Skiing

In Europe, cross-country skiing is one of the most popular aerobic activities. Of course, this sport requires snow and a certain amount of specialized equipment, but for those who can cross-country ski on a regular basis, studies show that it is one of the most effective cardiovascular fitness exercises.

Stretching	5–Minute Circle Exercises	10–Minute Circle Exercises	15–Minute Circle Exercises
• All stretching is passive and each exercise is held 5 to 6 seconds	• Jog in a circle 1 minute	• 15 jumping jacks	• Jog in a circle
• 3 single leg hugs (each leg)	• 7 bent knee sit-ups	• 7 knee dips (each leg)	• 10 knee dips with each leg
• 3 lateral trunk stretches	• Lateral shuffle in circle	• 15 jumping jacks	• Jog in a circle
• 3 sitting trunk stretches	• 10 side leg-lifts (each leg)	• Jog in a circle	• 5 bent knee sit-ups
	• 25 side hop-kicks	• 5 bent knee sit-ups	• 5 side leg-lifts (each leg)
	• 7 push-ups	• Jog backward in a circle	• 220-yard jog
	• Jog in a circle	• 10 back leg-lifts (one leg at a time)	• 220-yard walk
		• Jog in a circle	• Repeat stretching

Some general suggestions for using this exercise program are:

1. Stretch first to establish a pattern of regular stretching and to help eliminate possible soreness associated with the regular exercise program.

2. Start "too easy" rather than "too hard." You can always increase intensity after you determine your reaction to the exercise. You may wish to start out exercising for five or ten minutes and gradually progress to fifteen minutes.

3. If you exercise in a group, you may want to select a daily leader to choose the exercises. This can help motivate group members.

4. Vary the exercises daily but make sure all body parts are exercised.

5. Walk outside the circle if you find you need a slower pace. If the exercises are too difficult, start with what you can handle, but try to exercise continuously, even if it is just walking at first.

6. Use exercises appropriate for your individual needs. The ones listed are merely examples.

*Adapted from C. B. Corbin. "An Exercise Program for Large Groups," *The Physical Educator* 30 (March, 1973):46–47. Used by permission.

Dance Aerobics

Especially popular in recent years is dance aerobics. This type of aerobic activity is quite similar to continuous calisthenics except various dance steps are included with the regular calisthenics or other form of aerobic exercise. Dance aerobics is often accompanied by music and by preplanned choreography. A single routine may last for ten or fifteen minutes. If the routines are shorter, several may be done one after another to keep the activity continuous.

A typical dance aerobics routine includes calisthenics for flexibility, strength, and muscular endurance, together with dance steps and jogging, skipping, hopping, or some other cardiovascular activity. Books, records, audio and video tapes for dance aerobic routines are available from bookstores, music stores, and other sources. Some of the more well-known names for dance aerobics are Aerobic Dance, Rhythmic Aerobics, Jazzercise, and Dancercise.

Hiking and Backpacking

Like walking and jogging, hiking is an excellent form of exercise. Hiking has the advantage of an out-of-doors setting, often in a very scenic environment. It does require some equipment, such as a rucksack and good hiking shoes, but does not require highly specialized skills.

Backpacking is a form of hiking that usually covers longer distances and so involves an overnight stay, often in the mountains. When done continuously, backpacking is excellent for building muscular endurance as well as cardiovascular fitness. Like other aerobic activities, it can be very helpful in controlling body fatness. In recent years, it has become a very popular activity; nearly 11 million American adults report regular involvement in backpacking.

Jogging/Running

The aerobic activity that has rapidly grown in popularity in recent years among both adult men and women is jogging or running. Though there is no "official" distinction between jogging and running, those who run more than a few miles per day, who participate in races, and who are concerned about improving the time in which they run a certain distance, often prefer to be called runners rather than joggers. Fifteen to 20 million American adults report that they jog or run on a regular basis.

The major advantage of jogging/running is that it requires only a good pair of running shoes and very little skill. With effort, almost anyone can benefit from the activity and even improve performance if that is the goal.

There are some techniques that every jogger should be familiar with before starting a jogging program.

1. *Foot Placement*—The heel of the foot hits the ground first in jogging. Your heel should strike before the rest of the foot (but not vigorously) and then you should rock forward and push off with the ball of your foot. Contrary to some opinions, you should *not* jog on your toes. (A flat foot landing can be all right as long as you push off with the ball of the foot.) The toes should point straight ahead. The feet should stay under the knees and should *not* swing out to the sides as you jog.
2. *Length of Stride*—For efficiency, you should have a relatively long stride. Your stride should be at least several inches longer than your walking stride. If necessary, you may have to "reach" to lengthen your stride. Most older people find it more efficient to run with a shorter stride.
3. *Arm Movement*—While you jog, you should swing your arms as well as your legs. The arms should be bent at about 90 degrees and should swing freely and alternately from front to back. The arms should swing in the direction you are moving and not from side to side. Keep your arms and hands relaxed.
4. *Body Position*—While jogging, the upper body should be nearly erect. The head and chest should be held up and there should not be a conscious effort to lean forward as is the case in sprinting or fast running.

Those just beginning a jogging program should pay careful attention to the guidelines for exercise preparation outlined in Concept 4. Of course, for jogging/running to be effective in developing cardiovascular fitness, the heart rate must be elevated above threshold levels and into the target heart rate zone (see Concept 6).

Rope Jumping

Rope jumping is aerobic if done at a slow or moderate pace, but is anaerobic if done vigorously. One study shows that typical exercisers jump very briskly, and for this reason, cannot maintain the jumping continuously. Even those who are highly trained or who jump at a moderate pace find it difficult to continue this exercise long enough to build cardiovascular fitness because of leg fatigue, high heart rate, or loss of interest in the activity. To be most effective, a continuous routine involving several different jump steps should be used in combination with other forms of exercise. For example, rope jumping could be a part of a continuous calisthenics program or a dance aerobics routine.

TABLE 12.2 Achieving Fitness through Aerobic Exercise

Program Type	Cardiovascular Fitness	Strength and Muscular Endurance	Flexibility	Body and Fat Control	Skill-Related Fitness	Enjoyment or Fun[1]
Bicycling	***	**	*	***	*	**
Circuit Overload Training	**	***	*	**	*	**
Cooper's Aerobics	***	*	*	***	*	**
Continuous Calisthenics	***	**	***	***	*	**
Cross-Country Skiing	***	**	*	***	**	**
Dance Aerobics	***	**	***	***	*	**
Hiking and Backpacking	**	**	*	**	*	**
Jogging/Running	***	*	*	***	—	**
Rope Jumping	**	*	—	**	*	*
Swimming and Water Exercises	**	**	**	**	**	**
Walking	**	*	*	**	*	**

***Very Good   **Good   *Minimum   —Low

[1]Enjoyment and fun are relative, and for this reason, it is impossible to classify activities accurately. However, for the average person, some activities seem to be more enjoyable than others. The above listed classifications reflect the opinions of the typical person. *Any of the activities listed above can be fun and enjoyable for a given person in the right circumstances.*

Sports (Continuous)

As noted earlier in this concept, some activities that are at least partially anaerobic are considered aerobic if they are done at a pace that allows them to be done continuously. Many sports have extended rest periods and do not allow for continuous involvement. Some of the sports often considered good aerobic activities when performed continuously are basketball, handball, racquetball, and soccer. (For more information on sports, see Concept 15.)

Swimming and Water Exercises

The most recent exercise polls rank swimming as the first or second most popular form of regular exercise among adults. Most of those who swim for exercise swim laps or do water exercises. When done at a mild or moderate pace, both of these can be aerobic. When done continuously, these are excellent forms of exercise. Another popular but more formal program for this type of exercise is Aquadynamics prepared by the President's Council for Physical Fitness and Sports (see references).

Walking

Approximately one-quarter of all adult Americans report that they regularly walk for exercise. This popularity is probably due to the fact that the activity can be easily done by people of all ages and of all ability levels. Contrary to some opinions, walking can be a very good exercise for developing and maintaining good cardiovascular fitness and for helping to control body fatness. Of course, the exercise must be done in the target zone for it to be effective. Some regular walkers do not exercise often enough, hard enough, or long enough to reap optimal health benefits. Those who walk for exercise should walk briskly and continuously. They should follow the guidelines for preparing for exercise outlined in Concept 4, and vary their destination frequently to make the walk more interesting.

Different aerobic activities have different health-related benefits.

The health-related benefits of various aerobic activities are summarized in Table 12.2.

REFERENCES

Anshel, M. H. *Aerobics for Fitness.* Minneapolis: Burgess

Clement, D. B. "A Survey of Overuse Running Injuries." *Physician and Sportsmedicine* 9 (1981):47.

*Cooper, K. H. *The Aerobics Program for Total Well-Being.* New York: M. Evans, 1982.

*Corbin, C. B., and R. Lindsey. *Fitness for Life.* 2d ed. Glenview, IL: Scott, Foresman and Co., 1983.

Corbin, C. B. "Profiling for Flexibility." In *Clinics in Sports Medicine: Profiling,* edited by J. Nicholas and J. Herschberger. Philadelphia: Saunders Co., 1984.

Corbin, C. B., and R. Lindsey. *The Ultimate Fitness Book.* New York: Leisure Press, 1984.

Cureton, T. K. *Physical Fitness and Dynamic Health.* New York: Dial Press, 1965.

Getchell, B., and P. Cleary. "The Caloric Costs of Rope Skipping and Running." *Physician and Sportsmedicine* 8 (1980):56.

Harris, L., and Associates. *The Perrier Study: Fitness in America.* New York: Great Waters of France, 1979.

Research and Forecasts, Inc. *The Miller Lite Report on American Attitudes toward Sports.* Milwaukee: Miller Brewing Co., 1983.

*Schultz, P. "Walking for Fitness: Slow but Sure." *Physician and Sportsmedicine* 8 (1980):24.

Vickery, S. R., K. J. Cureton, and J. L. Langstaff. "Heart Rate and Energy Expenditure during Aqua Dynamics." *Physician and Sportsmedicine* 17 (1983):67.

13

STRENGTH AND ENDURANCE EXERCISES

CONCEPT 13

Strength exercises should be
performed against a near maximum resistance
using only a few repetitions.
Endurance exercises
require only a moderate resistance,
but a high number of repetitions.

INTRODUCTION

There are several kinds of strength and endurance exercises. Among the most popular are *isotonic calisthenics,* which require little or no special equipment; *isometric exercises,* which can be done in a small space; and *progressive resistance exercises (PRE),* which can be performed isotonically or isokinetically.

TERMS

Detailed descriptions of important strength and muscular endurance terms are presented in Concepts 7 and 8.

THE FACTS

Isotonic calisthenic exercises are among the most popular forms of exercise among adults.

Isotonic calisthenics, such as sit-ups and push-ups, are suitable for people of different ability levels, and can be used to improve both strength and muscular endurance. One disadvantage is that this type of exercise does little to increase strength unless more resistance is added. For example, doing a push-up will build strength to a point. However, once you can do several, adding more repetitions will only build muscular endurance, NOT strength. To develop additional strength, you can add more weights to increase the resistance or change the body position so there is a greater gravitational effect or more torque. For example, you can elevate your feet or wear a weighted vest while doing push-ups. Some isotonic calisthenics that you can do at home are illustrated on pages 95–98.

Weight training with "free weights" is a popular form of isotonic progressive resistance exercise.

Free weights are weights that are not attached to a machine or exercise device. They can be put on a bar so that the weight can be adjusted for different exercises as necessary to provide optimal resistance. Weight training with free weights is very popular because it can be done in the home with inexpensive equipment. Homemade weights can even be constructed from pieces of pipe and plastic bottles filled with water. Some of the exercises that are best for developing strength and muscular endurance are illustrated on pages 99–100.

The exercises suggested here should be performed as described until the person is able to increase the repetitions to approximately twenty-five. Additional weight should then be added. Muscles depicted in color are those primarily involved in the exercises.

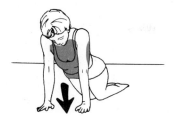

3. Bent Knee Let-downs

For those who cannot do bent knee push-ups.

Purpose

Develop muscles of the arms, shoulders, and chest.

Position

Same as a bent knee push-up position.

Movement

Slowly lower the body to the floor, keeping the body line straight; return to the starting position in any manner. Repeat.

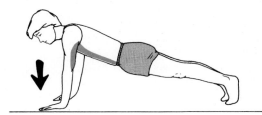

1. Full-length Push-ups

Purpose

Develop muscles of arms, shoulders, and chest.

Position

Take front-leaning rest position, arms straight.

Movement

Lower chest to floor. Press to beginning position in same manner. Repeat.

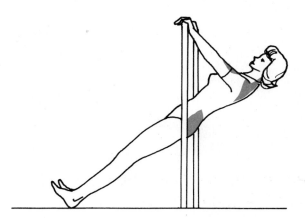

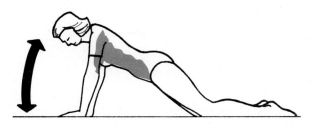

2. Bent Knee Push-ups

For those who cannot do full-length push-ups.

Purpose

Develop muscles of the arms, shoulders, and chest.

Position

Assume the push-up position, but rest the weight on the knees, not the feet.

Movement

Lower the body until the chest touches the floor; return to the starting position keeping the body straight. Repeat.

4. Modified Pull-ups

Purpose

Develop muscles of the arms and shoulders.

Position

Hang (palms forward and shoulder width apart) from a low bar (may be placed across two chairs), heels on floor, with the body straight from feet to head.

Movement

Pull up, keeping the body straight, touch the chest to the bar, then lower to the starting position. (Stronger persons may hang from a bar vertically and pull up.) Repeat.

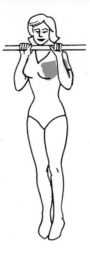

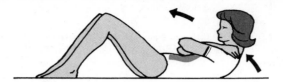

7. Bent Knee Sit-ups

Purpose

Develop the upper abdominal muscles and correct abdominal ptosis.

Position

Assume a hook-lying position with arms crossed and hands on shoulders.

Movement

Roll up, making elbows touch knees, then roll down to the starting position. Repeat. For more overload, place the hands on top of the head or place your index fingers by your ears (do not put hands behind neck and do not anchor feet).

5. Pull-ups (Chinning)

Purpose

Develop muscles of arms and shoulders.

Position

Hang from bar, palms forward, body and arms straight.

Movement

Pull up until chin is over bar. Repeat.

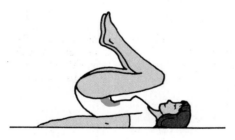

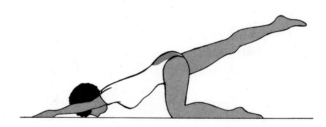

6. Reverse Sit-ups

Purpose

Develop the lower abdominal muscles and correct abdominal ptosis.

Position

Lie on the floor. Bend the knees, place the feet flat on the floor, and place arms at sides.

Movement

Lift the knees to the chest raising the hips off the floor; do not let the knees go past the shoulders. Return to the starting position. Repeat.

8. Leg Extension Exercise

Purpose

Develop muscles of the hips.

Position

Assume a knee-chest position, hands on floor with arms extended as far as possible.

Movement

Extend right leg upward in line with trunk, then lower. Continue repetitions. Repeat with other leg.

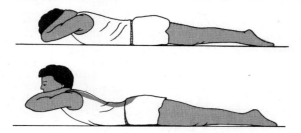

9. Upper Back Lift

Purpose

Develop muscles of the upper back. Correct kyphosis and round shoulders.

Position

Lie prone (face down) with hands clasped behind the neck.

Movement

Pull the shoulder blades together, raising the elbows off the floor. Slowly raise the head and chest off the floor by arching the upper back. Return to the starting position; repeat. Caution: Do not arch the lower back; lift only until the sternum (breast bone) clears the floor.

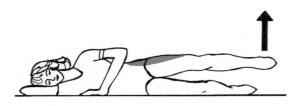

10. Side Leg Raises

Purpose

Develop muscles on outside of thighs.

Position

Lie on the side.

Movement

Raise the top leg toward the ceiling, then return. Do the same number of repetitions with each leg.

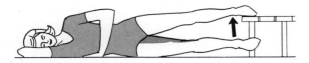

11. Lower Leg-lift

Purpose

Develop muscles on the inside of thighs.

Position

Lie on the side with the upper leg (foot) supported on a bench.

Movement

Raise the lower leg toward the ceiling; repeat. Roll to opposite side and repeat.

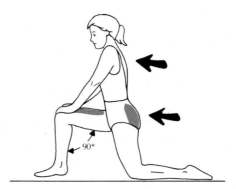

12. Forward Lunge

Purpose

Develop muscles of the legs and hips.

Position

Stand tall, feet together.

Movement

Take a step forward with the left foot, touching the right knee to the floor. The knees should be bent only to a 90° angle. Return to the starting position and step out with the other foot. Repeat, alternating left and right.

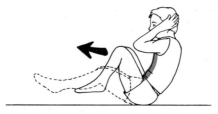

13. Sitting Tucks or "V Sit"

Purpose

Develop muscles of abdomen and legs.

Position

Sit on the floor so that the back and feet are off the floor. Interlock fingers on top of the head or extend arms forward for balance. Do not put hands behind neck.

Movement

Alternately draw the legs into the chest and extend the feet away from the body. Keep feet and back off the floor. Continue repeating.

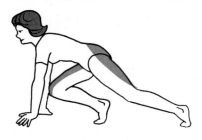

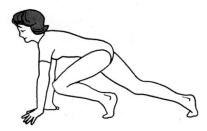

14. Stationary Leg Change

Purpose

Develop muscles of the legs and hips.

Position

Crouch on the floor with weight on hands, left leg bent under the chest, right leg extended behind.

Movement

Alternate legs; bring right leg up while left leg goes back. Repeat.

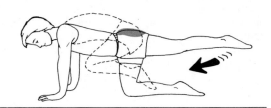

15. Knee-to-Nose Touch/Kneeling Leg Extensions

Purpose

Strength or endurance of gluteal muscles; stretch low back.

Position

Kneel on "all fours."

Movement

Pull knee to nose, then extend leg horizontally (do not go higher). Alternate legs; repeat.

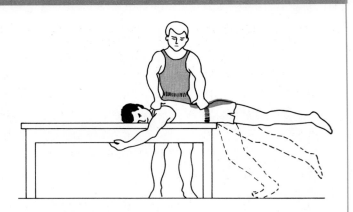

16. Lower Trunk Lift

Purpose

Low back and hip strength.

Position

Lie prone on bench or table with legs hanging over the edge.

Movement

Have a partner stabilize the upper back or grasp the edges of the table with hands. Raise the legs parallel to the floor and lower them. Do not raise past the horizontal or arch the back.

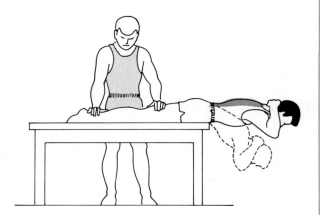

17. Upper Trunk Lift

Purpose

Develop upper back strength.

Position

Lie on a table or bench with the upper half of the body hanging over the edge.

Movement

Have a partner stabilize the feet while the trunk is raised parallel to the floor, then lower the trunk to the starting position. Place hands behind neck. Do not raise past the horizontal or arch the back.

The exercises suggested here should be performed as described until the person is able to increase repetitions. Muscles depicted in color are those primarily involved in the exercises.

1. Shoulder Shrug

Purpose

Strengthen the muscles of the shoulders.

Position

Stand with palms toward body, bar touching thighs, legs straight and feet together.

Movement

Lift shoulders (try to touch ears) then roll shoulders smoothly backward, down and forward. Repeat maximum number of times.

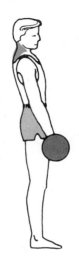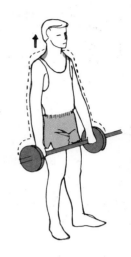

2. Military Press

Purpose

Strengthen the muscles of the shoulders and arms.

Position

Stand erect, bend elbows, palms forward at chest level, hands spread (slightly more than shoulder width). Bar touching chest, spread feet (comfortable distance), keep legs straight.

Movement

Move bar to overhead position (arms straight). Lower to chest position. Repeat.

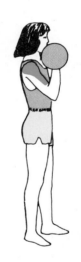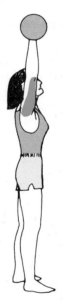

3. Half Squat

Purpose

Strengthen the muscles of the thighs and hips.

Position

Stand erect, feet turned out 45°. Rest bar behind neck on shoulders. Spread hands in a comfortable position.

Movement

Squat slowly, keeping back straight, eyes ahead. Bend knees to 90°; keep knees over feet. Pause, then stand. Repeat.

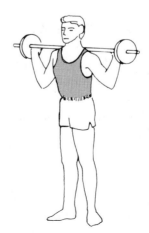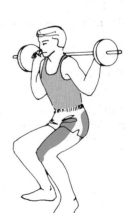

4. Biceps Curl

Purpose

Strengthen the muscles of the upper front part of the arms (biceps).

Position

Stand erect, palms forward; arms spread in order not to touch body; bar touching thighs. Spread feet in comfortable position.

Movement

Move bar to chin, keeping body straight and elbows forward of center line of body. Do not allow elbows to touch body. Lower to original position. Repeat.

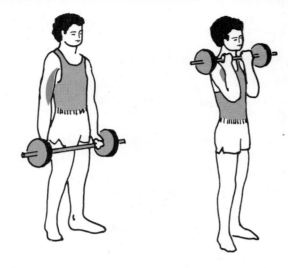

5. Triceps Curl

Purpose

Strengthen the muscles of the back part of the upper arms (triceps).

Position

Stand erect, elbows up, palms up. Rest bar behind neck on shoulders, hands near center of bar, feet spread.

Movement

Keep upper arms stationary. Raise weight overhead, return bar to original position. Repeat.

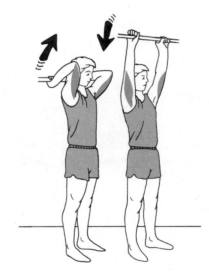

Exercise with "weight training machines" or "pulley exercisers" has become more popular and more accessible in recent years.

Weight training can be done on exercise machines and pulley devices. These have become more popular in recent years as lower-priced machines have been developed and exercise clubs have made them accessible to more people. These machines can be effective in developing strength and muscular endurance if used properly. They can save time because unlike free weights, the weight to be lifted can be changed easily and quickly. They are also safer since you are less likely to drop weights on machines. The kinds of exercises that can be done on these machines are more limited than those for free weights. Some good exercise using weight training machines and pulley exercisers are illustrated on pages 102–4.

6. Toe Raise

Purpose

Strengthen muscles of the legs (calf).

Position

Stand erect with front grip, hands wider than shoulder width apart, bar resting behind neck on shoulders. Rest balls of feet on two-inch block with heels on floor. Toes together, heels apart.

Movement

Rise on toes quickly, hold for one second. Lower heels to floor. Repeat. Keep toes in and heels out.

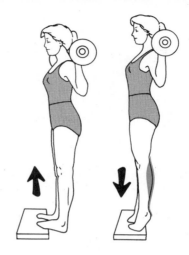

7. Pull to Chin

Purpose

Strengthen muscles of the shoulders and arms.

Position

Stand erect with a front grip (loose), hands together at center of bar, bar touching thighs, feet spread, head erect, eyes straight ahead.

Movement

Pull bar to chin. Keep bar close to body and elbows well above bar. Lower to extended position. Repeat.

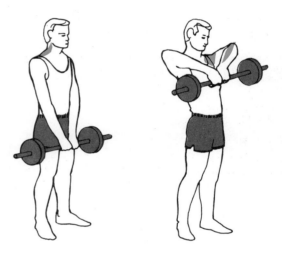

Isometric exercise is an effective and inexpensive way to build strength and muscular endurance.

Isometric exercise is an attractive form of exercise because it is effective in building strength and muscular endurance and can be done in the home, office, or car, in a limited space and with no costly equipment. All that is necessary to do many isometric exercises is a piece of rope or a towel and a doorway. It may be hard for some people to motivate themselves when performing isometrics because of the lack of movement involved. Also, isometric exercises will elevate blood pressure, and for that reason, those who have known cardiovascular problems should be under the supervision of a physician when involved in them. Recent evidence indicates that for normal, healthy individuals, isometrics do not cause cardiovascular problems. Some good isometric exercises that can be done in the home are illustrated on pages 105–10.

The exercises suggested here should be performed as described until the person is able to increase repetitions. Muscles depicted in color are those primarily involved in the exercises.

1. Biceps Curl (Low Pulley)

Purpose

Strengthen elbow flexor muscles on front of arm.

Position

Stand erect, arms at sides, palms up. Grasp bar.

Movement

Flex elbows, bringing bar to chest. Keep elbows pressed against sides. Lower; repeat.

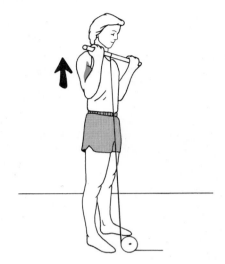

2. Seated Rowing (Low Pulley)

Purpose

Develop upper arms and shoulders.

Position

Sit facing pulley, feet braced and knees slightly bent. Grasp bar palm-up with hands shoulder width apart.

Movement

Pull bar to chest and return; repeat.

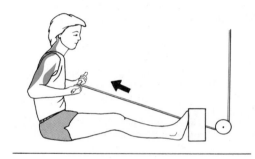

3. Leg Press

Purpose

Develop thigh and hip muscles.

Position

Sit on chair with feet on pedals, knees bent to right angle. Grasp handles.

Movement

Extend legs and return; repeat. Do not lock knees when legs straighten.

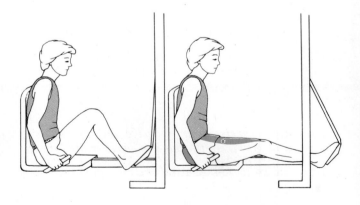

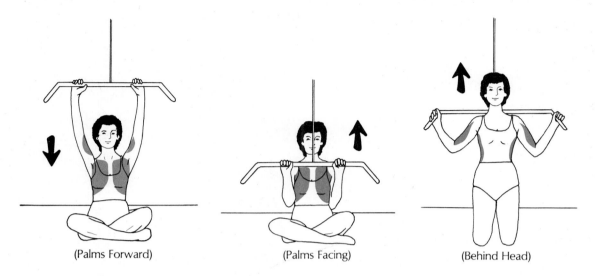

(Palms Forward)　　　　　(Palms Facing)　　　　　(Behind Head)

4. Lat Pull-down (High Pulley)

Purpose

Develop latissimus ("lat") and arm biceps.

Position

Tailor sit or kneel on both knees. Grasp bar with palms facing away from you, hands shoulder distance apart.

Movement

Pull bar down to chest and return; repeat.

Variations

Turn palms toward face; move hands out to ends of bar; pull bar behind head.

5. Triceps Curl

Purpose

Develop triceps and other muscles on back of arm.

Position

Stand erect. Grasp bar near center; palms down.

Movement

With elbows clamped against sides, pull bar down to thighs and return to chest height without moving elbows; repeat.

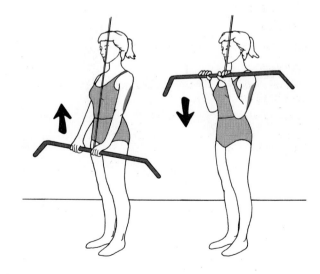

6. Bench Press

Purpose

Develop chest (pectoral) and triceps muscles.

Position

Lie supine on bench with feet on floor, or knees bent and feet flat on bench. Grasp handles at shoulder level.

Movement

Push bar up until arms are straight. Return; repeat. (Do not arch lower back.)

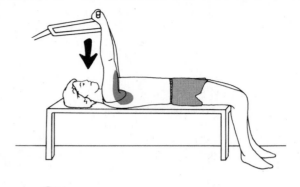

7. Ankle Press

Purpose

Develop the calf muscles.

Position

Sit at leg press station with legs straight. Grasp handles. Put ball of foot at lower edge of pedal.

Movement

Keeping legs straight, point toes by extending (plantar flexing) ankles. Return; repeat.

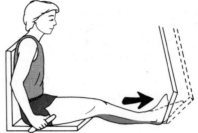

8. Knee Extension

Purpose

Develop thigh (quadriceps) muscles.

Position

Sit on end of bench with ankles hooked under padded bar. Grasp edge of table.

Movement

Extend knees. Return; repeat.

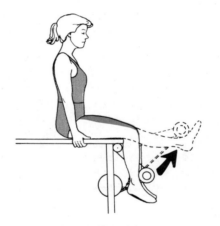

9. Hamstring Curl

Purpose

Develop hamstrings (muscles on back of thigh) and other knee flexors.

Position

Lie prone on bench with ankles hooked under padded bar. Rest chin on hands or grasp bench.

Movement

Flex knees as far as possible without allowing hips to raise. Return; repeat.

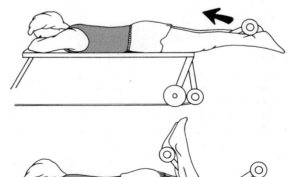

Isometric exercises are intended primarily to develop muscular strength and endurance. Eighteen different exercises for different body parts are presented here. You should select exercises for your program (if you choose isometric exercise) that meet your own personal needs. All of the following exercises should be held for five to eight seconds and should be repeated several times a day. Muscles depicted in red are those primarily involved in the exercises.

1. Chest Push

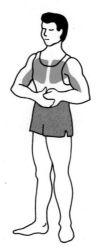

Purpose

Develop muscles of the chest and upper arms.

Position

Place left fist in palm of right hand. Keep hands close to chest, forearms parallel to floor.

Movement

Push hands together with maximum strength.

2. Fist Squeeze

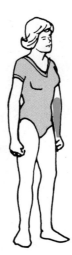

Purpose

Develop muscles of the lower arm.

Position

Arms extended at side.

Movement

Clench fists as hard as possible. Repeat.

3. Shoulder Pull

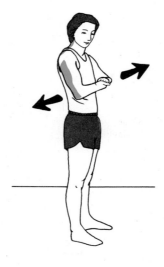

Purpose

Develop muscles of the upper back and arms.

Position

Cup hands and interlock fingers. Keep hands close to chest, forearms parallel to floor.

Movement

Attempt to pull hands apart with maximum force.

4. Neck Pull

Purpose

Develop muscles of the neck, upper back, and arms.

Position

Interlock fingers behind head, elbows pointing forward.

Movement

Force head backward. Pull hands forward with maximum strength.

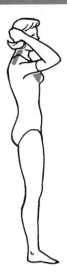

5. Leg Extension

Purpose

Develop muscles of shoulders, legs, and hips.

Position

Loop rope under feet. Stand on rope, feet spread shoulder width. Keep back straight. Bend knees, grasp both ends of rope, back erect, arms straight, and buttocks low.

Movement

Lift upward with maximum strength.

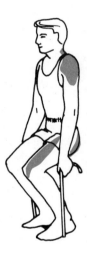

6. Overhead Pull

Purpose

Develop muscles of the arms.

Position

Fold rope in a double loop. Grasp rope overhead, palms outward. Extend arms.

Movement

Push outward at maximum force. Repeat with palms in.

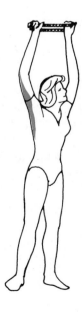

7. Curls

Purpose

Develop muscles on the front of the arms.

Position

Place rope loop behind thighs while standing in a half squat position. Grasp loop, palms up, shoulder width.

Movement

Lift upward with maximum strength. For reverse curls, repeat gripping with palms down.

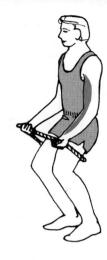

8. Foot Lift

Purpose

Develop muscles of legs.

Position

Stand on loop with left foot. Place loop around right ankle. Flex knee until taut.

Movement

Apply maximum strength upward. Repeat forward and to side with both feet.

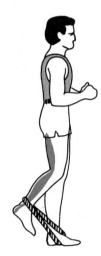

9. Military Press in Doorway

Purpose

Develop muscles of the arms and shoulders.

Position

Stand in doorway, face straight ahead, hands shoulder width apart, elbows bent.

Movement

Tighten leg, hip, and back muscles. Push upward as hard as possible.

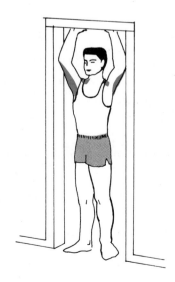

10. Arm Press in Doorway

Purpose

Develop muscles of the arms.

Position

Stand in doorway, back flat on one side of doorway, hands placed on other side.

Movement

Push with maximum strength.

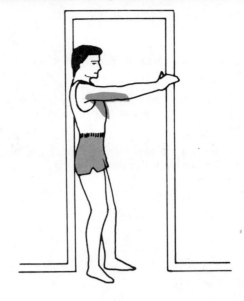

11. Leg Press in Doorway

Purpose

Develop muscles of the legs and hips.

Position

Sit in doorway facing side of door frame. Grasp molding behind head. Keep back flat on side of doorway, feet against other side.

Movement

Push legs with maximum strength.

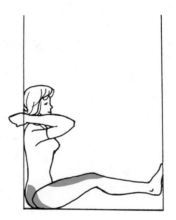

12. Wall Seat

Purpose

Develop muscles of the leg and hips.

Position

Assume half-sit position, back flat against wall, knees bent to 90°.

Movement

Push back against wall with maximum strength.

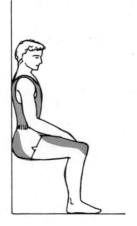

13. Triceps Extension

Purpose

Develop muscles of upper arm.

Position

Grasp towel at both ends. Hold left hand at small of neck, right hand over shoulder.

Movement

Pull towel with maximum force; repeat exercise, changing position of hands.

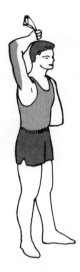

14. Leg Extension

Purpose

Develop muscles of top of upper leg.

Position

Place towel around right ankle, knee bent to 90° angle.

Movement

Grasp towel with both hands behind back, extend leg downward with maximum force. Repeat exercise, changing legs.

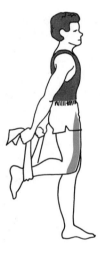

15. Waist Pull

Purpose

Develop muscles of the abdomen, chest, and arms.

Position

Grasp ends of towel, palms in, towel around back of waist, elbows flexed to right angle.

Movement

Pull forward on towel with maximum strength while contracting abdomen and flattening back.

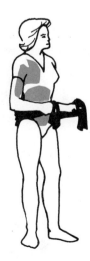

16. Bow Exercise

Purpose

Develop muscles of shoulders and upper back.

Position

Take archer's position with bow (towel) drawn, left elbow partially extended, right hand at chin, right arm parallel to floor.

Movement

Grasp towel and pull arms away from each other. Exchange positions of hands and repeat.

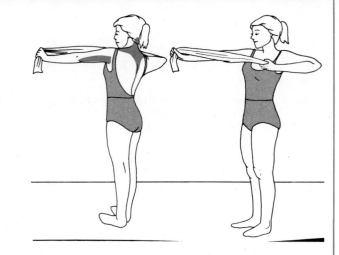

17. Gluteal Pinch

Purpose

Develop muscles of the buttocks.

Position

Lie prone, heels apart and big toes touching.

Movement

Pinch the buttocks together. Hold several seconds. Slowly relax; repeat several times.

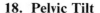

18. Pelvic Tilt

Purpose

Develop muscles of the abdomen and buttocks.

Position

Assume a supine position with the knees bent and slightly apart.

Movement

Press the spine down on the floor and hold for several seconds. Keep abdominals and gluteals tightened.

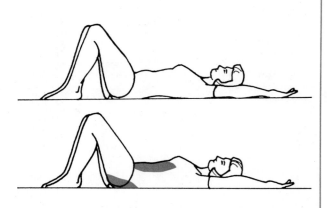

14
STRETCHING EXERCISES

CONCEPT 14

Stretching exercises
are designed to maintain or increase flexibility
by stretching the muscles
and other soft tissue around the joints.
This stretch may, in turn, prevent or alleviate
some musculoskeletal problems.

INTRODUCTION

There are many ways to stretch muscles and to exercise to improve flexibility (see Concept 9). The major types of muscle stretching exercises are static stretching, ballistic stretching, and PNF. These exercises can be done by yourself, using only your own muscles to stretch, or they can be done with the aid of gravity (body weight), or they can be done with the assistance of someone else. To develop flexibility, the soft tissues must be stretched beyond their normal limit.

TERMS

Detailed descriptions of important stretching and flexibility terms are presented in Concept 9.

THE FACTS

There is a correct way to perform stretching exercises.

Remember that while stretching may help to alleviate muscular soreness, it can also *cause* soreness, so "easy does it." Start below your threshold if you are unaccustomed to stretching a given muscle group and then work up to your target zone. The guidelines presented in Table 14.1 will help you to gain the most benefit from your exercises.

TABLE 14.1 Guidelines for Performing Stretching Exercises

1. Exercises that do not cause a muscle to lengthen beyond normal may maintain, but will not increase, flexibility.
2. To increase flexibility, the muscle must be "overloaded" (stretched beyond its normal length), but not to the point of pain.
3. Exercises must be performed for each muscle group and at each joint where flexibility is desired.
4. If ballistic stretching is used, precede it with static or PNF exercise.
5. Avoid ballistic exercises on previously injured muscles or joints.
6. Avoid ballistic toe touches in the presence of backaches.
7. If ballistic-stretches are used, the bounces should be gentle and probably should not exceed 10 percent of the normal antagonist static-stretch range of motion.
8. Avoid high risk stretching exercises (see Concept 19).

There are certain areas of the body that especially need to be stretched for good health and fitness.

Areas of the body that are most apt to need stretching include the muscles on the back of the legs (hamstrings) in order to prevent soreness, injury in sports, and referred back pain; the muscles on the inside of the thigh in order to prevent back, leg, and foot strain; the calf muscles in order to prevent soreness, and Achilles tendon injuries in jogging/running; the muscles on the front of the hip joint in order to prevent lordosis and backache; the low back muscles in order to help prevent back soreness and pain, as well as back injuries; and the muscles on the front of the chest and shoulders in order to prevent rounded shoulders and limited range of movement in the shoulder joint. The exercises pictured in this concept focus on these body areas.

SAMPLE FLEXIBILITY EXERCISES

These stretching exercises are intended primarily to develop flexibility. Fifteen exercises for different body parts are presented here. These exercises should be held for six to ten seconds. Muscles depicted in color are those primarily involved in the exercises.

1. Lower Leg Stretcher

Purpose

To stretch the calf muscles and Achilles tendon.

Position

Stand with the toes on a thick book or lower rung of a stall bar. Hold on to a support with hands.

Movement

Rise up on toes as far as possible and hold for several seconds. Relax and lower heels to floor as far as possible; hold. If ballistic-stretch is desired, bounce gently.

Note

Static stretch may alleviate sore calf muscles.

Contract   Relax and Stretch

2. Sitting Stretcher

Purpose

To stretch muscles on inside of thighs.

Position

Sit with the knees apart and the legs crossed at the ankles. Place the hands on the inside of the knees and resist while raising the knees.

Movement

Hold several seconds then relax and press the knees toward the floor as far as possible; hold.

Note

Useful for pregnant women or anyone whose thighs tend to rotate inward causing backache, knock-knees and flat feet.

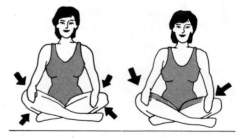

Contract, Relax, and Stretch

Certain stretching exercises are good for therapeutic purposes, as well as for fitness.

Stretching exercises can be prescribed specifically to alleviate pain. Usually, the same exercise, if done regularly, can prevent the condition that originally caused the pain. Examples of "therapeutic" exercises include exercise 1 (or some variation of it) to stretch the calf muscle. This will relieve muscle cramps in the lower leg. Exercise 6, Billig's exercise, can be used to relieve menstrual cramps (dysmenorrhea). The shin stretcher (exercise 11) will relieve soreness in the front of the lower leg (shin splints).

3. One-leg Stretcher

Purpose

To stretch lower back and hamstring muscles.

Position

Stand with one foot on a bench; keeping both legs straight.

Movement

Press down on bench with heel for several seconds, then relax and bend the trunk forward, trying to touch the head to the knee. Hold for a few seconds. Return to starting position and repeat with opposite leg. As flexibility improves, the arms can be used to pull the chest toward the legs.

Note

This is useful in relief of backache and correction of lordosis. If desired, bounce the trunk gently.

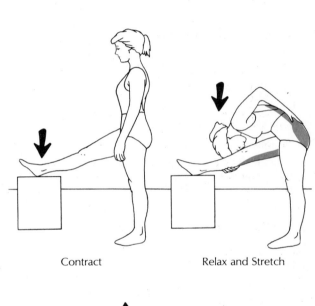

Contract   Relax and Stretch

4. Leg Hug

Purpose

To stretch lower back and gluteals.

Position

Hook-lying position.

Movement

Arch back and lift hips. Hold several seconds. Relax and pull knees to chest as hard as possible; hold.

Note

Useful for backache and lordosis (also see Concept 16).

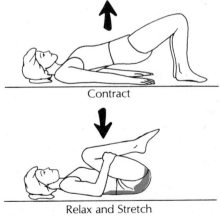

Contract

Relax and Stretch

5. Pectoral Stretch

Purpose

To stretch pectorals.

Position

Stand erect in doorway with arms raised shoulder height, elbows bent and hands grasping doorjambs; feet in front stride position.

Movement

Press forward on door frame with arm maximum contraction several seconds. Relax and shift weight forward on legs so muscles on front of shoulder joint and chest are stretched; hold.

Note

Useful to prevent or correct round shoulders and sunken chest.

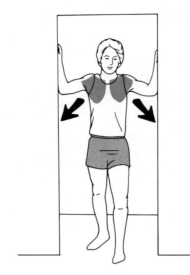

6. Billig's Exercise

Purpose

To stretch pelvic fascia, hip flexors, and inside of thigh.

Position

Stand with side to a wall and place the elbow and forearm against the wall at shoulder height. Tilt the pelvis backward tightening the gluteal and abdominal muscles.

Movement

Place opposite hand on hip and push the hips toward the wall. Push forward and sideward (45°) with the hips. Do not twist the hips. Hold. Repeat on opposite side.

Note

Useful for preventing some cases of dysmenorrhea.

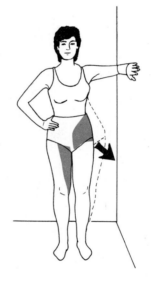

7. Lateral Trunk Stretcher

Purpose

To stretch trunk muscles.

Position

Stand with feet shoulder width apart.

Movement

Stretch left arm over head to right. Bend to right at waist reaching as far to right as possible with left arm and reach right arm as far as possible to the left; hold. Do not let trunk rotate. Repeat on opposite side. For less stretch, overhead arm may be bent at elbow.

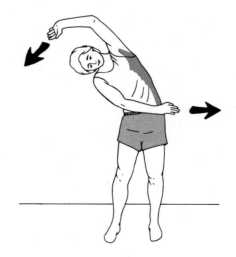

8. Iliopsoas Stretcher

Purpose

To stretch iliopsoas.

Position

Place right knee directly above right ankle and stretch left leg backward so knee touches floor. If necessary, place hands on floor for balance.

Movement

Press pelvis forward and downward; hold. Repeat on opposite side. Caution: Do not bend front knee more than 90°.

Note

Useful for those who have lordosis or lower back problems.

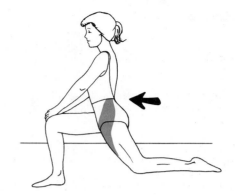

9. Neck Rotation

Purpose

To stretch neck rotators.

Position

Place palm of left hand against left cheek; point fingers toward ear and point elbow forward.

Movement

Try to turn head and neck left while resisting with left hand. Hold several seconds. Relax and turn head to right as far as possible; hold. Repeat.

Note

Useful for trigger points in neck and trapezius muscles.

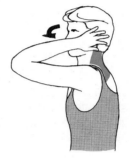
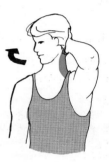

10. Arm Stretcher

Purpose

To stretch arm and chest muscles.

Position

Cross arms and turn palms of hands together. Raise arms overhead behind ears. Extend elbows.

Movement

Stretch as high as possible. Hold.

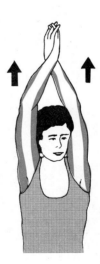

11. Shin Stretcher

Purpose

To stretch muscles on front of lower leg.

Position

Kneel on both knees, turn to right, and press down on right ankle with right hand.

Movement

Move pelvis forward. Hold. Repeat on opposite side.

Note

Stretches iliopsoas, as well as shin muscles; useful for muscle soreness (shin splints) in front of lower legs.

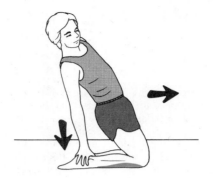

12. Wand Exercise

Purpose

To stretch front of shoulder and chest.

Position

Sit with wand grasped at ends. Raise wand overhead.

Movement

Bring it down behind shoulder blades. Keep spine erect. Hold. Hands may be moved closer together to increase stretch on chest muscles.

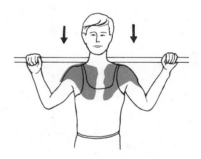

13. Hamstring Stretcher

Purpose

To stretch the muscles on the back of the thigh and behind the knee joint.

Position

Start in a hook-lying position. Bend right knee and grasp toes with right hand.

Movement

Place left hand on back of right thigh and bring knee toward chest; push heel toward ceiling. Repeat on left side.

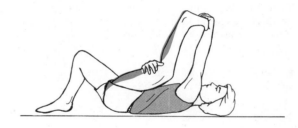

14. Calf Stretcher

Purpose

To stretch the calf muscles and Achilles tendon.

Note

This exercise is part of the sample warm-up included in Concept 4, and is described and illustrated on page 29.

15. Sitting Toe Touch

Purpose

To stretch the muscles of the lower back and the muscles of the back of the thigh (hamstrings).

Note

Several variations of this exercise are described and illustrated in Figure 9.1.

15
SPORTS, PREPLANNED, AND ANAEROBIC EXERCISE PROGRAMS

CONCEPT 15

Everyone, regardless of physical abilities, can find a sport or physical activity to enjoy for a lifetime.

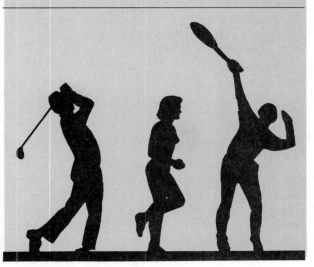

INTRODUCTION

There are many kinds of exercise and physical activity programs. Some of these, including aerobic exercise, strength and endurance training, and stretching, have been discussed in previous concepts (12, 13, and 14). Other popular and effective types of physical activity including sports, preplanned exercise programs, and anaerobic programs of exercise are discussed in this concept.

TERMS

Preplanned Exercise Programs—Preplanned exercise programs are exercise regimes planned by someone other than the person doing the exercise. Often they are designed for a large group of people rather than for one individual.

Lifetime Sport—A sport suitable for people of all ages; a sport that can be performed "from the cradle to the grave" (for a lifetime).

Sport—An activity that involves competition between teams or individuals and in which the goal is to beat the opponent or win the game. Except in the case of ties, there is a winner and a loser. Activities such as swimming, cycling, jogging/running are classified as sports by some writers, but since most adults do not perform these activities competitively, in this text, they are defined as aerobic activities rather than sports.

THE FACTS ABOUT SPORTS

Those sports in which youth are active are often not the activities performed by adults for a "lifetime."

Team sports are the most popular among school-age children. But the leading lifetime sports are bowling and tennis. However, many of the most popular lifetime activities are not even sports. Bowling is the only sport in the top five activities performed regularly by adults. The other four activities are walking, swimming, calisthenics, and bicycling. Only three of the top ten lifetime activities are sports. The top ten sports in which adults regularly participate (excluding swimming, cycling, and jogging/running) are listed in Table 15.1.

More and more adults favor involvement of their children in aerobic activities and lifetime sports.

While it is true that baseball, football, and basketball are still activities in which parents encourage their children's participation, especially boys, many now prefer their children to become involved in lifetime

117

TABLE 15.1 Achieving Fitness through Sports

Sport	Participants (in millions)	Cardiovascular	Muscular Endurance	Strength	Flexibility	Fat Control
Bowling	20.2	—	—	—	—	—
Tennis	14.0	**	**	*	*	*
Basketball	10.9	***	**	*	—	**
Softball	10.9	—	—	—	—	—
Baseball	9.3	—	—	—	—	—
Golf (walking)	7.8	*	*	—	*	*
Volleyball	7.8	*	**	*	*	*
Football	6.2	*	*	**	—	*
Frisbee	6.2	*	*	—	*	*
Table Tennis	6.2	—	—	—	*	—

***Very Good   **Good   *Minimum   —Low

sports or aerobic activities. Among the activities most preferred for boys are tennis, swimming, bicycling, jogging/running, and camping. Among those preferred for girls are tennis, bowling, softball, swimming, bicycling, walking, and dance aerobics.

Participation in sports can contribute to good health-related physical fitness.

The ten most popular sports performed on a regular basis by adults are presented in Table 15.1. Each has been assigned a value for building each of the health-related aspects of physical fitness.

Participation in a lifetime sport does not ensure good health-related physical fitness.

As seen in Table 15.1, many popular lifetime sports lack sufficient frequency, intensity, or time to improve health-related physical fitness. For example, bowling, softball, and baseball are fun for many people but do very little to improve fitness.

The way a person plays a sport affects the amount of fitness derived from it.

The way you play a sport will determine the fitness benefits derived from the activity. If you play basketball, you may just shoot baskets or play on half the court, or you may play a vigorous full-court competitive game. In tennis, you may just hit the ball back and forth, play a recreational game, or play a vigorous competitive game. The benefits illustrated in Table 15.1 are based on moderate recreational play. If you play less intensely or more vigorously, the benefits will vary accordingly.

Participation in lifetime sports can be a means of achieving physical fitness, but can also provide other valuable benefits as well.

One of the real benefits of regular participation in lifetime physical activities is improved health through improved cardiovascular fitness, muscular endurance,

strength, and flexibility. However, the participants may also derive personal satisfaction and meaning from the participation, and benefit from social interactions and the release of emotional tensions.

In many cases, a person needs to exercise to get fit for sports rather than play sports to get fit.

Many sports require a considerable amount of fitness, especially those involving vigorous competition, yet the sport may do relatively little to develop fitness. For example, you need considerable strength, muscular endurance, and flexibility to play football. However, football is not a particularly good activity for developing these aspects of fitness.

While most people learn recreational sports skills early in life, lifetime sports skills can be learned at any age.

Research evidence suggests that most skills are learned early in life. In fact, one study indicates that as many as 85 percent of all recreational skills are learned by the age of twelve. This does not mean that "old dogs cannot learn new tricks," but it does suggest a need to teach skills to children at an early age.

THE FACTS ABOUT PREPLANNED EXERCISE PROGRAMS

Preplanned exercise programs are a popular form of exercise.

The results of nationwide surveys in the United States and in Canada confirm that home calisthenics are among the most popular forms of exercise among adults. Preplanned programs are especially popular because someone else directs your performance.

TABLE 15.2   Achieving Fitness through Preplanned Exercise Programs

Program Type	Cardiovascular Fitness	Strength and Muscular Endurance	Flexibility	Body and Fat Control	Skill-Related Fitness	Enjoyment or Fun[1]
Aquadynamics	**	**	**	**	*	**
Dance Exercise[2]	***	**	***	***	*	**
XBX-5BX	*	***	**	*	—	*

***Very Good   **Good   *Minimum   —Low

[1]Enjoyment and fun are relative, and for this reason, it is impossible to classify activities accurately. However, for the average person, some activities seem to be more enjoyable than others. The above listed classifications reflect the opinions of the typical person. *Any of the activities listed above can be fun and enjoyable for a given person in the right circumstances.*

[2]All dance exercise classes are not "equal." If taught well by a professional, these rankings would be accurate.

There can be some problems in performing preplanned exercise programs.

Because preplanned exercise programs are planned by one person (or group) for individuals of many different levels of fitness, they may not be equally effective for all people who use them.

When selecting a preplanned exercise program, the following suggestions may be useful.

1. Find out who wrote the program. Is the person(s) an expert? What makes the person an expert? Look for a program written by someone with a good educational background in physical education, exercise physiology, or sports medicine. Programs written by movie stars and television celebrities are rarely sound.
2. Choose a program with more than one level of exercise. A good program will have exercises for beginning, intermediate, and advanced levels of fitness. This allows you to select a program appropriate to your needs. Be skeptical of programs that include one set of exercises for all people.
3. Make certain all of the exercises are "good" exercises. In Concept 17, some contraindicated or "bad" exercises are outlined. Avoid programs that include these exercises.
4. Choose a program that meets your needs. Since physical fitness includes many components, you need a program that includes exercises and activities for the fitness areas in which you need improvement.
5. Choose a program that you enjoy enough to continue on a regular basis. No matter how good a program is, if you don't do it, it won't work.
6. Choose a program that can be adapted to your needs as your fitness improves.

When performing a preplanned program, follow these suggestions.

1. Even in a multilevel program, you may have to make personal adjustments. You may already possess some fitness aspects but not in others. Adopting an advanced program for all components of fitness would not be in your best interest. You may need to do some exercises for an advanced level and others for a moderate or beginning level, depending upon your current fitness levels.
2. Many, if not most, preplanned exercise programs should be supplemented with extra exercise if total fitness is the goal. Some of the more popular preplanned programs are rated in Table 15.2. Those that are not "good" for a specific component of fitness may require supplemental exercises for the missing elements.
3. Alternate exercise programs from time to time. Variety may help keep your interest level up.

Aquadynamics

In Concept 12, water exercises were discussed. When done continuously, water exercises are a form of aerobic exercise. Aquadynamics is a set of preplanned water exercises developed by the President's Council for Physical Fitness and Sports. Those interested in this program should consult the appropriate reference at the end of this concept.

Dance Exercise

Though dance exercise was covered in Concept 12, it is an aerobic form of exercise and is included here because dance exercise routines are often preplanned. Dance exercise includes basic dance steps, exercises and calisthenics, and other forms of movement performed with music. Done properly, dance exercises can be an excellent form of exercise for building physical fitness and for having fun. Many books and records describing various dance exercise routines are available, some better than others. Before performing such preplanned exercise programs, make sure that the exercises included are good ones and that the programs are consistent with the guidelines described in this book.

Royal Canadian XBX and 5BX Programs

The Royal Canadian XBX and 5BX programs are progressive exercise plans designed to build total physical fitness. These plans, originally developed for use by The Royal Canadian Air Force, require eleven to twelve minutes a day. They were, like the Aerobics Program, originally designed to develop and maintain the physical fitness of military personnel. However, the programs have been widely received by the public.

The Canadian Air Force Program consists of two separate parts: 5BX for men and XBX for women, though either set of exercises is appropriate for either sex. These graduated programs are arranged so that a specific number of exercises and repetitions are performed, depending upon your initial fitness. The more fit people select exercises from a chart listing more difficult exercises, while the less fit people select exercises from a chart illustrating less difficult exercises.

The XBX plan contains four charts of ten exercises, each chart more difficult than the preceding one.

THE CANADIAN XBX AND 5BX EXERCISES (SAMPLE PROGRAM)*

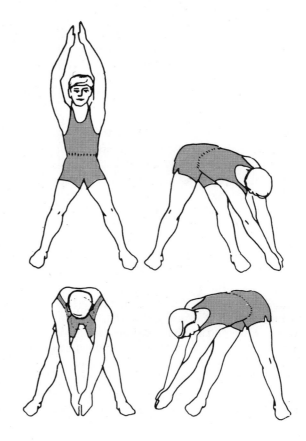

Perform each exercise the number of repetitions indicated.

Sample Program	Number of Repetitions
Exercise 1	10
Exercise 2	16
Exercise 3	12
Exercise 4**	24
Exercise 5**	26
Exercise 6**	28
Exercise 7	28
Exercise 8	22
Exercise 9	8
Exercise 10	140

1. **Toe Touching**
   Start. Stand erect, feet about sixteen inches apart, arms overhead. Bend down to touch floor outside left foot. Bob up and down to touch floor between feet. Bob again and bend to touch floor outside right foot. Return to starting position.
   Count. Each return to the starting position counts as one repetition.

2. **Knee Raising****
   Start. Stand erect, feet together, arms at sides. Raise left knee as high as possible, grasping behind the upper leg with hands. Pull leg against body. Keep straight throughout. Lower foot to floor. Repeat with right leg. Continue by alternating legs.
   Count. Left knee raise plus right knee raise counts as one repetition.

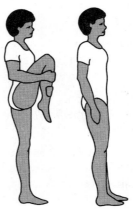

*Used by permission Royal Canadian Air Force, *Exercise Plans for Physical Fitness.* Queen's Printer, Ottawa, Canada: Revised U.S. Edition, 1962. By special arrangement with *This Week Magazine.*
**Exercises with double asterisks have been modified to improve them and to make them safer.

Each chart is divided into twelve fitness levels. The 5BX includes six charts of five exercises each and each chart is divided into twelve fitness "levels." Intensity of exercise increases progressively as you move from level to level and from chart to chart.

A sample from the Royal Canadian Program is shown here. It is one of the many included in the program, and is of moderate intensity. Some of the exercises have been modified to improve them. For example, the bent knee sit-up was substituted for the straight-leg sit-up because it is a better exercise for building abdominal strength and because it is not as likely to cause problems. The arm and leg-lift was substituted for a back arching exercise, and the arm circling and knee raising exercises were modified to make them safer. Finally, it is recommended that a supplemental cardiovascular fitness activity be included if cardiovascular fitness is an important goal. For more details, consult *Exercise Plans for Physical Fitness*. Be sure to look over each exercise carefully and to modify those that are dangerous using the information provided in Concept 17.

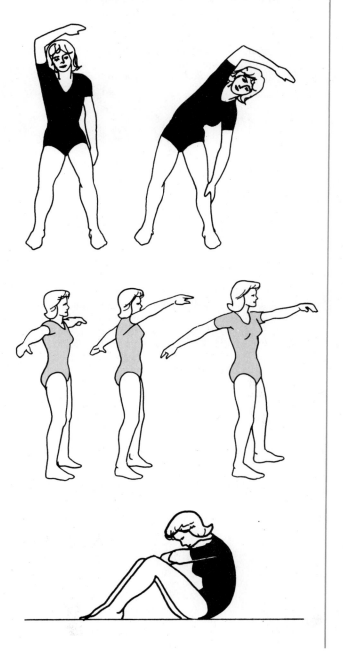

3. **Lateral Bending**
   Start. Stand erect, feet twelve inches apart, right arm extended over head, bent at elbow. Bend sidewards from waist to left. Slide left hand down leg as far as possible, and at the same time press to left with right arm. Return to starting position and change arm positions. Repeat to right. Continue by alternating to left, then right.
   Count. Bend to left plus bend to right counts as one repetition.

4. **Arm Circling****
   Start. Stand erect, feet twelve inches apart, arms at sides. Make large circles with arms in a windmill action—one arm following other and both moving at same time. Make backward circles only.
   Count. Each full circle by both arms counts as one repetition.

5. **Sit-ups****
   Start. Lie on back, knees bent and together, arms across chest. Roll shoulders and trunk forward to a sitting position. Return to starting position.
   Count. Each return to the starting position counts as one repetition.

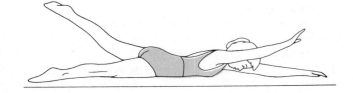

6. Arm and Leg-lift**

Start. Lie face down, legs straight and together; arms straight, together, and forward. First lift the left leg and the right arm. Return to starting position. Next lift the right leg and the left arm. Return to starting position. Keep the chin on the floor.

Count. Each return to the starting position counts as one repetition.

7. Side Leg Raising

Start. Lie on side with the legs straight along floor, top arm used for balance. Raise upper leg until it is perpendicular to floor. Lower to starting position.

Count. Each leg raise counts as one. Do half the number of repetitions raising the left leg. Roll to other side and do half with the right leg.

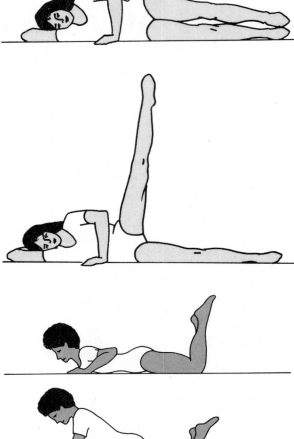

8. Modified Push-up

Start. Lie face down, hands directly under shoulders, knees on the floor. Raise body from floor by straightening it from head to knees. In the "up" position, the body should be in a straight line with palms of hands and knees in contact with floor. Lower to starting position. Keep head up throughout.

Count. Each return to the starting position counts as one repetition.

9. Leg-overs—Tuck

Start. Lie on back, legs straight and together, arms stretched sidewards at shoulder level, palms down. Raise both legs from floor, bending at hips and knees until in a tuck position. Lower legs to left, keeping knees together and both shoulders on floor. Twist hips and lower legs to floor on right side. Twist hips to tuck position and return to starting position. Keep knees close to abdomen throughout.

Count. Each return to the starting position counts as one repetition.

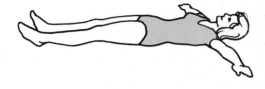
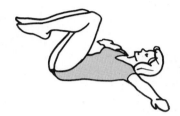
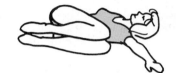

10. Run and Half Knee Bends

Start. Stand erect, feet together, arms at sides. Starting with left leg, run in place raising feet at least six inches from floor.

Count. Each time the left foot touches the floor counts as one repetition. After each fifty counts do ten half knee bends.

Half Knee Bends. Start with hands on hips, feet together, body erect. Bend at knees and hips, lowering body until thigh and calf form an angle of about 90 degrees. Do not bend knees past a right angle. Keep back straight. Return to starting position.

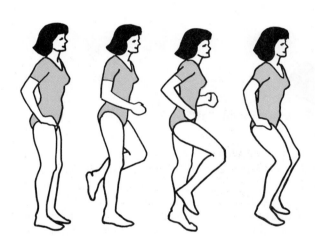

TABLE 15.3 Achieving Fitness through Anaerobic Exercise

Program Type	Cardiovascular Fitness	Strength and Muscular Endurance	Flexibility	Body and Fat Control	Skill-Related Fitness	Enjoyment or Fun[1]
Fartlek or "Speed Play"	***	**	—	***	—	*
Interval Training	***	**	—	***	—	*

***Very Good   **Good   *Minimum   —Low

[1]Enjoyment and fun are relative and for this reason it is impossible to classify activities accurately. However, for the average person some activities seem to be more enjoyable than others. The above listed classifications reflect the opinions of the typical person. *Any of the activities listed above can be fun and enjoyable for a given person in the right circumstances.*

THE FACTS ABOUT ANAEROBIC EXERCISE

Anaerobic exercise is excellent for building cardiovascular and other aspects of physical fitness.

The advantages and disadvantages of anaerobic exercise are outlined in Concept 6 (Table 6.1). Anaerobic exercise is especially useful for building cardiovascular fitness. The types of health-related fitness that can be developed into anaerobic exercise programs are rated in Table 15.3.

POPULAR ANAEROBIC EXERCISE PROGRAMS

Fartlek or "Speed Play"

Fartlek is one Swedish word for speed play. This exercise was developed in Scandinavia where pinewood paths follow curves of lakes, up and down many hills, where the scenery takes your mind off the task at hand. The idea is to get away from the regimen of running on a track and to enjoy the woods, lakes, and mountains. Because of the terrain, the pace is never constant. The uphill path requires slowing down, while a straight stretch or downhill trail allows for speed. In the "speed play," or fartlek system, you run easily for a time, a steady hard speed for a while, followed by rapid walking, then easy running broken with wind sprints, full speed uphill, and perhaps a fast pace for a while.

You can plan your own speed play program using your own course, which may include both uphill and downhill running with other variations. A sample program of moderate intensity is shown in Table 15.4.

TABLE 15.4 A Sample Speed Play Program*

1. Jog easily for 3 minutes.
2. Perform brisk calisthenics—no rest between exercises.
   a. Trunk stretch—With the feet spread, reach through the legs as far as possible. Hold for 8 seconds. Repeat 3 times.
   b. Do 5 to 10 bent-knee sit-ups. (See page 96.)
   c. Run in place for 50 steps.
   d. Do 5 to 10 push-ups or modified push-ups. (See page 95.)
   e. Do 10 side leg raises with each leg. (See page 97.)
3. Run 200 yards at 3/4 speed. Run on grassy area if possible.
4. Walk 200 yards.
5. Repeat 3 and 4.
6. Jog for 2 minutes.
7. Run 100 yards at 3/4 speed.
8. Walk 100 yards.
9. Repeat 7 and 8.
10. Jog for 2 minutes.

*If this *sample* program is too vigorous for your current level of fitness, try walking instead of jogging or running.

Interval Training Program

An interval training program involves repeated anaerobic running or swimming for short periods of time, separated by measured intervals of recovery jogging or stroking. (Developed by Gerschler of Germany, the stress of anaerobic running raises the heart rate to near maximal from which it drops to a moderate level during recovery.) This program controls distance, pace, number of reptitions, and recovery interval, allowing for a wide variety of programs of various intensities. Guidelines are presented in Concept 6 (Table 6.3).

Research suggests that short interval workouts should use maximum speed with rest intervals lasting from ten seconds to two minutes. These should be repeated eight to thirty times. Interval training having long intervals use 90 to 100 percent speed with rest intervals lasting from three to fifteen minutes. These should be repeated four to fifteen times. A sample short-interval program and a sample long interval running program are presented in Table 15.5. Using the guidelines in Concept 6, you can plan your own interval training program.

TABLE 15.5 Sample Interval Training Program (Moderate Intensity)

Short Intervals	Long Intervals
1. Do a flexibility and cardiovascular warm-up (see Concept 4).	1. Do a flexibility and cardiovascular warm-up (see Concept 4).
2. Run at 100% speed for 10 seconds (approximately 70 to 100 yards).	2. Run at 90% speed for one minute (approximately 300 to 500 yards).
3. Rest for 10 seconds by walking slowly.	3. Rest for 4 minutes by walking slowly.
4. Alternately repeat steps 2 and 3 until 20 runs have been completed.	4. Alternately repeat steps 2 and 3 until 5 runs have been completed.

REFERENCES

Anshel, M. H. *Aerobics for Fitness*. Minneapolis: Burgess, 1983.

*Cooper, K. H. *The Aerobics Program for Total Well-Being*. New York: M. Evans, 1982. (Contains information on aerobic dance and various sports.)

*Corbin, C. B., and R. Lindsey. *Fitness for Life*. 2d ed. Glenview, IL: Scott, Foresman, Inc., 1983.

Corbin, C. B., and R. Lindsey. *The Ultimate Fitness Book*. New York: Leisure Press, 1984.

Fitness Canada, *Canada Fitness Survey—Highlights*. Ottawa, Ontario, Canada: Government of Canada, 1983.

*Fox, E., D. Matthews, and J. Bairstow. *Interval Training for Lifetime Fitness*. New York: Dial Press, 1980.

Harris, L., and Associates. *The Perrier Study: Fitness in America*. New York: Great Waters of France, 1979.

Mahurin, J., and T. P. Martin. "Anaerobic Threshold: A Trainable Component of CV Fitness." *Motor Skills: Theory Into Practice* 6(1982):41.

Nash, J. B. *Philosophy of Recreation and Leisure*. Dubuque, IA: Wm. C. Brown Publishers, 1960.

O'Shea, J. P., C. Novak, and F. Gaulard. "Bicycle Interval Training for Cardiovascular Fitness." *Physician and Sportsmedicine* 10(1982):156.

President's Council on Physical Fitness and Sports. *Adult Physical Fitness*. Washington, D.C.: U.S. Government Printing Office, publication no. 017–000–00172–1. Copies available from Superintendent of Documents.

*President's Council on Physical Fitness and Sports. *Aquadynamics*. Washington, D.C.: U.S. Government Printing Office, publication no. 040–000–00360–6. Copies available from Superintendent of Documents.

Research and Forecasts, Inc. *The Miller Lite Report on American Attitudes toward Sports*. Milwaukee: Miller Brewing Co., 1983.

*Royal Canadian Air Force. *Exercise Plans for Physical Fitness*. Ottawa, Canada: Queen's Printer. Revised U.S. edition, published by Simon and Schuster, Inc., by special arrangement with *This Week Magazine*. Copies available from *This Week Magazine*, P.O. Box 77–E, Mt. Vernon, NY.

Snyder, E. E., and E. Spreitzer. "Adult Perceptions of Physical Education in the Schools and Community Sports Programs for Youth." *The Physical Educator* 40(1983):88.

16

EXERCISES FOR CARE OF THE BACK AND GOOD POSTURE

CONCEPT 16

Exercise plays an important role
in the prevention and correction of backaches
and poor posture.

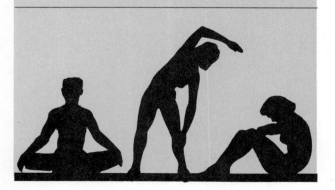

INTRODUCTION

The mechanics of back care and both static and dynamic postures are discussed in Concept 20. However, the vast majority of the population should do exercises similar to the samples included in this concept because backache and poor posture are so prevalent. Eighty percent of all Americans will see a physician about a backache during their lifetime. An estimated 75 million Americans have recurring back problems, and two million can't hold jobs as a result. Low back pain causes 93 million days of lost work per year and $10 billion in workers' compensation.

Incorrect postures, when standing, sitting, lying, or working, are responsible for many back problems. Compounding this are weak muscles that result from lack of exercise. Much can be done to prevent poor postures using proper education and proper exercise.

Treatment for painful spines ranges from surgical removal of a disc or fusion, to more conservative measures, such as injections, electrical stimulation, muscle relaxants, anti-inflammatory drugs, vapocoolant spray, bracing, traction, bed rest, heat, ice massage, and therapeutic exercise.

The exercises that follow are designed to strengthen or stretch certain muscles that are most often involved in back problems and most common in postural problems. (See Figure 16.1.) If you have had surgery or an injury, you should wait until your physician advises you to start exercising. If you have been inactive for a period of time, it would be wise to perform these exercises below your threshold level initially so as to avoid muscle soreness.

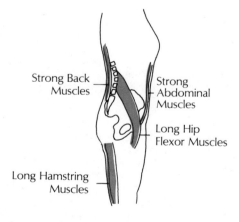

FIGURE 16.1 Muscles for Care of the Back and Good Posture

The exercises suggested here should be performed as described until the person is able to increase repetitions. Muscles depicted in color are those primarily involved in the exercise.

1. Bent Arm Lift

Purpose

To help prevent or correct round shoulders and kyphosis by strengthening adductors.

Position

Lie prone, arms in reverse T; forehead resting on floor.

Movement

Lift the arms vertically by contracting the muscles between the shoulder blades (adductors). Maintain the 90° angle at the elbow and the shoulder. Hold; relax and repeat. If the arms are pressed into the floor before being lifted, this is a PNF exercise, and range of motion may be greater.

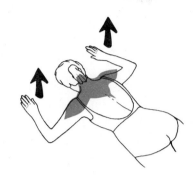

2. Straight Arm Lift

Purpose

To help prevent and correct round shoulders and kyphosis by strengthening adductors.

Position

Lie prone, arms extended overhead and held close to ears; forehead resting on floor.

Movement

Raise both arms as high as possible without lifting head. Hold; relax; repeat. Pressing downward on the floor before lifting may allow you to lift the arms higher.

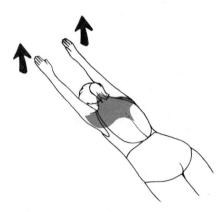

3. Wand Exercise

Purpose

To help prevent and correct round shoulders and kyphosis by stretching the muscles on the anterior side of the shoulder joint.

Position

Sit with wand grasped at ends. Raise wand overhead. Be certain that the head does not slide forward into a "poke neck" position. Keep the chin tucked and neck straight.

Movement

Bring wand down behind shoulder blades. Keep spine erect. Hold. Hands may be moved closer together to increase stretch on chest muscles.

Note

If this is an easy exercise for you, try straightening the elbows and bringing the wand to waist level in back of you.

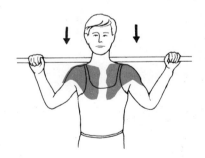

4. Lateral Trunk Exercise

Purpose

To help prevent and correct backaches by maintaining flexibility in the spine.

Position

Stand with feet shoulder width apart.

Movement

Stretch left arm overhead to right. Bend to right at waist reaching as far to right as possible with left arm and reach right arm as far as possible to the left; hold. Do not let trunk rotate. Repeat on opposite side.

Note

This exercise is made more effective if a weight is held in the hand opposite the side being stretched. More stretch occurs also if the hip on the stretched side is drooped and most of the weight borne by the opposite foot.

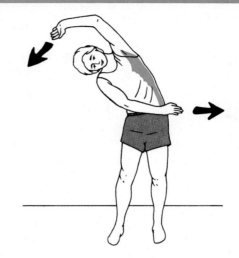

5. Lateral Neck Flexion

Purpose

To prevent or correct forward head cervical lordosis, as well as upper back and cervical trigger points.

Position

Sit erect.

Movement

Apply resistance to left side of head as you try to bend the head and neck sideward in that direction. This is an isometric strengthening exercise for the lateral flexors of the neck. Hold the contraction six seconds. Repeat to threshold, and then exercise the right side of the neck using the right hand as resistance. For neck exercises, it is probably best to use less than a maximal contraction. This is particularly true in the presence of arthritis, degenerated discs, and injury.

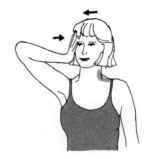

6. Neck Flexion Exercise

Purpose

To prevent or correct forward head or cervical lordosis, as well as upper back and cervical trigger points.

Position

Place hands on forehead.

Movement

Resist forward flexion. Keep the chin tucked to avoid the forward head position. This isometric exercise strengthens the neck and head flexors.

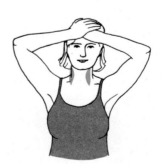

7. Neck Extension Exercise

Purpose

To prevent or correct forward head or cervical lordosis, as well as upper back and cervical trigger points.

Position

Place hands on back of head.

Movement

Apply resistance on back of head and isometrically push the head backward, keeping the neck straight. This strengthens the head and neck extensor muscles.

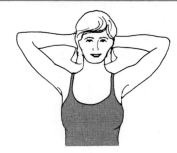

8. Neck Rotation Exercise

Purpose

This PNF exercise strengthens and stretches the neck rotators. It should always be done with the head and neck in axial extension (good alignment). It is particularly useful for relieving trigger point pain and stiffness.

Position

Place palm of left hand against left cheek; point fingers toward ear and point elbow forward.

Movement

Try to turn head and neck while resisting with left hand. Hold several seconds. Relax and turn head to right as far as possible; hold. Repeat.

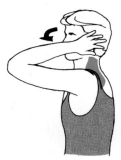
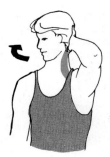

9. Bent Leg Stretcher

Purpose

To help prevent or correct backache caused in part by short hamstrings.

Position

Sit on the floor with the feet against the wall or an immovable object. Bend left knee and bring foot close to buttocks. Clasp hands behind back.

Movement

Bend forward from hips, keeping lower back as straight as possible. Let bent knee rotate outward so trunk can move forward. Use static or gentle ballistic-stretch to lengthen hamstring and calf muscles.

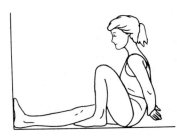
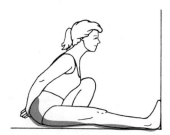

10. Iliopsoas Stretcher

Purpose

To help prevent or correct forward pelvic tilt and lumbar lordosis or backache.

Position

Place knee directly above right ankle and stretch left leg backward so knee touches floor. If necessary, place hands on floor for balance.

Movement

Press pelvis forward and downward; hold. Repeat on opposite side. Caution: Do not bend front knee more than 90°.

Note

This exercise uses the weight of the body to stretch the flexor muscles on the front of the hip joint, particularly the iliopsoas group.

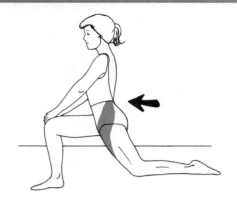

11. Low Back Stretcher

Purpose

To help prevent or correct lumbar lordosis and backache.

Position

Supine position.

Movement

Draw one knee up to the chest and pull it down tightly with the hands, then slowly return to the original position. Repeat with the other knee. Do not grasp knee; grasp thigh. If a partner or a weight stabilizes the extended leg, the iliopsoas on that leg will also be stretched.

Note

This same exercise may be done on a table with one leg hanging over the edge approximately one-third of the length of the thigh. If a partner, weight, or strap stabilizes the leg, the iliopsoas will be stretched more effectively.

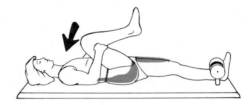

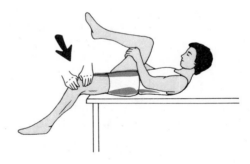

12. Knee-to-Chest Exercise

Purpose

To prevent or correct lordosis and backache; the fetal stretch.

Position

Bring both knees to chest and grasp thighs.

Movement

Pull knees to chest and curl both pelvis and upper body off of floor. Hold for 30–60 seconds. Stretches lumbar muscles and gluteals (hip extensors).

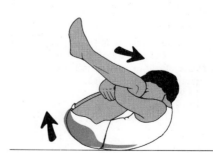

13. Straight Leg Back Flattener

Purpose

To help prevent or correct lordosis and backache.

Position

Supine with knees bent.

Movement

Draw one knee to the chest, then extend the knee and point the foot toward the ceiling; hold. Return to the starting position by drawing the knee back to the chest before sliding the foot to the floor. Repeat with other leg (stretches lumbar muscles).

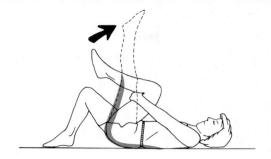

14. Leg-up Exercise

Purpose

To help prevent or correct lordosis and backache (advanced exercise).

Position

Supine with knees bent.

Movement

Draw both knees to the chest, then extend both legs toward the ceiling, keeping the lower back flat. Return to the starting position by drawing the knees to the chest before placing the feet on the floor (stretches lumbar muscles).
(Note: This is a more strenuous exercise and the weak person should not attempt it until the other exercises have been performed for three or four weeks.)

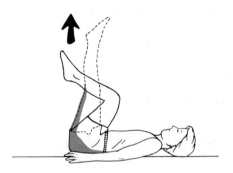

15. Pelvic Tilt

Purpose

Help prevent or correct lumbar lordosis, abdominal ptosis, and backache.

Position

Supine with knees bent.

Movement

Tighten the abdominal muscles and try to flatten the lower back against the floor. At the same time, tighten the hip and thigh muscles. Hold, then relax. Breathe normally during the contraction, do not hold the breath (strengthens abdominals).

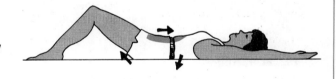

16. Trunk Curl

Purpose

To help prevent or correct lumbar lordosis, abdominal ptosis, or backache.

Position

Supine with the knees bent.

Movement

Roll the head and neck forward, then the shoulders. Roll as far forward as possible without lifting the lower back off the floor. Hold. Return to start and repeat (strengthens abdominals).

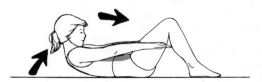

17. Sit-up

Purpose

To help prevent or correct lumbar lordosis, abdominal ptosis, or backache.

Position

Assume a hook-lying position with arms crossed and hands on shoulders.

Movement

Roll up, making elbows touch knees, then roll down to the starting position. Repeat. For more overload, place hands on top of head or place index fingers by ears (do not put hands behind neck and do not anchor feet).

Note

If you are weak, start in the sitting position and gradually curl down. Stop and hold and return to sit, gradually getting lower until full sit-up can be done.

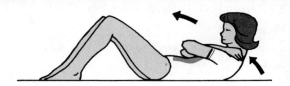

18. Gluteal Lift

Purpose

To help prevent and correct lordosis and forward pelvic tilt.

Position

Supine with knees bent and feet close to buttocks.

Movement

Contract gluteals, lifting buttocks off the floor as high as possible without raising the back off the floor above the waistline. Hold; relax; repeat. Strengthens hip extensor muscles, particularly the gluteus maximus. Do not allow the lower back to arch.

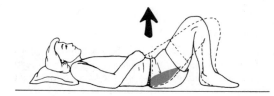

19. Wall Slide

Purpose

To help prevent or correct poor spinal alignment by teaching the feel of flattening the neck and back and tilting the pelvis.

Position

Stand with heels 4–6 inches from wall, arms at sides.

Movement

Flatten neck and lumbar region to wall by flexing knees and sliding down wall until spine can be forced against it. Slide up wall, maintaining flat spine. Walk away from wall, keeping curves flat. Return to wall and check alignment. Repeat with hands behind neck and elbows touching wall. Repeat with arms at sides and sandbag on head. Repeated flexion and extension of the knees can develop strength in the quadriceps muscles on the front of the thigh.

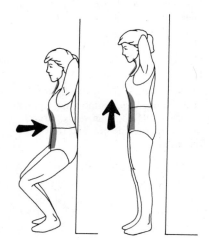

Testing for Back Weakness and Muscular Imbalance

Test 1—Back to wall
Stand with your back against a wall, with head, heels, shoulders, and calves of legs touching the wall as shown in the diagram. Try to flatten your neck and the hollow of your back by pressing your buttocks down against the wall. Your partner should just be able to place a hand in the space between the wall and the small of your back. If this space is greater than the thickness of his/her hand, you probably have lordosis with shortened lumbar and hip flexor muscles.

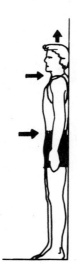

Test 2—Supine leg-lift
Lie on your back with hands behind your neck. The partner on your right should stabilize your right leg by placing his/her left hand on the knee. With the right hand, your partner should grasp your left ankle and raise your left leg as near to a right angle if possible. In this position (as shown in the diagram), your lower back should be in contact with the floor. Your right leg should remain straight and on the floor throughout the test. If your left leg bends at the knee, short hamstring muscles are indicated. If your back arches and/or your right leg does not remain flat on the floor, short lumbar muscles or hip flexor muscles (or both) are indicated. Repeat the test on the opposite side.

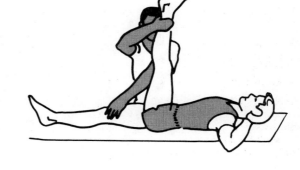

Test 3—Knee to chest
Lie on your back on a table or bench with your left leg extended beyond the edge of the table (approximately one-third of the thigh off the table). Bring your right knee to your chest and pull it down tightly with your hands. Your lower back should remain flat against the table as shown in the diagram. Your left thigh should remain on the table. If your left thigh lifts off the table while your right knee is hugged to chest, a tight hip flexor (iliopsoas) on that side is indicated. Repeat on the opposite side.

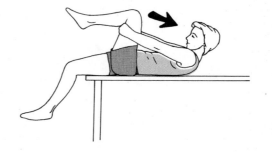

CHART 16A.1 Rating for Back ''Health''

Rating	Number of Tests Passed
Good	3
Fair	2
Poor	0–1

CHART 16B.1 Posture Evaluation

Side View	Points	Back View	Points
Head forward	_____	Tilted head	_____
Sunken chest	_____	Protruding scapulae	_____
Round shoulders	_____	Symptoms of scoliosis:	
		Shoulders uneven	_____
Kyphosis	_____	Hips uneven	_____
Lordosis	_____	Lateral curvature of spine (Adams position)	_____
Abdominal ptosis	_____	One side of back high (Adams position)	_____
Hyperextended knees	_____		
Body lean	_____		

Total score _____

CHART 16B.2 Posture Rating Scale

Classification	Total Score
Excellent	0–2
Very good	3–4
Fair	5–7
Poor	8–11
Very poor	12 or more

REFERENCES

Belkin, S. C., and H. H. Banks. *Backaches*. Tufts-New England Medical Center, Inc. Wellesly: Arandel Publishing Co., 1978.

*Kornfeld, J. "Getting Aggressive About Conservative Therapy for Back Pain." *Medical World News*. July 5, 1982.

Section Three
IMPORTANT FITNESS
FACTORS

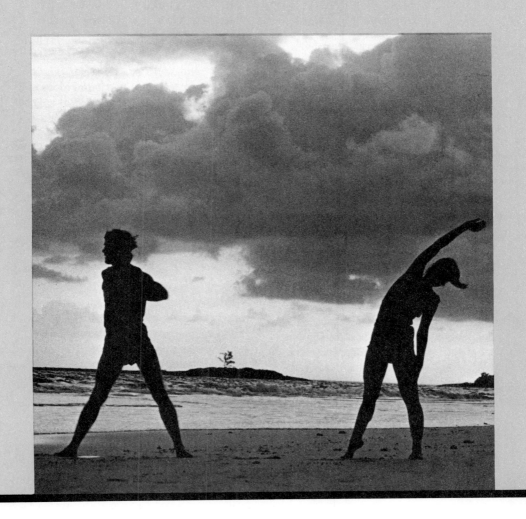

17
EXERCISE CAUTIONS

CONCEPT 17

Some exercises should be used with caution or
not used at all because they are
"high risk" exercises or because they may cause
more harm than good.

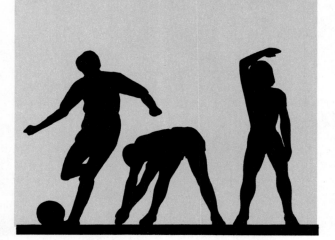

INTRODUCTION

There are literally thousands of exercises to choose
from—some good, some bad, and some of little con-
sequence. In some exercises, there are certain inherent
hazards that can and should be minimized with proper
technique, knowledgeable instructors, proper equipment, appropriate apparel, and careful adherance to the
principles mentioned in the first four concepts. As a
general rule, when in doubt, don't do it. There is always
a safe and effective alternative exercise for any specific
muscle group.

TERMS

Dehydration—Excessive loss of water from the body,
    usually through perspiration, urination, or evapo-
    ration.
Hyperventilation—"Overbreathing;" forced, rapid, or
    deep breathing.
Epiglottis—The lidlike structure that closes the en-
    trance to the windpipe.
Lumbar—Lower back region.
Pyriformis Syndrome—Muscle spasm and nerve en-
    trapment in the pyriformis muscle of the buttocks
    region causing pain similar to sciatica.
Sciatica—Pain along the sciatic nerve down the but-
    tocks and back of the leg.
Valsalva Maneuver—Exerting force with the epi-
    glottis closed, thus increasing pressure in the thorax
    and raising arterial pressure. When released, arte-
    rial pressure drops rapidly, blood vessels expand and
    are then filled, causing a lag in blood flow to the left
    ventricle. Peripheral arterial blood pressure then
    drops and dizziness or fainting occurs.

THE FACTS

*As a general rule, exercises that stretch the pos-
terior upper back and neck should be avoided.*
(See pages 138–39.)

It has been estimated that 80 percent of the population
has forward head and kyphosis (hump back). Exercises
that tend to promote or aggravate these conditions by
further stretching already elongated muscles and ligaments should be avoided. Examples of such exercises
include:

1. Shoulder stands, such as:
   a. the plough
   b. the plough shear
   c. vertical "bicycling"
2. Sit-up with the hands behind the neck (note: hands
   may be placed on top of head or fingers may be
   placed beside ears to avoid pull on neck).

As a general rule, exercises that cause hyperextension in the lower back should be avoided. (See pages 138–39.)

There are better ways of strengthening the back than by arching (hyperextending) it. Hyperextension stretches the abdominals, which are usually too elongated to begin with, and may also cause backache, myofascial trigger points, and even herniated discs. Examples of contraindicated exercises include:

1. Back bends
2. Straight-leg lifting
3. Straight-leg sit-ups
4. Prone or all-fours leg-lifts
5. Prone swan (back arch)
6. Backward trunk circling

Exercises that cause hyperextension of the neck should be avoided. (See pages 138–39.)

Tipping the head backward during any exercise, such as is done in neck circling, can pinch arteries and nerves at the base of the skull and result in dizziness or myofascial trigger points. It also aggravates arthritis and degenerated discs. Therefore, backward tilting of the head is not recommended for many people.

Exercises that cause muscle imbalance should be avoided.

Frequently, one set of muscles is overdeveloped while opposing muscles are neglected. This causes misalignment of the body. A common example is the overuse of exercises to strengthen the pectorals (chest muscles) while neglecting the rhomboid and trapezius muscles between the shoulder blades. This results in round shoulders.

Some common stretching exercises are classified as high risk because of their potential for causing injury.

Examples of high risk exercises include:

1. Hurdler's stretch—May cause strain in the groin and laxity of the medial ligament of the bent knee. Also puts great stress on the cartilage of the bent knee.
2. Standing toe touches, especially ballistic toe touches—May overstretch the muscles and ligaments of the lumbar region and the knee, as well as the joint capsule and cartilage of the knee. These are especially hazardous for a person with back problems.
3. Ballet stretches "at the bar" when the extended leg is raised ninety degrees or more and the trunk is bent over the leg—Some experts believe this can lead to sciatica and pyriformis syndrome, especially in the person who has limited flexibility.
4. Shin stretches and quadriceps stretches where the knee is hyperflexed 120 degrees or more—As frequently performed when these muscles are stretched, the knee joint is apt to be flexed too far and perhaps even rotated as the participant either grasps the foot and pulls it backward or sits on the foot. This may damage the knee by tearing the cartilage or by stretching the ligaments.

Stressing the knee joint when it is flexed more than ninety degrees may damage its structure. (See pages 138–39.)

Deep-squatting exercises may harm the knee joint by stretching the ligaments and irritating the synovial membrane (also see preceding fact).

Repeatedly rising on the toes and heels may weaken the long arch.

Tiptoeing exercises will develop the calf muscles, but at the same time, they will stretch the muscles and ligaments that help support the long arch of the foot. "Heel walking" may have the same effect—that is, it may develop strong muscles while further weakening the arch. The potential harm is lessened if these exercises are performed with the toes turned in slightly.

Isometric exercises may be harmful to some people.

Isometric exercise has its advantages (see Concept 7), but studies have shown it may be more dangerous to heart patients than isotonic exercise, since it may cause irregular heartbeats and a marked rise in blood pressure. Isometric exercise (along with weight training) for preadolescents is also questionable because their growth centers (epiphyses) in the bones have not closed.

There are many safe and effective exercises that should be substituted for unsafe or high risk exercises.

Some examples of "good" exercises that can be substituted for the "bad" (questionable) exercises are listed in Table 17.1 on page 140. There are also dozens of other good alternatives that are not listed in this table. A physical educator, physical therapist, or corrective therapist could advise you on some of these alternatives.

Some exercise equipment is potentially harmful.

Most exercise equipment is safe when used properly, but there is still the potential for abuse. One piece in particular is very difficult to use safely—the "slimming wheel." This wheel, with a handle passing through its axis, is used in a push-up type exercise and is advertised as a back and abdomen strengthener. Unfortunately, the wheel is difficult to control and may roll too rapidly, causing the users to fall flat on their faces. When this occurs, the abdominals may be overstretched and hemorrhaging of that muscle may develop.

BAD EXERCISES

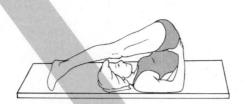

1. **Plough**

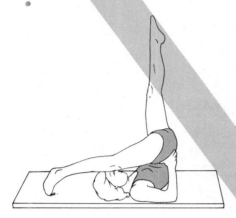

2. **Plough Shear**

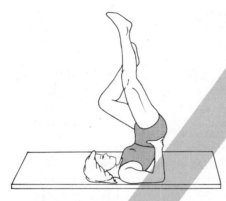

3. **Shoulder Stand Bicycle**

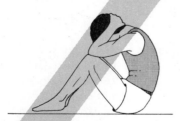

4. **Hands-Behind-the-Head Sit-up**

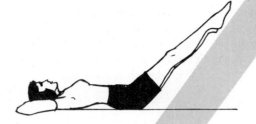

5. **Double Leg-lift**

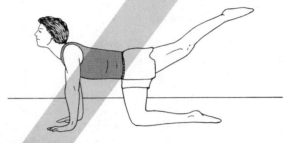

6. **Back Arching/Neck Arching**

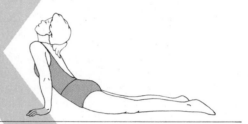

7. **Back Arching/Abdominal Stretch**

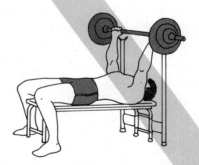

8. **Back Arching**

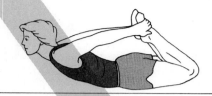

9. Back Arching/Abdominal Stretch

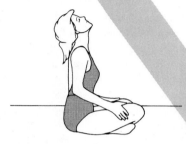

10. Neck Hyperextension

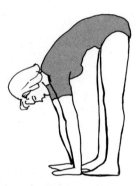

11. Standing Toe Touch

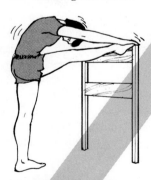

12. Ballistic Ballet Bar Stretch

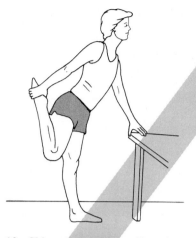

13. Shin and Quadriceps Stretch

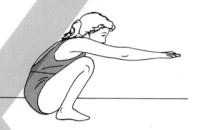

14. Deep Knee Bends

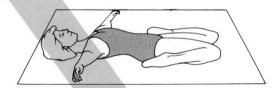

15. The Hero

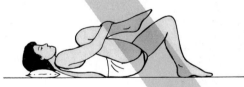

16. Knee Pull-down

TABLE 17.1 Good Alternatives To Bad Exercises

Bad Exercises	Good Alternative Exercises
A. Concept 17, nos. 1, 2, 3 plough, plough shear, and shoulder stand bicycle	Concept 13, no. 8 — kneeling leg extension Concept 16, no. 19 — axial extension of neck Concept 14, no. 3 — hamstring stretch
B. Concept 17, no. 4 — hands-behind-the-head sit-up	Concept 13, no. 7 — sit-up, hands by ears or on head
C. Concept 17, no. 5 — double leg-lift	Concept 13, no. 13 — sitting tucks Concept 13, no. 6 — reverse sit-up Concept 13, no. 17 — modified leg-lift Concept 15, no. 14 — double leg extension
D. Concept 17, nos. 6, 7, 8, 9 — back arching	Concept 13, no. 9 — upper back lift Concept 13, no. 16 — lower trunk lift Concept 13, no. 17 — upper trunk lift Concept 13, no. 31 — bench press with knees bent and feet on bench Concept 13, no. 15 — knee-to-nose touch with horizontal extension
E. Concept 17, no. 10 — neck hyperextension	Concept 14, no. 9 — PNF neck rotation Concept 16, nos. 5, 6, 7 — neck lateral flexion, neck extension, neck flexion Concept 19, no. 1 — neck stretch
F. Concept 17, nos. 11, 12 — standing toe touch, ballistic ballet bar stretch	Concept 14, no. 13 — hamstring stretch Concept 16, no. 9 — bent leg stretcher
G. Concept 17, nos. 13 and 15 — shin and quadriceps stretch	Concept 14, no. 11 — shin stretcher
H. Concept 17, no. 14 — deep knee bend	Concept 13, no. 12 — kneeling Concept 13, no. 14 — stationary leg change
I. Concept 17, no. 16 — knee pull-down	Concept 16, no. 11 — low back stretcher Concept 16, no. 12 — fetal stretch

Jogging is an excellent exercise for cardiovascular conditioning, weight control, and improvement of a variety of conditions; however, reasonable caution should be observed.

Jogging has been used successfully in rehabilitating cardiac patients and those with pulmonary emphysema; in assisting reducing diabetics; in relaxing insomniacs, the emotionally disturbed, and migraine patients; and in reducing the discomfort accompanying arthritis in the legs and back. Like many other exercises, jogging should not be done without a physician's approval for those with arthritis, osteoporosis, and heart and circulatory diseases. It is *not* harmful to women, although some women may need to wear a special bra as a comfort measure. Jogging can cause shin splints, blisters, and foot, ankle, knee, and hip problems. Using the proper footwear and learning how to jog correctly will minimize these hazards. If you have poor leg or foot alignment, you would be wise to jog only three to six days per week since studies show that the risk of injury is greatest for those who jog everyday. The same fitness levels will result with less risk of injury.

Dehydration, a hazard in certain sports and exercise situations, is a serious medical problem.

Dehydration can impair performance and lead to illness, heat stroke, and even death. Weight losing gimmicks that cause dehydration, such as high protein/low carbohydrate diets, steam baths, or plastic sweat suits, are dangerous, especially for athletes (e.g., wrestlers trying to "make weight"). Exercisers subjected to heat stress should weigh themselves before and after exercises and replace the water-weight loss. Water should not be restricted during exercise. The person who regularly exercises under heat stress conditions may benefit from drinking a quart of milk and two eight-ounce glasses of orange juice per day. It is *not* necessary to take salt tablets because most people already consume three or four hundred times the daily salt requirement. Sweating releases more water than it does salt from the body, thus increasing, rather than decreasing, the body's salt concentration.

You are more susceptible to heat stroke if you are obese, older, have had previous heat strokes, or are dehydrated, poorly conditioned, or not adjusted to a warmer climate.

When exercising out-of-doors in cold weather, certain precautions should be taken.

During cold-weather exercising, stay warm, but don't wear bulky clothes that interfere with movement. Wear a thin absorbent layer next to the skin and two removable layers on top of that, such as a sweat suit and windbreaker. This outfit enables you to peel off layers as you become warm from the exercise. Do wear a cap and mittens (they are warmer than gloves) and wool socks. Change clothes immediately after coming indoors.

Breathing cold air will not freeze the lungs, but it does slow the heart. Those with heart disease should be wary of exercising in extreme cold.

Some people can be allergic to exercise.

It is rare, but there is a shocklike syndrome associated with vigorous exercise known as "exercise-induced anaphylaxis." This syndrome can occur in anyone, whether a beginner or a well-conditioned athlete. The syndrome's symptoms include itching, swelling of the throat, and generalized swelling. Treatment is the same as for allergic reactions to insect bites—an injection of epinephrine. Since an occurrence of this syndrome is rare, an emergency kit is probably not necessary equipment, but it is a good idea to always exercise with a partner. If you experience the symptoms, seek emergency care immediately.

There are times when you should not exercise, but pregnancy is not one of them.

Regular exercise is important, but you should not exercise when your body temperature is above 100°F. Certain diseases or injuries are also aggravated by exercise. Extreme temperatures and humidity should discourage most people, and smog alerts certainly should be heeded.

Pregnant women, contrary to some beliefs, can exercise and even jog safely, but they should first consult their physician, as should anyone with disease or injury or who is regularly taking medication.

Exercise can alter the effect of drugs on the body, as well as the effect of certain disorders.

The effect of drugs used to treat thyroid disease may be altered by exercise. Likewise, patients taking certain medicine for asthma and collagen diseases may not be able to normally perform exercises that require moderate or heavy exertion. Exercise alters the effect of nonsteroidal analgesics and anti-inflammatory drugs (like aspirin). During exercise, these drugs can cause increased oxygen consumption and increased carbon dioxide production, as well as promote sweating and dehydration. Muscle relaxants may cause depression and hinder coordination.

There is some evidence that anabolic androgenic steroids enhance performance when taken in massive doses. There is, however, clear-cut evidence that these steroids have serious side effects, including hepatitis, carcinoma, and myeloid leukemia. It is best to consult your physician about any drugs you are taking before beginning an exercise program.

Too much exercise can result in "overtraining."

Overworking—doing too much, too soon—so that there is not enough time for recovery between workouts will lead to weight loss, depression, insomnia, increased resting heart rate, decreased work capacity, poorer performance, and loss of enjoyment and of motivation. When these symptoms occur, cut back on the intensity, frequency, or duration of your training.

The valsalva maneuver should be avoided when exerting great force in weight lifting, calisthenics, or isometrics.

Dizziness, blackouts, and inguinal hernias may result from the valsalva maneuver. This can be prevented in weight lifting by avoiding hyperventilation, squatting as briefly as possible, and as rapidly as possible raising the weight to a position where it can be supported while breathing normally. In all activities, breathe normally! Do *not* hold your breath during exercise.

Commercial establishments, such as health clubs, reducing salons, and aerobic dance centers, may not employ personnel qualified to prescribe exercise programs.

Studies indicate that many commercial enterprises do not employ properly trained instructors. Those who are qualified to advise you about exercise have college degrees and four to eight years of study in such courses as anatomy, physiology, kinesiology, preventive and therapeutic exercise, and physiology of exercise. These qualified individuals are physical educators, corrective therapists, and physical therapists. On-the-job training, a good physique or figure, and good dancing ability are not sufficient qualifications for teaching or advising about exercise.

REFERENCES

American College of Sports Medicine. "Position Stand on the Use of Anabolic-Androgenic Steroids in Sports." *Sports Medicine Bulletin* (1984):1.

American College of Sports Medicine. "Weight Loss in Wrestlers: Position Stand of American College of Sports Medicine." In *P. E. Conditioning and Physical Fitness,* edited by P. E. Allsen. Dubuque, IA.: Wm. C. Brown Publishers, 1978.

Anderson, S. D. "Drugs Affecting the Respiratory System with Particular Reference to Asthma." *Medicine and Science in Sports and Exercise* 13(1981):259.

Basmajian, J. V. *Therapeutic Exercise.* 3d ed. Baltimore: Williams and Wilkins, 1984.

Beaulieu, J. E. "Developing a Stretching Program." *Physician and Sportsmedicine* 9(1981):59.

Blackburn, S. E., and I. G. Portney. "Electromyographic Activity of Back Musculature during Williams' Flexion Exercises." *Physical Therapy* 61(1981):878.

Day, R. O. "Effects of Exercise Performance on Drugs in Musculoskeletal Disorders." *Medicine and Science in Sports and Exercise* 13(1981):272.

*Dominguez, R. H., and R. S. Gajda. *Total Body Conditioning.* New York: Charles Scribners Sons, 1982.

Hage, P. "Exercise and Pregnancy Compatible, M. D. Says." *Physician and Sportsmedicine* 9(1981):23.

Johnson, G. T. "House Call." *Register.* Santa Ana, CA: April, 1980.

Kaufman, W. C. "Cold Weather Clothing for Comfort or Heat Conversion." *Physician and Sportsmedicine* 10(1982):71.

Kavanaugh, T. "Postcoronary Joggers Need Precise Guidelines." *Physician and Sportsmedicine* 4(1976):63.

*Kelly, D. L. "Exercise Prescription and the Kinesiological Imperative." *Journal of Health, Physical Education, Recreation and Dance* 53(1982):18.

Kendall, F. P., and E. K. McCreary. *Muscles: Testing and Function.* 3d ed. Baltimore: Williams and Wilkins, 1983.

Kuntzleman, C. "Winter Fitness Guide." *Family Weekly* (January 23, 1983):15.

*Lindsey, R., B. Jones, and A. V. Whitley. *Fitness for Health, Figure/Physique, Posture.* 5th ed. Dubuque, IA: Wm. C. Brown Publishers, 1983.

Maitland, G. D. *Vertebral Manipulation.* Boston: Butterworth, 1977.

McGlynn, G. H. "A Reevaluation of Isometric Strength Training." *Journal of Sports Medicine and Physical Fitness* 12(1972):258.

Mirkin, G. quoted in *Sports Medicine Technology* 1(1983):2. "Overtraining of Athletes: A Round Table." *Physician and Sportsmedicine* 11(1983):93.

Powles, A. C. P. "The Effect of Drugs on the Cardiovascular Response to Exercise." *Medicine and Science in Sports and Exercise* 13(1981):252.

Rasch, P. J. *Weight Training.* 4th ed. Dubuque, IA: Wm. C. Brown Publishers, 1982.

Ricci, B., M. Marchetti, and F. Figura. "Biomechanics of Sit-Up Exercises." *Medicine and Science in Sports and Exercise* 13(1981):54.

Shefer, A. quoted in "Exercise Can Provoke Allergic Reaction." *Atlanta Journal* (February 1980).

Smith, M. "What Arnold Schwarzenegger Hath Wrought." *Los Angeles Magazine* (January 1980):162.

Stevenson, E. "Double Leg Raising." *CAHPERD Journal Times* 44(1982):18.

Stevenson, E. "The Mad Cat." *CAHPERD Journal Times* 44(1982):23.

Stevenson, E. "The Sit-Up." *CAHPERD Journal Times* 44(1982):17.

Stevenson, E. "Specificity of Exercise." *CAHPERD Journal Times* 45(1982):6.

Stevenson, E. "Head Circling." *CAHPERD Journal Times* 45(1983):6.

Stevenson, E. "The Shoulder Stand." *CAHPERD Journal Times* 45(1983):19.

Sutton, J. R. "Drugs Used in Metabolic Disorders." *Medicine and Science in Sports and Exercise* 13(1981):266.

Sutton, J. R. "The Effects of Drugs on Exercise Performance." *Medicine and Science in Sports and Exercise* 13(1981):246.

Sweeney, G. D. "Drugs—Some Basic Concepts." *Medicine in Sports and Exercise* 13(1981):247.

Weltman, A., and G. Stamford. "Exercising Safely in The Winter." *Physician and Sportsmedicine* 10(1982):130.

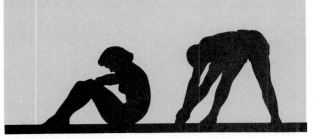

18
EXERCISE AND NUTRITION

CONCEPT 18

The basic nutritional needs
of exercisers or athletes compared to those
of sedentary people
do not differ except for caloric requirements.
Although there are special considerations
for athletes/exercisers,
many of their dietary practices are faddish,
unsound, and even dangerous.

INTRODUCTION

In spite of the fact that nutrition is an advanced science, many myths and misconceptions prevail. These are propagated by commercial interests. Product sales are advanced by the public's, and even physicians' and educators', superstition and ignorance of the true facts. Superstition seems to thrive particularly among athletes and coaches. Such misconceptions can lead to imbalanced diets, high cost, and disappointment over the influence on performance.

Some current theories and practices are discussed in this concept, and an attempt is made to dispel some myths about the diets of athletes and others who engage in regular physical activity.

Because nutrition affects us all, it is important that we are knowledgeable about the subject. It is far too complicated to cover even the fundamentals in these pages; therefore, the reader is encouraged to enroll in a nutrition course taught by a registered dietician, or to study reliable books on the subject, such as those listed in the references at the end of this chapter.

TERMS

Cellulose—Indigestible fiber (bulk) in foods.
Dehydration—Excessive loss of body fluids (e.g., through perspiration, diarrhea, or urination).
Kilogram—A metric unit of weight equaling 2.2046 pounds.
"Making Weight"—Quick loss or gain in weight so an athlete (usually a wrestler) can compete in a given weight category.

THE FACTS

The amount and kind of food you eat affects your size, strength, and fitness.

There are about forty to forty-five nutrients in food that are essential for the body's growth, maintenance, and repair. These are classified into carbohydrates, fats, proteins, vitamins, minerals, and water. The first three of these provide energy, which is measured in calories.

The Food and Nutrition Board of the National Academy of Sciences—National Research Council has established a "recommended daily allowances" (RDA) for each nutrient. To help assure that you select foods containing the essential elements, they have classified foods into groups, each of which should be included in the daily diet. The quantity of nutrients recommended varies with age and other considerations; for example, a young, growing child needs more calcium than an adult, and a pregnant woman needs more calcium than other women.

TABLE 18.1 Recommended Food Selections for Good Health

Food Group	Amount for Adults	Special Role in Diet
1. Milk, cheese, ice cream, and other dairy products	• 2 or more servings	• Protein, calcium and other minerals, vitamins
2. Meat, poultry, fish, eggs (alternates: nuts, dried beans, peas)	• 2 or more servings	• Protein, iron and other minerals, B vitamins

3. All vegetables and fruits, including potatoes
 	
   a. Green and yellow vegetables
   b. Citrus fruits, tomatoes, raw cabbage, etc.
	• 4 or more servings	• Minerals, vitamins, fiber, iron, vitamin A, folacin, vitamin C

4. Grain products — bread, flour, cereals, baked goods (perferably whole-grain or enriched)	• 4 or more servings	• Inexpensive source of energy, iron, vitamin B

The specified number of servings from each of the food groups on a daily basis will provide a well-balanced diet for most people, including exercisers/athletes.

See Table 18.1, "Recommended Food Selections for Good Health," for information on the four food groups and the recommended number of daily servings.

The number of calories needed per day depends on such factors as age, sex, size, muscle mass, glandular function, emotional state, climate, and exercise.

A moderately active college-age woman needs about 2,000 calories per day, while a moderately active man of the same age needs about 2,800 calories. A female athlete in training might burn 2,600 to 3,500; a male athlete in training may expend 3,500 to 6,000 calories. If weight remains at the optimum, the caloric content of the diet is correct. If weight varies from optimal, the caloric content of the diet may need to be altered.

Athletes and active people do not need relatively more protein than nonathletes or inactive people.

Protein needs vary with age, size, and other factors such as pregnancy, but the well-balanced diet includes about sixty grams of protein per day. This is well over the minimum needed and is adequate for most people. The recommended protein intake is about one gram per kilogram of body weight, or 10 to 15 percent of the total calories per day.

Athletes or active people frequently consume more calories than nonathletes or inactive people, and for this reason, consume more protein (assuming that they eat a balanced diet). Because protein is not an important source of energy, and because high quality protein is provided by all meats, milk, eggs, and cheese, there is no need to supplement the athlete's or active person's diet with protein. Consequently, there is no reason for athletes to gorge themselves on beefsteak or to take supplemental proteins, such as "protein energizers" or "protein powerizers," if they eat a balanced diet.

Fat should be eaten only in moderate to low amounts.

Humans need some fat in their diet because fats are carriers of vitamins E, K, D, and A; are a source of essential linoleic acid; make food taste better; and provide a concentrated form of calories.

Fat has twice the calories per gram as carbohydrates, but does not provide twice the energy. High fat diets provide no special benefits for the athlete. Most popular weight loss diets are high in protein; unfortunately, that usually means lots of meat and, therefore, lots of fat. Most Americans consume about 40 percent of their calories in fats, but this amount should probably be reduced to about 25 percent to cut down on obesity and high blood fat levels. High fat also means high cholesterol, a coronary heart disease risk factor. (Cholesterol intake should be less than 300 milligrams per day.) It is recommended that one-half to two-thirds of the fat in the diet be saturated or polysaturated. As discussed in Concept 6, aerobic exercise is believed to reduce the levels of these blood lipids.

Breakfast is an important meal.

Numerous studies have shown that skipping breakfast impedes performance because blood sugar drops in the long period between dinner the night before and lunch the following day. About one-fourth of the day's calories should be consumed at breakfast.

For the athlete or active person, food should be taken at four-to-six-hour intervals throughout the day for good performance. Skipping meals or snacking during the day and eating one big meal in the evening may adversely affect performance.

There is no scientific basis for eliminating milk from the athlete's diet.

Milk does *not* cause "cotton mouth." A dry mouth is due to decreased saliva flow caused by dehydration or an emotional state. Milk does *not* decrease speed, "cut wind," produce sour stomach, or interfere with performance unless the individual has a milk intolerance.

"Quick energy" foods eaten just before events of short duration do not enhance performance.

Ingesting honey, glucose, or other sweets just prior to short-term performance does not provide the athlete with a burst of energy. The body will use its own energy reserves. The carbohydrates eaten will help replace the energy used in the performance.

No carbohydrates should be eaten one and one-half to two hours before an endurance event since this may produce a physiological effect leading to premature exhaustion of the glycogen stores.

"Carbohydrate loading" may improve performance in long endurance events, but is not without hazard.

The normal recommended daily allowance of carbohydrate is 55 to 60 percent of the total caloric intake. Carbohydrates provide most of the energy used in heavy exercise and endurance events exceeding thirty to sixty minutes, such as in marathon runs. Several studies have supported a procedure called "carbohydrate loading." For example, before an endurance event, days one through three, limit carbohydrate intake and deplete the body of glycogen by engaging in severe exercise. On days four through six, load the body with carbohydrates. Increase your carbohydrate intake to 80 percent of your total caloric intake and taper off exercise or rest. On day seven, eat a light meal three to four hours before the event—then perform the event. This regime will not make a person run faster, but he or she may be able to run longer at a given speed.

Most experts recommend that the glycogen depletion stage (days one through three) be omitted and replaced by a high carbohydrate diet and rest for one to two days before the event. Depletion can cause hypoglycemia and elevate cholesterol and blood lipids. We do not know the effect of repeated depletion and loading, but done for only a week, there are probably no harmful effects. Carbohydrate loading is most suitable for those in events that exceed one hour and involve high energy expenditure, such as running, swimming, cycling, cross-country skiing, and tournament play in soccer, tennis, or handball. Carbohydrate loading may be harmful to those with diabetes, hypertriglyceridemia, muscle enzyme deficiencies, or kidney disorders.

The timing may be more important than the makeup of the preevent meal.

It is probably best to eat about three hours before competition or heavy exercise to allow time for digestion. Generally, the athlete can make his or her food selection on the basis of past experience. Tension, anxiety, and excitement are more apt to cause gastric distress than is food selection. It is generally accepted that fat intake should be minimal because it digests more slowly;

"gas formers" should probably be avoided; and proteins and high cellulose foods should be kept to a moderate amount prior to prolonged events to avoid urinary and bowel excretion. Two or three cups of liquid should be taken to ensure adequate hydration.

As previously mentioned, carbohydrates should not be ingested within an hour or two of an event because they may cause an insulin response that results in weakness and fatigue. Sometimes they cause stomach distress, cramps, or nausea.

It should be noted that the excitement associated with competition is probably the main reason for having a special diet before participation. Since many people who exercise regularly usually are not competing, there is little reason to alter normal diet before regular exercise. Likewise, there is no need to delay exercise for long periods after the meal if exercise is moderate and noncompetitive.

"Health foods," tonics, and supplements will not contribute to health, fitness, weight control, or athletic performance (also see Concept 17 regarding drugs).

The Food and Drug Administration labels the health food racket as the most widespread quackery in the United States. Whether athletic or sedentary, the individual on a well-balanced diet does *not* benefit from special organic foods, phosphate, alkaline salts, additional vitamins, choline, lecithin, wheat germ, honey, gelatin, aspartates, brewer's yeast, gelatin, royal jelly, or any other supplement, unless specifically prescribed for a medical purpose by a physician.

Vitamins are not drugs and do not contain energy. Most people who take supplemental vitamins do not need them. There is no chemical difference between natural and synthetic vitamins, but the vitamins in food contain other associated nutrients, especially minerals. Megadoses of vitamins may even be harmful. Athletes most often abuse B complex, C, and E, as well as minerals. If you have a balanced diet, none of these will increase performance. (B_{15} [pangamic acid] is **not** a vitamin; it is a fraud and may be harmful.)

Fad diets are not a satisfactory means to long-term weight reduction and may adversely affect the health.

There are hundreds of fad diets and diet books, but nutritionists warn that there is no scientific basis for drastic juggling of food constituents. Such diets are usually unbalanced and may result in serious illness or even death, especially for the obese person who is already apt to be suffering from a number of health disorders. Fad diets cannot be maintained for long periods of time; therefore, the individual usually regains any lost weight. Constant losing and gaining may be more harmful than the original obese condition.

Crash diets that bring about weight loss by dehydration of only 5 percent in forty-eight hours have been shown to reduce the individual's working capacity by as much as 40 percent. The practice of "making weight" in athletics, whether by dehydration, induced vomiting, or starvation diets, is dangerous to health and should be condemned (see Concept 10 on weight control and Concept 17 on dehydration).

Caffeine use during or prior to exercise needs more research.

Some research has shown that caffeine has a beneficial effect on the rate of lipid metabolism, leading to the theory that it may enhance work output in some endurance events. Much more research is needed, however. On the other hand, caffeine may cause insomnia, restlessness, ringing in the ears, abnormal heart beat, and diuresis in some people. Most experts recommend that caffeine be omitted from the pregame meal or during activity.

Exercise goes hand in hand with nutrition in health maintenance.

"Eat right and get plenty of exercise" is a common prescription. The benefits of exercise specifically include the following: it can reduce blood lipids, burn excess calories to reduce weight (see Table 10.2), help prevent or improve cardiac heart disease, increase high-density lipoproteins that may protect against heart disease, train the heart muscle, reduce high blood pressure, have an insulin effect for the diabetic, reduce blood glucose, and reduce psychic stress and tension.

REFERENCES

American Alliance of Health, Physical Education, Recreation and Dance. *Nutrition for Athletes.* Washington, D.C., 1980.

Barrett, Stephen. *The Health Robbers.* Philadelphia: George F. Stickley Co., 1980.

"Common Sense Approach to Athletic Training." *Sports Medicine Digest* 5 (1983).

Darden, Ellington. *Nutrition and Athletic Performance.* Pasadena, CA: Athletic Press, 1976.

Haskell, W., J. Scala, and J. Whittam. *Nutrition and Athletic Performance.* Palo Alto, CA: Bull Publishing Co., 1982.

Herbert, Victor, and Stephen Barrett. *Vitamins and Health Food Robbers: The Great American Hustle.* Philadelphia: George F. Stickley Co., 1981.

Lindsey, R., B. J. Jones, and A. V. Whitley. *Fitness.* Dubuque, IA: Wm. C. Brown Publishers, 1983.

Moore, M. "Carbohydrate Loading: Eating Through the Wall." *Physician and Sportsmedicine* 9 (1981):97.

Nutrition References and Book Reviews. Rev. ed. Chicago: Chicago Nutrition Assoc., 1981. $8.00.

"Nutrition Update." *Sports Medicine Digest* 5 (1983).

Serfas, R. C. "Nutrition for the Athlete Update," *Contemporary Nutrition,* 7 (1982):1.

Sherman, G., et al. "Effects of Exercise Diet Manipulation on Muscle Glycogen and Its Subsequent Utilization during Performance." *International Journal of Sports Medicine* 2 (1981):114.

Sports Medicine Technology 1 (1983):2.

*Williams, M. H. *Nutrition for Fitness and Sport.* Dubuque, IA: Wm. C. Brown Publishers, 1983.

*Wink, Dorothy. *Nutrition.* 2d ed. Reston, VA: Reston Publishing Co., 1983.

CHART 18A.1 Diet Record

Day _____			
Breakfast Food	**Amount**	**Calories**	**Nutrition**
			Dairy group ☐ ☐ Meat/Fish/Eggs ☐ ☐ Vegetables/Fruits ☐ ☐ ☐ ☐ Breads/Cereals ☐ ☐ ☐ ☐
Lunch Food	**Amount**	**Calories**	**Nutrition**
			Dairy group ☐ ☐ Meat/Fish/Eggs ☐ ☐ Vegetables/Fruits ☐ ☐ ☐ ☐ Breads/Cereals ☐ ☐ ☐ ☐
Dinner Food	**Amount**	**Calories**	**Nutrition**
			Dairy group ☐ ☐ Meat/Fish/Eggs ☐ ☐ Vegetables/Fruits ☐ ☐ ☐ ☐ Breads/Cereals ☐ ☐ ☐ ☐
Snack Food	**Amount**	**Calories**	**Nutrition**
			Dairy group ☐ ☐ Meat/Fish/Eggs ☐ ☐ Vegetables/Fruits ☐ ☐ ☐ ☐ Breads/Cereals ☐ ☐ ☐ ☐
Total Calories for Day			

CHART 18A.2 Activity Record

Day _____				
Activity	Minutes	Calories per Minute per Pound	Weight in Pounds	Total Calories Used
				Total for Day

19
STRESS, TENSION, AND RELAXATION

CONCEPT 19

Mental and physical health are affected by an individual's ability to avoid or adapt to stress, emotional factors, and tension.

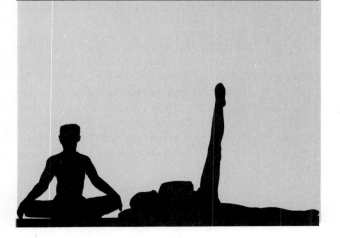

INTRODUCTION

Stress can trigger an emotional response that, in turn, evokes the autonomic nervous system to a "fight or flight" response. This adaptive and protective device stimulates the ductless glands to hypo- or hyperactivity in preparation for what is perceived as a threat or assault on the whole organism. In some instances, this "alarm reaction" of the body may be essential to survival, but when evoked inappropriately or excessively, it may be more harmful than the effects of the original stressor.

TERMS

Adaptation—The body's efforts to restore normalcy.

Alarm Reaction—The body's warning signal that a stressor is present.

Anxiety—A state of apprehension with a compulsion to do something; excessive anxiety is a tension disorder with physiological characteristics.

Chronic Fatigue—Constant state of entire-body fatigue.

Neuromuscular Hypertension—Unnecessary or exaggerated muscle contractions; excess tension beyond that needed to perform a given task. Also called hypertonus.

Physiological Fatigue—A deterioration in the capacity of the neuromuscular system as the result of physical overwork and strain. Also referred to as "true fatigue."

Psychological Fatigue—A feeling of fatigue usually caused by such things as lack of exercise, boredom, or mental stress that results in a lack of energy and depression. Also referred to as "subjective" or "false" fatigue.

Relaxation—The release or reduction of tension in the neuromuscular system.

Stress—The nonspecific response of the body to any demand made upon it.

Stressor—Anything that produces stress or increases the rate of wear and tear on the body.

THE FACTS

All living creatures are in a continual state of stress (some more; some less).

There are many kinds of stressors. Environmental stressors include heat, noise, overcrowding, climate, and terrain. Physiological stressors may be such things as injury, infection, or disease. Mental effort can be a stressor, as can physical effort.

Psychosocial stimuli are probably the most common stressors affecting humans. These include "life-change events," such as a change in work hours or line of work, family illnesses, problems with superiors, deaths of relatives or friends, and increased responsibilities. In school, the pressures of grades, term papers, and oral presentations may induce stress.

Too little stress is undesirable.

Stress is not always harmful. Moderate stress may enhance behavioral adaptation and is necessary for maturation and health. It stimulates psychological growth. It has been said that "freedom from stress is death" and "stress is the spice of life."

Too much stress or an inability to adapt appropriately to stress is harmful.

Cumulative clinical evidence has demonstrated a link between stress and disease and death. Between 50–70 percent of all illnesses are linked to stress response. Some mental and physical conditions that can be psychosomatic (or stress-caused) include high blood pressure and heart disease; psychiatric disorders, such as depression and schizophrenia; indigestion; colitis; ulcers; headaches; insomnia; diarrhea; constipation; increased blood clotting time; increased cholesterol concentration; diuresis; edema; and low back pain. Even serious diseases, such as cancer, can be influenced by the person's state of mind.

Individuals react and adapt differently to different stressors.

What one person finds stressful may not be for others, and stress affects people differently. It mobilizes some to greater efficiency, while it confuses and disorganizes others. For example, skydiving or riding a roller coaster would be fun for some people, but for others it would be very stressful.

An individual's response to stress depends upon the intensity of the threat, the type of situation in which it occurs, and such personal variables as cultural background, tolerance levels, past experience, and personality. You can't make a racehorse out of a turtle and vice versa. The individual's capacity to adapt is not a static function, but fluctuates with energy, drive, and courage.

Individuals tend to adapt best to moderate stress.

You would expect mild stress to produce mild adaptations, and strong stress to produce strong adaptive responses, but this is not so. High levels of threat tend to evoke ineffective, disorganized behavior. Figure 19.1 shows this relationship between stress and adaptive responses.

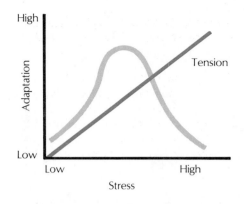

FIGURE 19.1 Stress and Adaptive Responses

Stress can be self-induced and pleasurable or unpleasurable.

Some people may deliberately place themselves in stressful situations; for example, athletes place themselves under maximum strain; lawyers and surgeons are challenged by difficulties; pregnancy imposes psychological and physiological stress on a woman. Self-induced stress may also be an unpleasant but necessary interlude that cannot be avoided. For example, there is a risk of falling that is necessary in learning to ride a bicycle.

Occupations are common sources of stress and some are more stressful than others.

One study found that the twelve most stressful jobs were laborer, secretary, inspector, clinical lab technician, office manager, foreman, manager/administrator, waiter/waitress, machine operator, farm owner, miner, and painter. Air traffic controller is currently considered one of the most stressful jobs. Business and industry often hire psychologists to counsel employees for occupational stress to help reduce absenteeism, boredom, and the number of accidents and resignations.

Neuromuscular hypertension may be both a cause and an effect of stress.

Tension is a primary index of stress. Anxiety is an emotional response caused by stressors that is manifested in muscular tension. Muscular tension may also be physical in origin, resulting from overuse of a muscle group. This tension can cause muscle spasms and pain that, in turn, become additional stressors. Trigger points and the myofascial pain syndrome that lead to backache and headache are good examples of muscular tension.

Some tension is normally present in muscles and contributes to the adjustment of the individual to the environment.

Some tension is needed to remain awake, alert, and ready to respond. In fact, a certain degree of tension aids some types of mental activity. It appears that each individual has an optimum level of tension to facilitate the thought process. However, too much tension can inhibit some types of mental activity and physical skills (such as those requiring accuracy and steadiness in held postures).

Fatigue and neuromuscular hypertension are closely related.

High levels of tension are a source of fatigue. Fatigue from lack of rest or sleep, emotional strain, pain, disease, and muscular work may produce too much muscle tension. Fatigue may be either psychological or physiological in origin, but both can result in a state of exhaustion or chronic fatigue with muscle tenseness.

Excessive tension can be avoided or relieved by proper "coping strategies."

Psychologists say stressful situations must be recognized and people trained to withdraw psychologically to a state of reflection, meditation, or relaxation. "Moderation in all things" may still be a helpful maxim. Work must be balanced with rest. Provision should be made for recreational activities and diversions. Diversions may be even more important than rest, since stress on one system helps to relax another. This may range from a temporary change from one task to another (e.g., from studying to lawn mowing), or a change of scenery, a change in job, a vacation, or even retirement. The approach to life may even need to be altered.

Some methods of relieving tension are less desirable or are not recommended.

There is no magic cure for stress or tension, but there are a variety of therapeutic approaches. Some treatments are less desirable than others because they act only as "crutches" or "fire extinguishers" and do not get at the root of the problem. Hypnosis may lead to fantasy and dependency. Alcoholic beverages, tranquilizers, and painkillers may give temporary relief and may be prescribed by the physician as part of the treatment, but do not resolve the problem and may even mask the symptoms or cause further problems. Drugs do not provide a long-term solution to chronic tension.

The primal scream, EST, transactional analysis, psychoanalysis and other popular methods are useful but do not teach techniques for reducing physical tension and increasing body relaxation.

There are several satisfactory methods of releasing tension through techniques of conscious relaxation.

In some way not fully understood, certain involuntary bodily functions can be controlled by an act of will (voluntarily). Relaxation of the muscles is a skill that can be learned through practice just as other muscle skills are learned.

Conscious relaxation techniques usually employ the "Three Rs" of relaxation: (1) reduce mental activity, (2) recognize tension, and (3) reduce respiration.

Some examples of these systems are described here:

1. *Jacobson's Progressive Relaxation Method*—You must recognize how a tense muscle feels before you can voluntarily release the tension. In this technique, contract the muscles strongly and then relax. Each of the large muscles is relaxed first, and then later the small ones. The contractions are gradually reduced in intensity until no movement is visible. Always, the emphasis is placed on detecting the feeling of tension as the first step in "letting go," or "going negative." Jacobson emphasizes the importance of relaxing eye and speech muscles, since he believes these muscles trigger reactions of the total organism more than other muscles. A sample contract-relax exercise routine for relaxation is presented on page 153.
2. *Autogenic (self-generated) Relaxation Training*— Several times daily, the individual lies down in a quiet room and, with eyes closed, passively concentrates on preselected phrases. This technique has been used to focus on heaviness of limbs, warmth of limbs, heart regulation, breathing regulation, and coolness in the forehead. It evokes changes opposite to those produced by stress.

    Transcendental Meditation (TM), as used by the Eastern religions, falls into this category. The individual sits quietly and attempts to block out distracting thoughts by mentally repeating a personal, secret word or phrase. Research has shown that those who are skilled in this technique can decrease oxygen consumption, change the electrical activity of the brain, slow the metabolism, decrease blood lactate, lower body temperature, and slow the heart rate.

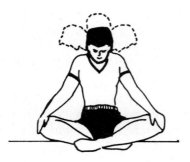

1. Neck Stretch—Roll the head slowly in a half circle, first right and then left. Close your eyes and feel the stretch. Do *not* make a full circle by tipping the head back. Repeat several times.

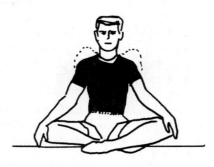

2. Shoulder Lift—Hunch the shoulders as high as possible and then let them drop. Repeat several times. Inhale on the lift; exhale on the drop.

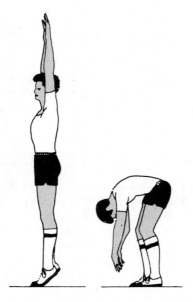

3. Trunk Stretch and Drop—Stand and reach as high as possible; tiptoe and stretch every muscle, then

collapse completely, letting knees flex and trunk, head, and arms dangle (see trunk swing illustration). Repeat two or three times.

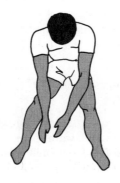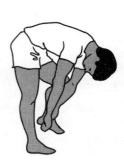

4. Trunk Swings—Following the trunk drop (described above), bounce gently with a minimum of muscular effort. Set the trunk swinging from side to side by shifting the weight from one foot to the other, letting the heels come off the floor alternately. Then with a slight springing movement of the lower back, gently bob up and down, keeping the entire body (especially the neck) limp.

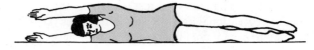

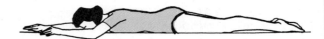

5. Tension Contrast—With arms extended overhead, lie on your side. Tense the body as "stiff as a board," then "let go," and relax, letting the body fall either forward or backward in whatever direction it loses balance. Continue "letting go" for a few seconds after falling and allow yourself to feel like you are still "sinking." Repeat on the other side.

CONTRACT-RELAX EXERCISE ROUTINE FOR RELAXATION*

1. Hand and forearm—Contract your hand, making a fist; relax.

2. Biceps—Flex the elbow and contract your biceps; relax.

3. Forehead—Raise your eyebrows and wrinkle your forehead; relax.

4. Cheeks and nose—Make a face; wrinkle your nose and squint; relax.

5. Jaws—Clench your teeth; relax.

6. Lips and tongue—With teeth apart, press lips together and press tongue to roof of mouth; relax.

7. Neck and throat—Push head backward while tucking chin, pushing against floor or pillow if lying; if sitting, push against high chair back; relax.

8. Shoulders and upper back—Hunch shoulders to ears; relax.

9. Abdomen—Suck in abdomen; relax.

10. Thighs and buttocks—Squeeze your buttocks together and push your heels into the floor (if lying) or against a chair rung (if sitting); relax.

11. Calves—Pull instep and toes toward shin; relax.

12. Toes—Curl toes; relax.

*Note: Eventually, you should progress to a combination of muscle groups and gradually eliminate the "contract" phase of the program.

3. *Biofeedback-Autogenic Relaxation Training—* Biofeedback training utilizes machines that monitor certain physiological processes of the body and provide visual or auditory evidence of what is happening to normally unconscious bodily functions. When combined with autogenic phrases, subjects have learned to relax and reduce the electrical activity in their muscles, lower blood pressure by increasing the temperature of their hands, decrease heart rate, change their brain waves, and decrease headaches, asthma attacks, and some psychosomatic disorders.

4. *Imagery*—Thinking autogenic phrases, you can visualize such feelings as "sinking into a mattress or pillow," or you can think of being a "limp, loose-jointed puppet with no one to hold the strings." You can imagine being a "half-filled sack of flour resting on an uneven surface" or pretend to be "a sack of granulated salt left out in the rain, melting away." Some people seem to respond better to the concept of "floating" than to feeling "heavy," but whatever the image you wish to conjure, imagery is a form of self-hypnosis that helps to take your mind off anxieties and distractions, and at the same time, releases unwanted tension in the muscles using "mind over matter."

Exercise is one of the best ways to relieve stress and aid muscle tension release.

Exercise is especially useful to relieve white-collar job stress. Hans Selye believes physical fitness serves as a sort of "inoculation against stress." (Selye 1977) Stretching exercises and rhythmical exercises, especially, aid in relaxation.

Some good relaxation exercises are illustrated in the box on page 152.

Massage, heat, and deep breathing aid relaxation of tense muscles.

Gentle effleurage, a type of massage; heat in the form of a hot bath (or shower or sauna); and deep breathing with prolonged exhalation, when combined with conscious relaxation techniques described in this concept, are effective for most people.

LAB RESOURCE MATERIALS (FOR USE WITH LAB 19A, PAGE 239, AND 19C, PAGE 243)

TABLE 19A.1 Stressful Life Events*

Event	Score	Event	Score
Death of spouse	100	Son/daughter leaves home	29
Divorce	73	Trouble with in-laws	29
Marital separation	65	Outstanding achievement	28
Jail term	63	Spouse begins work	26
Death of close family member	63	Start or finish school	26
Personal injury/illness	53	Change in living conditions	25
Marriage	50	Revision of personal habits	24
Fired from work	47	Trouble with boss	23
Marital reconciliation	45	Change in work hours, conditions	20
Retirement	45	Change in residence	20
Change in family member's health	44	Change in schools	20
Pregnancy	40	Change in recreational habits	19
Sex difficulties	39	Change in church activities	19
Addition to family	39	Change in social activities	18
Business readjustment	39	Mortgage/loan under $10,000	18
Change in financial status	38	Change in sleeping habits	16
Death of close friend	37	Change in number of family gatherings	15
Change in number of marital arguments	35	Change in eating habits	15
Mortgage/loan over $10,000	31	Vacation	13
Foreclosure of mortgage/loan	30	Christmas season	12
Change in work responsibilities	29	Minor violation of law	11

This test is adapted from the Social Readjustment Scale devised by Thomas Holmes and Richard Rahe. Used by permission.

CHART 19A.1 Rating Scale for Stressful Life Events

Rating	Score	Implication for Illness
Low stress	150 or less	This indicates that a person has a 35% chance of getting a stress-related disease in the next two years.
Moderate stress	151–300	51% chance of getting a stress illness in the next two years.
High stress	301 or higher	80% chance of getting a stress illness in the next two years.

Evaluating Muscular Tension

A trained person can diagnose neuromuscular hypertension by observation and by manual testing. While there is insufficient time in this course to master either the technique of relaxing or the techniques of evaluation, it is possible to learn the procedures for both.

1. Following the procedure outlined here, look for visual signs of tension outlined in section A of Chart 19C.1. Place a check mark in the appropriate column.
2. Quietly and gently, the tester should grasp the subject's right wrist with his or her fingers, and slowly raise it about three inches from the floor, letting it hinge at the elbow; then let the hand drop. Observe the signs of tension outlined in section B of Chart 19C.1. Record results.
3. After all visual and manual symptoms have been recorded on the chart, determine the total number of symptoms checked yes.
4. Find your total score on Chart 19C.2 to determine your rating.

CHART 19C.1 Signs of Tension

	No	Yes
A. Visual Symptoms		
Frowning	☐	☐
Twitching	☐	☐
Eyelids fluttering	☐	☐
Breathing	☐	☐
shallow	☐	☐
rapid	☐	☐
irregular	☐	☐
Mouth tight	☐	☐
Swallowing	☐	☐
B. Manual Symptoms		
Assistance (subject helps lift arm)	☐	☐
Resistance (subject resists movement)	☐	☐
Posturing (subject holds arm in raised position)	☐	☐
Perseveration (subject continues upward movement)	☐	☐

Total number of yes checks _____

CHART 19C.2 Tension-Relaxation Rating Scale

Classification	Total Score
Excellent (relaxed)	0
Very good (mild tension)	1–3
Fair (moderate tension)	4–6
Poor (tense)	7–9
Very poor (marked tension)	10–12

REFERENCES

Benson, Herbert. *The Relaxation Response.* New York: Avon, 1975.

Brown, B. B. *Stress and the Art of Biofeedback.* New York: Harper and Row, 1977.

*Fisher, D. D. *I Know You Hurt but There's Nothing to Bandage.* Beaverton, OR: Touchstone Press, 1978.

Geba, B. H. *Breathe Away Your Tension.* New York: Random House, 1973.

Graham-Bonnalie, F. E. *The Doctor's Guide to Living with Stress.* New York: Drake Publisher, Inc., 1972.

Gunderson, E., and R. Rahe, eds. *Life Stress and Illness.* Springfield, IL: Charles C. Thomas, Publisher, 1974.

Hollis, M. *Practical Exercise Therapy,* 2d ed. Boston: Blackwell Scientific Publications, 1981.

"How to Deal with Stress on the Job." *U.S. News and World Report* (March 13, 1978):80.

*Jacobson, E. *Anxiety and Tension Control.* Philadelphia: J. B. Lippincott Co., 1964.

Kahn, C. "The Golden Rule of Health." *Family Health* (April 1978):40.

Lenz, F. P. *Total Relaxation.* Indianapolis: Bobbs-Merrill Co., Inc., 1980.

Lindsey, R., B. Jones, and A. V. Whitley. *Fitness for Health, Figure/Physique, Posture.* 5th ed. Dubuque, IA: Wm. C. Brown Publishers, 1983.

Menninger, R. W. "Coping with Life's Strains." *U.S. News and World Report* (May 1, 1978):80.

Monaghan, J., and C. D. Meyer. "Surviving Stress." Santa Ana, CA: *The Register* (July 10–14, 1983).

Pollock, M., J. Willmore, and S. M. Fox. *Health and Fitness through Physical Activity.* New York: John Wiley and Sons, 1978.

Rosen, Gerald. *The Relaxation Book.* Englewood Cliffs, NJ: Prentice-Hall, Inc., 1974.

*Selye, H. *Stress without Distress.* Philadelphia: J. B. Lippincott, 1974.

Selye, H. "Secret of Coping with Stress." *U.S. News and World Report* (March 21, 1977):51.

Taylor, L. P. *Electromyometric Biofeedback Therapy.* Los Angeles: Biofeedback and Advanced Therapy Institute, Inc., 1981.

Travell, J. G., and D. G. Simons. *Myofascial Pain and Dysfunction.* Baltimore: Williams and Wilkins, 1983.

Woodworth, R. S., and H. Schlosberg. *Experimental Psychology.* 3d ed. London: Methuen, 1972.

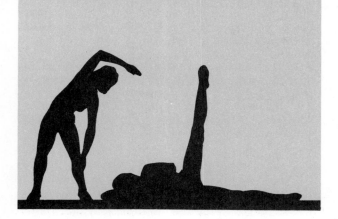

20
BODY MECHANICS

CONCEPT 20

Since the human body is a system of

weights and levers, its efficiency and

effectiveness at rest or in motion

can be improved by the application of sound

mechanical and anatomical principles.

INTRODUCTION

"Body mechanics" is the application of physical laws to the human body. The bones of the body act as levers or simple machines, with the muscles supplying the force to move them. Therefore, mechanical laws can be applied to body use to aid in performing more and better work with less energy while avoiding strain or injury.

This concept focuses on three aspects of body mechanics. The first part of the concept discusses the mechanics of body alignment while sitting or standing (*static postures*). The second part of the concept emphasizes the *prevention of low back and neck pain* through proper body mechanics. The third section of the concept stresses *dynamic postures* for the activities in daily living.

TERMS

Center of Gravity—The center of the mass of an object.

Effectiveness—The degree to which the purpose is accomplished.

Efficiency—The relationship of the amount of energy used to the amount of work accomplished.

Head Forward—The head is thrust forward in front of the gravity line; also called "poke neck."

Herniated Disc—The soft nucleus of the spinal disc protrudes through a small tear in the surrounding tissue; also called prolapse.

Hyperextended Knees—The knees are thrust backward in a locked position.

Kyphosis—Increased curvature (flexion) in the upper back; also called "hump back."

Linear Motion—Movement in a straight line.

Lumbar Lordosis—Increased curvature (hyperextension) in the lower back (lumbar region), with a forward pelvic tilt; commonly known as "swayback."

Myofascial Trigger Points—See Concept 9 terms.

Posture—The relationship of body parts, whether standing, lying, sitting, or moving. "Good posture" is the relationship of body parts that allows you to function most effectively, with the least expenditure of energy and with a minimum amount of strain on muscles, tendons, ligaments, and joints.

Referred Pain—Pain that appears to be located in one area, while in reality it originates in another area.

Round Shoulders—The tips of the shoulders are drawn forward in front of the line of gravity.

Ruptured Disc—Spinal disc crushed from a severe blow or jolt.

Sciatica—Pain radiating down the sciatic nerve in the back of the hip and leg.

Scoliosis—A lateral curvature with some rotation of the spine; the most serious and deforming of all postural deviations.

THE FACTS ABOUT STATIC POSTURES

Good posture has aesthetic benefits.

The first impression one person makes on another is usually a visual one. Good posture can help convey an impression of alertness, confidence, and attractiveness.

There is probably no one best posture for all individuals, since body build affects the balance of body parts. But in general, certain relationships are desirable.

In the standing position, the head should be centered over the trunk, the shoulders should be down and back, but relaxed, with the chest high and the abdomen flat. The spine should have gentle curves when viewed from the side, but should be straight as seen from the back. When the pelvis is tilted properly, the pubis falls directly underneath the lower tip of the sternum. The knees should be relaxed, with the kneecaps pointed straight ahead. The feet should point straight ahead and the weight should be borne over the heel, on the outside border of the sole, and across the ball of the foot and toes.

Clinical evidence cited by physicians and opinions of educators indicate that poor posture can cause a number of health problems.

For example:

1. Protruding abdomen and lumbar lordosis may contribute to painful menstruation, susceptibility to back injury, and backache.
2. A forward position of the head can result in headache, dizziness, and neck, shoulder, and arm pain.
3. Rounded shoulders may impair respiratory capacity.
4. Hyperextended knees may predispose a person to knee injury.
5. Unbalanced postural lines can cause excessive tension in muscle groups, produce joint strain, stretch ligaments, damage joint cartilage, and become a factor in arthritic changes.
6. Poor posture creates mechanical stresses that perpetuate myofascial trigger points.

If one part of the body is out of line, other parts must move out of line to balance it, thus increasing the strain on muscles, ligaments, and joints.

The body is made in segments that are held balanced in a vertical column by muscles and ligaments. If gravity or a short muscle pulls one segment out of line, other portions of the body will move out of alignment to compensate, producing worse posture, more stress and strain, and possible deformity of the musculoskeletal system (Fig. 20.1).

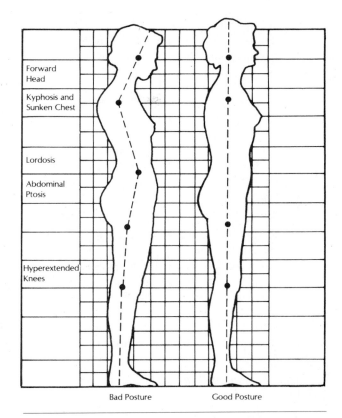

FIGURE 20.1 Comparison of Bad and Good Posture

There are many causes of poor posture, including hereditary, congenital, and disease conditions, as well as certain environmental factors.

Some factors that may contribute to poor posture include ill-fitting clothing, chronic fatigue, improperly fitting furniture (including poor beds and mattresses), emotional and personality problems, poor work habits, lack of physical fitness due to inactivity, and lack of good posture knowledge.

Approximately 80 percent of the adult population suffers from acquired foot defects.

Most foot defects are acquired and are preventable. They are most often caused by improperly fitting shoes and socks; excessive hard use (such as in athletics); long standing or walking on hard surfaces; obesity or rapid weight gain (as in pregnancy); and improper bearing of weight through poor foot and leg alignment.

Exercises for the correction of postural deviations are generally based on the assumption that if the problem is a functional deformity, regardless of the factors causing it, muscular imbalance will be present.

If the muscles on one side of a joint are stronger than the muscles on the opposite side of that joint, the body part is pulled in the direction of the stronger muscles. Corrective exercises are usually designed to strengthen the long, weak muscles and to stretch the short, strong ones in order to have equal pull in both directions. For example, persons with lumbar lordosis may need to strengthen the abdominals and stretch the lower back muscles.

THE FACTS ABOUT BACK AND NECK ACHES

Poor posture, especially lordosis, can cause back strain and pain and make the back more susceptible to injury.

The forward tilt of the pelvis may cause the sacral bone or one of the lumbar vertebrae to press on nerve roots with consequent low back pain and sciatica. To be on the safe side, some authorities advise those who have lordosis and weak abdominals to eliminate all exercises that hyperextend the spine. Incidence of lordosis is about the same for men as it is for women, except that women experience an added back strain during pregnancy, and high heels may also contribute to spinal strain.

The neck is probably strained more frequently than the lower back.

The neck is constructed with the same curve and has the same mechanical problems as the lower back. The postural fault of "head forward" places a chronic strain on the posterior neck muscles. Tension in these muscles can lead to myofascial trigger points, causing headache or referred pain in the face, scalp, shoulder, arm, and chest.

The overwhelming majority of back and neck aches are avoidable. A common cause of backache is muscular strain, frequently caused by poor body mechanics in daily activities or during exercise.

When lifting improperly, there is great pressure on the lumbar discs and severe stress on the lumbar muscles and ligaments. Many popular exercises place great strain on the back (see Concept 16). Sleeping flat on the back or abdomen on a soft mattress can also cause lower back strain.

Muscular fatigue and weak muscles are frequent causes of backache.

Backache has been referred to as a "hypokinetic disease," meaning that it is caused by insufficient exercise. Lack of exercise results in weak muscles that are easily strained and fatigued. Sedentary workers are particularly susceptible to spinal strain, and weak abdominal and back muscles are especially to blame. If the abdominals are weak, the pelvis is apt to tilt forward, causing lordosis.

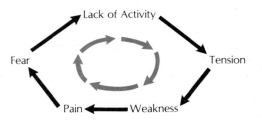

FIGURE 20.2 The Viscious Cycle of Back Pain

Most people agree excessive muscle tension is a contributing factor in painful spines.

Backaches may be precipitated by a minor injury or strain that sets off a muscle spasm; this causes pain, worry, excitement, fear, and stimulation of already hypersensitive muscular areas, referred to as "trigger points." These tender, painful spots occur frequently in the neck, shoulders, back, and hip as a result of constant tension, strain, or muscle spasm. When these tense muscles shorten, lose elasticity, and are weakened by lack of exercise, the "low back syndrome" occurs. With a weak back, the mildest movement can trigger back pain.

Back pains may result from "referred pain" caused by muscle tension in other areas. In some cases, the pain is "referred" from the back of the legs if the hamstring muscles have been overstretched or injured.

There is no such thing as a "slipped disc."

Disc problems are frequently misunderstood. Vertebral discs may herniate or rupture, but they do not slip. Disc material pressure on nerves causes pain, and a protective reflex (muscle spasm) occurs to protect it. This causes more pain, beginning a vicious cycle (Fig. 20.2). The discs in the lumbar area are subjected to greater pressure, partly because they are at the bottom of the spine. Therefore, they are more apt to be damaged by severe jolts or strains.

Most backaches can be prevented or alleviated by good sense, proper exercise, and relaxation.

Several "good sense" suggestions for taking care of the back are listed here:

1. Avoid the swayback position at all times by taking such precautions as the following:
   a. To relieve back strain during prolonged standing, try to keep the lower back flat by propping one foot on a stool, bar, or rail; alternate feet occasionally (see Fig. 20.3). (Dentists, beauticians, barbers, and store clerks are particularly susceptible to back problems because they must stand to work.)

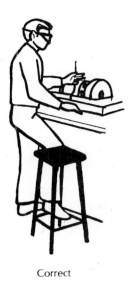
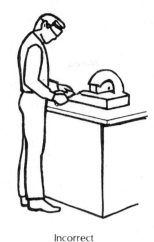

Correct   Incorrect

FIGURE 20.3 Standing Work Postures

b. When sitting, use a hard chair with a straight back, placing the spine against it; keep one or both knees higher than the hips by crossing the legs (alternate sides) or by using a foot rest and keeping the knees bent.

c. When driving a car, place a hard seat-and-backrest combination over the seat of the automobile; pull the seat forward so the legs are bent when operating the pedals.

d. When lying, keep the knees and hips bent; avoid lying on the abdomen. When lying on the back, a pillow or lift should be placed under the knees.

e. Avoid lifting and carrying improperly. Especially avoid bending over or straightening up while twisting the trunk.

2. To prevent neck strain, avoid the head forward position. The forward thrust is apt to occur in such activities as card playing, sewing, studying, and watching television. Sleeping on a high pillow may also cause back or neck strain.

3. Do corrective exercises to strengthen the abdominal muscles and stretch the lower back muscles. Avoid exercises that strain or arch the lower back (see Concepts 16 and 17).

4. General exercises, involving the entire body, are important in preventing weak muscles and lack of flexibility.

5. Warm up before engaging in strenuous activity.

6. Get adequate rest and sleep. Avoid pushing yourself mentally or physically to the point of exhaustion.

7. Vary the working position by changing from one task to another before feeling fatigued. When working at a desk, get up and stretch occasionally to relieve tension.

8. Sleep on a firm mattress or place a three-fourths-inch-thick plywood board under the mattress.

9. Avoid sudden, jerky back movements.

10. The smaller the waistline, the lesser the strain on the lower back. Avoid being overweight.

THE FACTS ABOUT DYNAMIC POSTURE: LIFTING AND CARRYING

The best method for lifting or carrying a given object depends upon its size, weight, shape, and position in space. However, there are some general principles that are applicable in all situations.

1. *Stand close to the object and assume a wide base.* Stand in a forward-backward stride position with the object at the side of the body, or assume a side-stride position with the object between the knees. The purpose of lifting from this position is to allow you to lift straight upward from a stable position, utilizing the most efficient leverage.

2. *Keep the back straight and bend at the hips and knees. Squat, do not bend, regardless of how light the object may be.* The back was never meant to be used as a lever for lifting. Orthopedists constantly caution against leaning forward to pick up objects without bending the knees because of the strain placed on the muscles and joints of the spine. This kind of back strain can occur when improperly making a bed or when lifting a child out of a crib. When bending from the waist, the body's center of gravity is higher than when squatting, thus the bending posture is less stable as well as more injurious than the squatting position.

3. *Lower your body only as far as necessary, directly downward, keeping the hips tucked.* Squatting lower than is necessary is a waste of energy, but more importantly perhaps, deep knee bends can damage the structures of the knee joints. The deeper the flexion, the greater the twist on the joint and the greater the tension in the leg muscles.

4. *Grasp the object and lift with your leg muscles, keeping the object close to the center of the body's gravity.* The leg muscles are the strongest in the body, and if the back is kept erect, use of the legs for lifting allows a maximal force to be applied to the load without wasting energy.

5. *Push or pull heavy objects, if this can be done efficiently, rather than lifting them.* Theoretically, it takes about thirty-four times more force to lift than to slide an object across the floor. The size, shape, and friction of the object determine whether or not it is feasible to push or pull it.

6. *Carry the object close to the body's center of gravity and no higher than waist level (except when carrying on the shoulder, head, or back).* When objects are carried in front of the body above the level of the waist, you must lean backward to balance the load, producing an undesirable arch in the lower back. Carrying loads at the midline of the body, such as in a knapsack or on the head or shoulders, is effective in reducing the stress on the skeletal system.

7. *Divide the load if possible, carrying half in each arm. If the load cannot be divided, alternate the load from one side of the body to the other.* When walking with the weight carried on one side of the body, the force on the opposite hip is much greater than when the load is distributed on both sides. This is true even when the bilateral load is twice as great as the unilateral load. If the weight must be carried on only one side, the opposite arm should be raised to counterbalance the load and to help keep the center of gravity over the base.

8. *Avoid arching the back when lifting and lowering an object from overhead. Any lift above waist level is inefficient.* Occasionally, you must reach overhead to lift an object from a high shelf. To avoid back strain, climb a ladder or stand on a stool so you don't have to raise your arms overhead. If this is not practical, reach for the object with your weight on the forward foot, and then step backward on the rear foot as the object is lowered.

9. *Do not try to lift or carry burdens too heavy for you.* The most economical load for either a man or a woman is about thirty-five percent of his or her body weight. Obviously, with strength training, you can safely lift a greater load.

THE FACTS ABOUT DYNAMIC POSTURES: PUSHING AND PULLING

The choice to push or to pull depends upon the nature of the task.

When deciding whether to push or pull, you must consider such factors as desired direction, type of movement, distance to be moved, and friction. If a downward force is desired, pushing would be best. If an upward force is desirable, pulling is probably better. Pushing tends to increase friction because of the downward force, but may offer better control since the object is closer to the person.

Pushing and pulling are forms of lifting; therefore, the same mechanical principles may be applied.

When pushing or pulling, the back should be kept as straight as possible, a wide stance should be used, and the leg muscles should do the work rather than the back or arms. You may alternate the working muscles by changing positions occasionally. That is, face forward, then backward, then sideward.

Force should be applied as nearly as possible in the desired line of direction.

If linear motion is desired, you should apply force at the center of the object's gravity and push or pull in the desired direction by leaning from the hips in that direction. To move an object horizontally, the upward and downward components of the push or pull should be reduced to a minimum. When pulling, increasing the length of the handle reduces the vertical component.

If there is a great deal of friction, the force should be applied below the object's center of gravity. Sufficient force should be applied continuously to keep the load moving, since it takes more force to start an object moving (overcoming inertia) than to keep it going.

When rotary motion is desired, apply force away from the center of gravity of the object.

Objects that are too heavy or too awkward to be moved as a whole, such as a refrigerator or couch, can be moved by applying force alternately at one end and then the other, so that a pivoting or "walking" action is employed to rotate the object.

THE FACTS ABOUT DYNAMIC POSTURES: SAVING ENERGY DURING WORK

When working with the arms in front of the body, a pulling motion is easier than a pushing motion.

The pulling motion uses the stronger flexor muscles, while a pushing motion employs the seldom used extensors that are usually weaker. Thus, counterclockwise circular movements are easier for the right hand, and clockwise circular movements easier for the left hand.

Organize work to avoid stooping or unnatural positions.

1. Sideward flexion of the trunk is more strenuous than forward trunk flexion.
2. Avoid constant arm extension, whether forward or sideward.
3. Whenever possible, sit while working but stand occasionally.
4. The arms should move either together or in opposite directions. When the conditions allow, use both hands in opposite and symmetrical motions while working.
5. Tools most often used should be the closest to reach.
6. When working with the hands, the workbench or kitchen cabinet should be about 5 to 10 cm (2 to 4 inches) below the waist. The office desk should be about 74 to 78 cm (29 to 30 inches) high for the average man and about 70 to 74 cm (27 to 29 inches) high for the average woman.

Some types of arm movements are more accurate than others.

Horizontal movements are more precise than vertical ones. Circular movements are better than zigzag ones. Movements toward the body are easier to control than those away from the body. Rhythmic movements are more accurate and less tiring than abrupt movements.

REFERENCES

Belkin, S. C., and H. H. Banks. *Backaches*. Tufts-New England Medical Center, Inc. Wellesly: Arandel Publishing Co., 1978.

*Calliet, R. *Neck and Arm Pain*. 2d ed. Philadelphia: F. A. Davis Company, 1981.

*Calliet, R. *Low Back Pain Syndrome*. 3d ed. Philadelphia: F. A. Davis Company, 1981.

Calliet, R. *Soft Tissue Pain and Disability*. Philadelphia: F. A. Davis Company, 1977.

Daniels, L., and C. Worthingham. *Therapeutic Exercise*. 2d ed. Philadelphia: W. B. Saunders Company, 1977.

Fisk, J. W. *The Painful Neck and Back*. Springfield: Charles C. Thomas Publisher, 1977.

Keim, H. A., and W. H. Kirkaldy-Willis. "Low Back Pain." *Clinical Symposia* 32(1980):6.

Kornfield, J. "Getting Aggressive about Conservative Therapy for Back Pain." *Medical World News* (July 5, 1982).

Kottke, F. J., G. K. Stillwell, and J. F. Lehmann. *Krusen's Handbook of Physical Medicine*. 3d ed. Philadelphia: W. B. Saunders Company, 1982.

Kraus, H. "Ecology and Backaches." *Journal of Physical Education* 69(1972):111.

Kreighbaum, E., and K, M. Barthels. *Biomechanics*. Minneapolis: Burgess Publishing Company, 1981.

Lindsey, R., B. Jones, and A. V. Whitley. *Fitness for Health, Figure/Physique, Posture*. 5th ed. Dubuque, IA: Wm. C. Brown Publishers, 1983.

Luttgens, K., and K. F. Wells. *Kinesiology*. 7th ed. Philadelphia: Saunders College Publishing, 1982.

Sherrill, C. *Adapted Physical Education and Recreation*. Dubuque, IA: Wm. C. Brown Publishers, 1981.

Stanitski, C. L. "Low Back Pain in Young Athletes." *Physician and Sportsmedicine* 10(1982):77.

Travell, J. G., and D. G. Simons. *Myofascial Pain and Dysfunction*. Baltimore: Williams and Wilkins, 1983.

*Williams, P. C. *Low Back and Neck Pain: Causes and Conservative Treatment*. Springfield, IL: Charles C. Thomas Publisher, 1974.

21
HYPOKINETIC DISEASE RISK FACTORS

CONCEPT 21

There are many factors that contribute to increased risk of hypokinetic disease. Many of these are controllable.

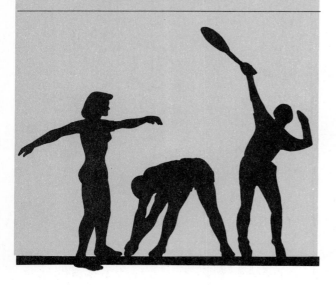

INTRODUCTION

As the name indicates, hypokinetic diseases and conditions are caused or compounded by a lack of regular exercise. Such hypokinetic conditions as heart disease and back pain, however, are caused by many factors other than lack of exercise. These factors associated with hypokinetic conditions are called "risk factors." It cannot be proven that all risk factors cause hypokinetic disease, but the link between them is strong. Some risk factors such as sex and age cannot be altered. They are predetermined by heredity and the passing of time. Other factors can be controlled by modifying your lifestyle. You can do something about these.

TERMS

Blood Lipids—Fats in the bloodstream, including cholesterol and triglicerides.

Diastolic Blood Pressure—Commonly referred to as resting blood pressure, it is the lower of the two blood pressure readings. It occurs just before the heartbeats that increase the pressure.

Hypertension—Another word for high blood pressure.

Hypokinetic Disease or Condition—A disease or condition associated with physical inactivity.

Risk Factor—A factor or circumstance that relates to the increased risk of acquiring a disease or medical condition; in this case, increased risk of hypokinetic conditions such as heart disease and back pain.

Systolic Blood Pressure—Commonly referred to as working blood pressure, systolic blood pressure is the higher of the two blood pressure readings. It is the pressure necessary to force movement of the blood through the artery and is measured (usually the brachial artery on the inside of the upper arm) just after the heart beats, forcing a surge of blood through the artery.

THE FACTS

There are many risk factors associated with hypokinetic diseases and conditions.

Some of the major risk factors associated with hypokinetic disease, especially heart disease and back pain, are presented on the next page.

Certain risk factors cannot be altered by changes in lifestyle.

There is nothing you can do about some risk factors, such as age, heredity, and sex. For example, an older male with a family history of heart disease has a higher risk of heart disease than a young female without a history of heart disease. If you possess risk factors you cannot control, it is especially important that you do what you can to alter those that you can control.

Some risk factors can be altered by changing your lifestyle.

Risk of hypokinetic conditions can be reduced by controlling body fatness; altering diet to include good basic foods low in fat and salt; following your doctor's advice to control existing medical conditions (including taking medicine as prescribed); exercising regularly; eliminating smoking; avoiding excessively stressful situations; and learning how to cope effectively with stress. The person at risk must make lifestyle changes in order to effectively reduce the incidence of hypokinetic disease.

Altering risk factors can help reduce the risk of more than one adverse condition at the same time.

By altering the risk factors that are controllable, you can reduce the risk of several hypokinetic conditions. For example, controlling body fatness reduces the risk of diabetes, hypertension, and back problems. Altering your diet can reduce the chances of developing high levels of blood lipids, and thus reduce the risk of atherosclerosis.

Risk reduction does not guarantee freedom from disease.

Reducing risk alters the probability of disease, but does not assure disease immunity.

HYPOKINETIC DISEASE RISK FACTORS

Factors That Cannot Be Altered

1. *Age*—As you grow older, your risk of hypokinetic diseases increases. For example, the risk of heart disease is approximately three times as great after sixty as before. The risk of back pain and ulcer disease is considerably greater after forty.

2. *Heredity*—Those people who have a family history of hypokinetic disease are more likely to develop a hypokinetic condition. Heart disease, hypertension, ulcers, back problems, obesity, high blood lipid levels, and other problems have been shown to be more prevalent among those who have a family history of these conditions than among those with no family history. Black Americans are 45 percent more likely to have high blood pressure than whites, and so suffer strokes at an earlier age and with more severe results than whites.

3. *Sex*—Men have a higher incidence of many hypokinetic conditions than women. Although the number of women who experience heart disease is increasing, they still have only about half the incidence of the disease as do men. The incidence of heart disease increases sharply in women after menopause.

Factors That Can Be Altered

4. *Body Fatness*—Having too much body fat is considered by many to be a hypokinetic condition because it may limit your ability to function efficiently and effectively. Even those who do not classify overfatness as a hypokinetic condition agree that it does increase the risk of other hypokinetic conditions. For example, loss of fat can result in relief from symptoms of adult-onset diabetes; can reduce problems associated with certain types of back pain; and can reduce the risks of surgery.

5. *Diet*—There is a clear association between hypokinetic disease and certain types of diets. The excessive intake of saturated fats, such as animal fats, is linked to atherosclerosis and other forms of heart disease. Excessive salt in the diet is associated with high blood pressure.

6. *Diseases*—People who have one hypokinetic disease are more likely to develop a second, or even a third, condition. For example, if you have diabetes, atherosclerosis, or high blood pressure, your risk of having a heart attack or stroke increases dramatically. People with poor posture have a high risk of experiencing back pain and those with too much body fat have a greater than normal risk of diabetes. Although you may not be entirely able to alter the extent to which you develop certain diseases and conditions, reducing your risk and following your doctor's advice can improve your "odds" significantly.

7. *Regular Exercise*—As noted throughout this book and especially in Concept 3, regular exercise can help reduce the risk of hypokinetic disease.

8. *Smoking*—Smokers have a much higher risk of developing and dying from heart disease than nonsmokers. The risk of heart attack is twice as great among young smokers as among young nonsmokers. (Most striking is the difference in risk between older women smokers and nonsmokers.) Smokers have five times the risk of heart attack. Smoking is also associated with increased risk of high blood pressure, cancer, and several other medical conditions. Apparently the more you smoke, the greater the risk. Stopping smoking, even after years, can significantly reduce the hypokinetic disease risk.

9. *Stress*—There is evidence that people who are subject to excessive stress are predisposed to various hypokinetic diseases including heart disease and back pain. Statistics indicate that hypokinetic conditions are common among those in certain high-stress jobs and those having "Type A Personality" profiles.

Some risk factors are present at a very early age.

It is never too early to begin controlling hypokinetic disease risk factors. Studies of very young children show that even these youngsters exhibit early-stage symptoms of atherosclerosis, Type A personality traits, obesity, and even high blood pressure. Establishing healthy lifestyles early in life can be effective in reducing the risk of hypokinetic disease.

It is never too late to begin altering risk factors.

More than one person has said, "It's too late for me," implying that eliminating a risk factor is of little value. This is just not true! For example, eliminating smoking can result in an almost immediate decrease in risk of heart disease and cancer. The same is true for other risk factor modifications.

LAB RESOURCE MATERIALS (FOR USE WITH LAB 21, PAGE 247)

Heart Disease Risk Factor Questionnaire*

Circle the appropriate answer to each question.

	Risk Points				
	1	2	3	4	Score
Unalterable Factors					
1. How old are you?	30 or less	31–40	41–54	55+	_____
2. Do you have a history of heart disease in your family?	none	grandparent with heart disease	parent with heart disease	more than one with heart disease	_____
3. What is your sex?	female		male		_____
				Total Unalterable Risk Score	_____
Alterable Factors					
4. What is your percent of body fat?	F =17%↓ M=14%↓	22%↓ 17%↓	27%↓ 19%↓	28%↑ 20%↑	_____
5. Do you have a high-fat diet?	no	slightly high in fat	above normal in fat	eat a lot of meat, fried and fatty foods	_____
6. What is your blood pressure? (systolic or upper score)	120↓	121–135	136–155	155↑	_____
7. Do you have other hypokinetic diseases?	no	ulcer	diabetes	both	_____
8. Do you exercise regularly?	4–5 days a week	3 days a week	less than 3 days a week	no	_____
9. Do you smoke?	no	cigar or pipe	less than 1/2 pack a day	more than 1/2 pack a day	_____
10. Are you under much stress?	less than normal	normal	slightly above normal	quite high	_____

Total Alterable Risk Score _____

Grand Total Risk Score _____

*Adapted from Stone, W. J. CAD Risk Factor Scoring Scale. Tempe, Arizona: State University, 1984.

CHART 21.1 Heart Disease Risk Rating Scale

Rating	Unalterable Score	Alterable Score	Total Score
Very High	9 or More	21 or More	31 or More
High	7–8	15–20	26–30
Average	5–6	11–14	16–25
Low	4 or Less	10 or Less	15 or Less

REFERENCES

*American Heart Association. *1983 Heart Facts Reference Sheet.* Dallas: American Heart Association, 1983.

American Heart Association. *Putting Your Heart into the Curriculum.* Dallas: American Heart Association, 1983.

Corbin, C. B. and R. Lindsey. *The Ultimate Fitness Book.* New York: The Leisure Press, 1984.

*Gilliam, T. B., et al. "Exercise Programs for Children: A Way to Prevent Heart Disease?" *Physician and Sportsmedicine* 10(1982):96.

Stone, W. J. "Exercise and Long-Term CV Risk Reduction in Corporate Executives." *Health Education* 14(1983):26.

Stone, W. J. *Lab Manual for Exercise Physiology.* Tempe, AZ: Arizona State University, 1983.

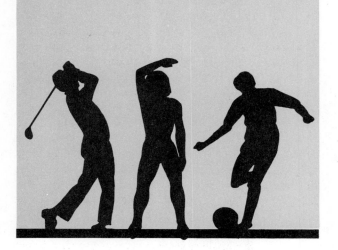

22
EXERCISE FOR A LIFETIME

CONCEPT 22

Exercise can contribute to physical fitness, good health, and an improved quality of life for people of all ages.

INTRODUCTION

In our culture, some think activity is only appropriate for children and youth. Yet research evidence indicates that *all people need* regular physical activity.

TERMS

Acquired Aging—The acquisition of characteristics commonly associated with aging but that are, in fact, caused by immobility or inactivity.

Time-Dependent Aging—The loss of function resulting from growing older.

THE FACTS: PHYSICAL ACTIVITY FOR CHILDREN

The risk factors associated with hypokinetic disease begin to develop very early in life.

The most recent research evidence indicates that the risk factors of such hypokinetic conditions as coronary heart disease and back pain begin to evidence themselves very early in life. Fat deposits on the walls of the arteries have been found in school-age children, and too many children are overfat. Tests of the fitness components that promote good posture and a healthy back show that a large percentage of children are physically unfit. This is, in part, due to the fact that children are not as active as you might expect. All children do *not* voluntarily engage in vigorous activity. Usually, the children most likely to need exercise are the ones most likely to avoid it.

Children, even very young children, are quite capable of vigorous physical activity. However, the optimal time for development of high levels of health-related fitness occurs after the beginning of adolescence.

Children can exercise regularly. The typical child needs several hours of large muscle activity daily. For their body size, children can perform as well as young adults, but should not be expected to compete with adolescents and young adults (because of their smaller size and because they are not mature emotionally).

A healthy child cannot physiologically injure his or her heart with physical exercise.

Parents should not be concerned about the old wives' tale that suggests that exercise for children will result in heart damage. Research has dispelled this myth. At the same time, children are not miniature adults and programs of exercise for health-related fitness, including cardiovascular fitness, should be designed to meet both the physical and psychological needs and interests of children. Too much too soon may breed dislike for any type of physical activity.

✳ *Children should be exposed to a wide variety of physical activities in order to establish a basis for a lifetime of activity.*

Recent research indicates that nearly all Americans have had some physical education during their school years. Nevertheless, only 40 percent of all schoolchildren have physical education in the elementary school. Most skills are learned by age twelve or by the end of the sixth grade. For this reason, it is important that children not specialize in one activity too early, thus allowing more time to learn as many activities as possible during the school years. Just as a child learning to read must first learn the alphabet and grammar, in physical activity the child should be exposed to many fundamental activities early in life so that he or she can take advantage of more than one lifetime activity in adulthood.

Certain types of activities, particularly weight training and weight lifting, are not recommended for preadolescents.

Although there is evidence that children can build muscle as a result of overload training, the best current information suggests that this type of training program should start after bone growth is relatively complete.

THE FACTS: PHYSICAL ACTIVITY FOR THE ADOLESCENT

Like children, adolescents are often physically unfit.

As previously noted, during the teen years, the potential for health-related fitness improvement is great. However, the results of physical fitness tests indicate that many teenagers never achieve optimal fitness levels. Regular exercise and sound nutrition is especially important during this age period.

It is during adolescence that exercise contributes the most dramatic improvements in health-related physical fitness.

During adolescence, hormonal changes occur that promote dramatc increases in cardiovascular fitness and strength with regular exercise. Fitness in both boys and girls can improve significantly at this age with regular exercise.

Adolescence is a time when the social aspects of sports competition and participation can provide great satisfaction for both the participant and the spectator.

Because adolescence is a social age, and because sports and sporting events are social experiences, sports can be a significant part of the life of the adolescent. However, for a lifetime of exercise, the adolescent should be encouraged to become involved in sports as a participant, as opposed to becoming only a spectator.

Adolescence is a good time to refine lifetime sports skills.

Most skills are learned during childhood, but it is during adolescence that lifetime sports skills are refined. Adolescents acquire the health-related, as well as the skill-related, fitness necessary to refine and become efficient in sports skills. They should be exposed to a variety of skills that can be used for a lifetime.

THE FACTS: PHYSICAL ACTIVITY FOR ADULTS (AGE 17 PLUS)

It is during young adulthood that the greatest potential for high level fitness and physical performance exists.

For many people, "their best level of fitness" will be achieved during the school years because they become less active after this time. However, with continued regular exercise, fitness and performance will reach peak levels in the young adult years.

The activity level of adults does more than contribute to personal fitness.

Parents who are active are more likely to have fit and active children than parents who are sedentary. The regular activity in which adults engage is important to personal fitness, but also appears to promote active lifestyles among children. Active-women role models are especially important for young girls.

Most of the limitations on adults in exercise are self-imposed.

Of those who do not exercise regularly, it is their own lack of fitness from years of inactivity that makes them feel unable to participate. While one of five American adults has been told by a physician to exercise, rarely does a physician suggest inactivity except for short periods of time for a specific ailment.

The "weekend" adult athlete may create, rather than solve, exercise problems.

A "weekend athlete" exercises, sometimes vigorously, only on the weekend. This person may avoid exercise during the "busy" weekdays and attempt to "make up" for a week of inactivity on Saturday or Sunday. To be effective, exercise must be regular (at least three times a week). Vigorous exercise done only one day a week can be dangerous because the weekly exercise is not sufficient to produce improvements in fitness. Thus, the unfit person may be exercising when the body is unprepared.

Being "too busy" is not a good excuse for inactivity.

The most common reason for inactivity among adults is, "I can't take the time." If business or other obligations make such weekday activities as golf or tennis impossible, then walking, jogging, or calisthenics are appropriate. These activities take relatively little time, and if planned properly, can provide important fitness and health benefits. After the inactive person has had a heart attack or some other hypokinetic disease, he or she will have more free time than is really wanted. Exercise may be as important as food and, like meals, should be scheduled on a regular basis.

THE FACTS: PHYSICAL ACTIVITY FOR OLDER ADULTS

Adults are never "too old" to begin exercising.

Physical fitness for old age should begin in the early years in order to enjoy maximum benefits. If this does not occur for one reason or another, a person is never too old to begin exercising. Studies conducted over a period of years indicate that properly planned exercise for older people is not only safe, but that older men and women are *not* significantly different from youth in their abilities to improve fitness through exercise.

Regular exercise can significantly delay the aging process.

One researcher suggests that "exercise is the closest thing to an antiaging pill now available" (Butler 1975, p. 67). Another indicates that continued mental and physical activity is ". . . the only antidote for aging that I know" (Klump 1975, p. 93).

There is a difference between "acquired aging" and "time-dependent aging."

Forced inactivity in young adults can cause losses in function (acquired aging) that are very much like those that are generally considered to occur with aging (time-dependent aging). Studies suggest that aging is a product of a sedentary lifestyle. In Africa, Asia, and South America, where older adults (age sixty-five and older) maintain an active lifestyle, individuals do not "acquire" many of the characteristics commonly associated with aging.

In our culture, middle-aged and older people are encouraged (and sometimes compelled) to reduce their physical activity to the extent that they cannot continue to function on their own.

In our society, the attitude toward older people is often one of overprotection, placing the person in a dependent position. A spokesperson for the President's Council for Physical Fitness and Sports suggests that ". . . a state of physical fitness enhances the quality of life for the elderly by increasing independence. The ability to 'go places and do things' without being dependent on others provides a strong psychological lift which is conducive to good mental health" (Conrad 1975, p. 83).

One famous active American, H. G. "Dad" Miller, a golfer who made a hole in one at the age of 100, said, "We don't stop exercising because we get old—we get old because we stop exercising."

Participation in regular activity has benefits other than improved physical health and fitness.

A general feeling of "well-being" is frequently reported to be one of the real benefits of regular fitness for older people. Nervous tension, which detracts from the feeling of well-being, is a problem for many older adults. One recent study showed that exercise can be more effective than tranquilizers in the treatment of nervous tension in older people.

Participation in regular physical activity has many physical health benefits for the older adult.

In addition to the exercise health benefits already presented in this book, older people can enjoy other benefits from regular physical activity.

1. "The syndrome of shaky hand and tottery gait is responsible in a large degree for much of the dependency of the aged. The treatment (for this condition) is physical exercise" (Swartz 1975, p. 7). (Merely fifteen minutes of exercise a day will not do it, rather there must be a shift from a sedentary to an active lifestyle.)
2. Active older adults have fewer illnesses and fewer early deaths than do those who are inactive.
3. Reductions in physical working capacity, which is the most obvious result of aging, does not occur in older men who engage in regular exercise.
4. Regular exercise can help older adults in the "War with Gravity." With time, if muscles are not kept fit, gravity can cause a "bay window" or protruding abdomen, sagging shoulders, poor posture, and joint immobility. These problems result from lack of strength, muscular endurance, and flexibility, but can be forestalled with regular activity.
5. Bones that are not used tend to decalcify. Regular exercise for older adults can delay bone decalcification.
6. Regular exercise can forestall the decline in circulatory function. In addition, increases in atherosclerosis, blood pressure, and EKG abnormalities that occur with age can be prevented with appropriate, regular exercise.

7. Decreased skeletal muscle, gain in body fat, decrease in oxygen-use capacity, and decreased respiratory function can be postponed with regular exercise.

Older adults can participate in a variety of sports and physical activity.

It has been shown that with appropriate, progressively maintained exercise, older adults can participate in most sports for a lifetime. For example, one eighty-five-year-old man regularly plays handball, and the increased participation in masters (over fifty) classifications in track and field, swimming, and tennis are well documented. Bowling is the leading participant sport in the United States and is well suited for older people. Golf is another activity well suited for older Americans. For those who do not wish to choose a sport, walking, jogging, bicycle riding, swimming, and calisthenics are forms of physical activity that are widely used by people of all ages.

REFERENCES

*American Academy of Pediatrics. "Weight Training and Weight Lifting: Information for the Pediatrician." *Physician and Sportsmedicine* 11(1983):157.

Butler, R. N. "Psychological Importance of Physical Fitness." *Testimony on the Physical Fitness of Older People.* Washington, D.C.: National Association for Human Development, 1975.

Conrad, C. C. "Physical Fitness for the Elderly." *Testimony on the Physical Fitness of Older People.* Washington, D.C.: National Association for Human Development, 1975.

*Corbin, C. B., ed. *A Textbook of Motor Development.* 2d ed. Dubuque, IA: Wm. C. Brown Publishers, 1980.

*Corbin, D. E., and J. Metal-Corbin. *Exercise and Dance for Older Americans.* Dubuque, IA: Eddie Bowers and Co., 1983.

deVries, H. A. *Physiology of Exercise.* 3d ed. Dubuque, IA: Wm. C. Brown Publishers, 1980.

deVries, H. A. "What Research Tells Us Regarding the Contributions of Exercise to the Health of Older People." *Testimony on the Physical Fitness of Older People.* Washington, D.C.: National Association for Human Development, 1975.

Elrich, H. "Exercise and the Aging Process." *Testimony on the Physical Fitness of Older People.* Washington, D.C.: National Association for Human Development, 1975.

Gilliam, T. B., et al. "Physical Activity Patterns Determined by Heart Rate Monitoring in 6–7-Year-Old Children." *Medicine and Science in Sports and Exercise* 13(1981):65.

*Gilliam, T. B. "Exercise Programs for Children: A Way to Prevent Heart Disease?" *Physician and Sportsmedicine* 10(1982):96.

Harris, L., and Associates. *The Perrier Study: Fitness in America.* New York: Great Waters of France, 1975.

Hazzard, W. "Preventative Gerontology: Strategies for Healthy Aging." *Postgraduate Medicine* 72(1983):279.

Hollozy, J. O. "Exercise, Health, and Aging: A Need for More Information." *Medicine and Science in Sports and Exercise* 15(1983):1.

*Klump, F. "Overcoming Overprotection of the Elderly." *Physician and Sportsmedicine* 4(1976):107.

Klump, F. "Physical Activities and Older Americans." *Testimony on the Physical Fitness of Older People.* Washington, D.C.: National Association for Human Development, 1975.

Lamb, L. L. "Staying Youthful and Fit." *Testimony on the Physical Fitness of Older People.* Washington, D.C.: National Association for Human Development, 1975.

Londeree, B. R., and M. L. Moeschberger. "Effects of Age and Other Factors on Maximal Heart Rate." *Research Quarterly for Exercise and Sports* 53(1983):297.

Montoye, H. J., et al. "Bone Mineralization in Tennis Players." *Scandinavian Journal of Sport Science.* 2(1980):26.

Pangrazi, R. P., et al. "From Theory to Practice: A Summary." *Motor Development: Theory into Practice.* Monograph 3(1981):65.

Radd, A. "Statement on Physical Fitness and the Elderly." *Testimony on the Physical Fitness of Older People.* Washington, D.C.: National Association for Human Development, 1975.

Research and Forecasts, Inc. *The Miller Lite Report on American Attitudes toward Sports.* Milwaukee: Miller Brewing Co., 1983.

Spirduso, W. W. "Exercise and the Aging Brain." *Research Quarterly for Exercise and Sports* 54(1983):208.

Swartz, F. C. "Statement on Physical Fitness and the Elderly." *Testimony on the Physical Fitness of Older People.* Washington, D.C.: National Association for Human Development, 1975.

Section Four
PLANNING FOR FITNESS

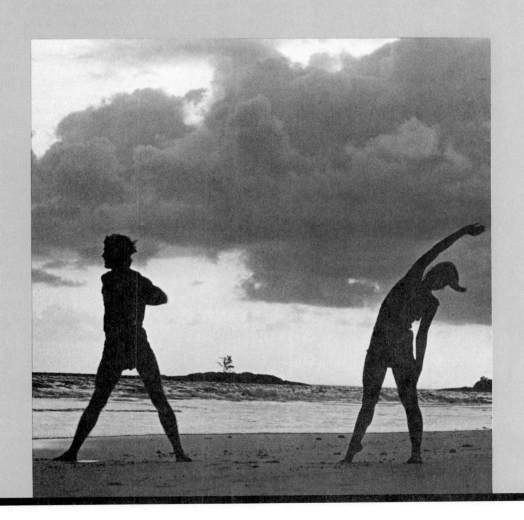

23
ENJOYING EXERCISE

CONCEPT 23

Exercise is for everyone.
No matter who you are, there is some form of
exercise that you can enjoy.

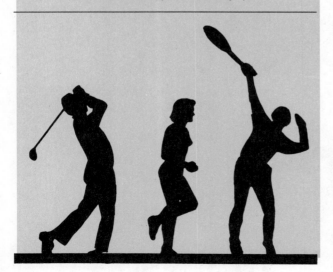

INTRODUCTION

Many adults are now participating in a variety of physical activities on a regular basis. However, roughly 64 million American adults over the age of eighteen do not exercise during their leisure time. Of those who are active, many spend only a few minutes a week participating in the activity. One reason is that many do not enjoy exercise; they feel that it is "just not for them."

All people, regardless of age, sex, or ability, can enjoy exercise if they carefully choose activities, carefully perform the activities, and follow some basic guidelines for making physical activities fun.

TERMS

Catharsis—The release or purifying of emotions; in this book, the release of stress and tension.
Mental Practice—Imagining the performance of a skill without physically performing it.
Overlearning—Practicing a skill over and over many times in an attempt to make the skill a "habit."
"Paralysis by Analysis"—Overanalysis of skill behavior. This occurs when more information is supplied than the performer can really use or when concentration on too many details of a skill results in interference with performance.
Skill Analysis—Breaking the performance of a skill into component parts and critically evaluating each phase of the performance.

THE FACTS

Those who are prepared for exercise are likely to enjoy it.

If you are sore, injured, or afraid of irritating a medical problem, exercise can become something to fear rather than something to enjoy. It is especially important to be well prepared for exercise. Review the information in Concept 4 to make sure you are well prepared before you begin regular exercise. Consider the following factors: be medically ready, start slowly, warm-up before and cool-down after exercise, and dress properly for exercise.

Having a "positive" attitude may enhance exercise enjoyment.

As noted in Concept 1, there are many reasons people do and do not exercise regularly. Earlier you assessed your own feelings concerning physical activity. You may want to reassess them at this time (Lab 24). If you can determine the reasons you especially enjoy activity, you can focus on them, and if you can determine those things you dislike about exercise, you may be able to change your attitudes so that active participation is more enjoyable. All people do not exercise for the same reasons. Consider your feelings about physical activity as you select activities as part of your exercise program.

Selecting "personalized" physical activities can help make exercise more enjoyable.

There is no such thing as a single best activity for all people. Everyone has different abilities and feelings about exercise. There are, however, some factors that are useful in selecting personalized activities *just* for you.

1. *Some people especially enjoy social activities.* If you are a social person, you may want to consider group activities. In fact, exercising in a group can sometimes help motivate you. Friends can encourage each other and make exercise something to enjoy.

2. *Competition may or may not make exercise fun.* Some people especially enjoy competition. Others, however, avoid competitive activities because they have not had success in competitive games. Whatever the benefits of regular physical activity, none should be exaggerated to the point of detracting from a fuller life. Overemphasis on sports can cause anxiety and even a type of neurosis. In fact, people who create stress for themselves by being excessively competitive may increase their chances of getting stress-related diseases.

3. *Variety may enhance exercise enjoyment.* Some people enjoy doing the same basic activities day in and day out, year after year. Others like a change from time to time. You may want to consider a variety of activities to keep your exercise interesting.

4. *Self-criticism may reduce exercise enjoyment.* If an activity makes you angry with yourself, it may decrease your enjoyment of the activity. Improving your skills may reduce self-criticism. Selecting an activity that requires less skill may also reduce self-criticism. Jogging/running, walking, cycling, swimming, and home calisthenics are quite popular because they do not take a great amount of physical skill, and they do not produce as much self-criticism as other activities. It is good to remember that most people are far more critical of their own abilities than they are of the abilities of others.

5. *What "feels good" to others may not "feel good" to you.* Choose an activity that "feels good" to YOU. Sometimes you find yourself doing those things others do, or others want you to do. You should, however, select activities that "feel good" to you, regardless of what others do.

A person does not have to be a "great" performer to enjoy sports and physical activity for a lifetime.

Many Americans discontinue participation in physical activity as they get older because they "are not very good at sports." There are many different types of sports and activities and each requires different abilities. Failure in the past does not mean that you cannot find enjoyment in sports in the future. Some activities require coordination; some require agility and balance; while others may require health-related physical fitness, such as cardiovascular fitness, strength, and flexibility; and still others require daring or ability to use strategy.

Skill proficiency in a sport and selection of a partner of similar ability are both important for the enjoyment of the sporting experience.

Those who have some skill in an activity are more likely to participate in that activity than those with little or no skill. For this reason, it is advisable to practice and perhaps seek instruction to enhance enjoyment of a lifetime activity. People with greater skill are more likely to get involved because they are more likely to be successful. However, there is another way to increase satisfaction from sports participation. Research indicates that you must be 65 to 75 percent as good as your partner if either of you is to enjoy the activity. For this reason, it is not only advisable to improve your skills, but you should find a playing partner or group of similar ability.

There are certain guidelines that can be followed to help you learn and enjoy lifetime sports and physical activities.

1. *When learning a new activity, concentrate on the "general idea" of the skill first; worry about details later.* For example, a diver who concentrates on pointing the toes and keeping the legs straight at the end of a "flip" may land flat on his or her back. To make it "all the way over," concentration should be on merely doing the flip. When the "general idea" is *mastered,* then concentrate on details.

2. *The beginner should be careful not to emphasize too many details at one time.* After the "general idea" of the skill is learned, the learner can begin to focus on the details, one or two at a time. Concentration on too many details at one time may result in "paralysis by analysis." For example, a golfer who is told to keep the head down, the left arm straight, the knees bent, etc., cannot possibly concentrate on all these details at once. As a result, neither the details nor the "general idea" of the golf swing are performed properly.

3. *In the early stages of learning a lifetime sport or physical activity, it is not wise to engage in competition.* Beginners who compete are likely to concentrate on "beating their opponent" rather than learning a skill properly. For example, in bowling, the beginner may abandon the newly learned hook ball in favor of the "sure thing" straight ball. This may make the person more successful immediately, but is not likely to improve the person's bowling skills for the future.

4. *To be performed well, lifetime sports skills must be "overlearned."* Oftentimes, when you learn a new activity, you begin to "play the game" immediately. The best way to learn a skill is to "overlearn it," or practice it until it becomes "habit." Frequently, game situations do not allow you to overlearn skills. For example, it is not a good time to learn the tennis serve during a game since there may be only a few opportunities to serve. For the beginner, it would be much more productive to hit many services (overlearn) with a friend until at least the "general idea" of the serve is well learned. Further, the beginner *should not* sacrifice speed to concentrate on serving for accuracy. Accuracy will come with practice of a properly performed skill.

5. *Once the "general idea" of a skill is learned, an analysis of the performance may be helpful.* Being careful not to overanalyze, it may be helpful to have a knowledgeable person help locate strengths and weaknesses. Movies and videotapes of performances have been shown to be of help to learners.

6. *When "unlearning" an old (incorrect) skill and learning a new (correct) skill, performance may get worse before it gets better.* Frequently, a performer hopes to unlearn a "bad habit" so as to be able to "relearn" the new or correct skill. For example, a golfer with a "baseball swing" may want to learn the correct golf swing. It is important for the learner to understand that the score may worsen during the relearning stage. As the new skill is overlearned, skill will improve, as will the golf score.

7. *Mental practice may aid skill learning.* Mental practice may benefit performance of motor skills, especially if the performer has had previous experience in performing the skill. Mental practice might be used for golf, tennis, and other sports when the performer cannot participate regularly because of weather, business, or lack of time.

8. *For beginners, practicing in front of other people may be detrimental to learning a skill.* Research indicates that an audience may inhibit the beginner's learning of a new sports skill. This is especially true if the learner feels that his or her performance is being evaluated by someone in the audience.

Women can enjoy and benefit from the same activities as men.

In the past, many sports and physical activities were considered appropriate for men only. The benefits of regular exercise are similar for men and women, so there is no reason why both cannot choose to become involved in enjoyable activities.

To enjoy physical activities, give yourself a chance to succeed.

Some people avoid exercise because they see it as a source of failure. If done properly, anyone can succeed in exercise. As already noted, practice and becoming skilled in an activity can enhance your chances of success. Some other suggestions are listed here.

1. *Set realistic goals for yourself.* Set small and realistic goals at first. Gradually increase your expectations, but only after your performance increases. If you set your goals too high, you increase the chances of failure.

2. *Do not equate success with winning.* Sports psychologists agree that one problem experienced by many adults is that they cannot enjoy competitive activities unless they win. Though most people enjoy winning, it must be realized that only 50 percent of the participants in most activities can win. Playing well and enjoying playing also makes you a "winner."

3. *Avoid comparing yourself and your accomplishments to those of other people.*

4. *Consider long-term improvement over time as a successful accomplishment.*

5. *Try using a handicap system when competing with those of unequal skill.* Such systems as those used in golf and bowling can be adapted for other activities to help "even up" the competition.

The "psychological benefits" of exercise can be a source of enjoyment to those who exercise.

Although some studies have indicated that participation in highly competitive athletics may not contribute to character development or good sportmanship, there is evidence that those who are involved in regular exercise throughout life reap both social and emotional benefits. Some of the psychological benefits are presented in Concepts 2 and 3; others are listed here.

1. Participation in physical activity can provide a "catharsis," or emotional release, from the pent-up tensions of regular, daily activity.

2. Physically fit individuals are more likely to try new leisure time activities, which can provide for a meaningful social life.

3. Those who exercise regularly are more likely to have good physical health, which in turn contributes to good mental health.

4. As noted in a previous concept, people who suffer from psychological depression can benefit from regular exercise. Regular exercise and fitness are associated with a sense of well-being. If you exercise regularly, you can develop what some call a "positive addiction" to exercise. A positive addiction is a need to do something for which the consequences are positive.

Movement has meaning.

Movement is a means to many ends. Through movement, you perform work, achieve health and physical fitness, and accomplish other useful objectives. However, movement can be an end in itself. Those who have performed a dance, played a game, or jogged a mile realize that the mere performance of any of these tasks is an accomplishment in itself. Movement and physical activity do not always have to be purposeful; you can derive satisfaction merely from your involvement in a movement experience.

LAB RESOURCE MATERIALS (FOR USE WITH LAB 23, PAGE 251)

CHART 23.1 The Physical Activity Questionnaire

The term "physical activity" in the following statements refers to all kinds of activities, including sports, formal exercises, and informal activities, such as jogging and cycling. Check your answers first, and then read the directions for scoring at the end of the questionnaire.

	Strongly Agree	Agree	Undecided	Disagree	Strongly Disagree	Score
1. Doing regular physical activity can be as harmful to health as it is helpful.	☐	☐	☐	☐	☐	_____
2. One of the main reasons I do regular physical activity is because it is fun.	☐	☐	☐	☐	☐	_____
3. Participating in physical activities makes me tense and nervous.	☐	☐	☐	☐	☐	_____
4. The challenge of physical training is one reason why I participate in physical activity.	☐	☐	☐	☐	☐	_____
5. One of the things I like about physical activity is the participation with other people.	☐	☐	☐	☐	☐	_____
6. Doing regular physical activity does little to make me more physically attractive.	☐	☐	☐	☐	☐	_____
7. Competition is a good way to keep a game from being fun.	☐	☐	☐	☐	☐	_____
8. I should exercise regularly for my own good health and physical fitness.	☐	☐	☐	☐	☐	_____
9. Doing exercise and playing sports is boring.	☐	☐	☐	☐	☐	_____
10. I enjoy taking part in physical activity because it helps me to relax and get away from the pressures of daily living.	☐	☐	☐	☐	☐	_____
11. Most sports and physical activities are too difficult for me to enjoy.	☐	☐	☐	☐	☐	_____
12. I do not enjoy physical activities that require the participation of other people.	☐	☐	☐	☐	☐	_____
13. Regular exercise helps me look my best.	☐	☐	☐	☐	☐	_____
14. Competing against others in physical activities makes them enjoyable.	☐	☐	☐	☐	☐	_____

Score the physical activity questionnaire as follows:

1. For items 1, 3, 6, 7, 9, 11, and 12 give one point for strongly agree, two for agree, three for undecided, four for disagree, and five for strongly disagree. Put the correct number in the blank to the right of these statements.
2. For items 2, 4, 5, 8, 10, 13, and 14 give five points for strongly agree, four for agree, three for undecided, two for disagree, and one for strongly disagree. Put the correct number in the blank to the right of each statement.
3. Determine each of the following seven scores by adding the numbers to the right of the items listed here (two numbers for each score).

			Score
a. Health and fitness score	Item 1 _____ + Item 8	_____ =	_____
b. Fun and enjoyment score	Item 2 _____ + Item 9	_____ =	_____
c. Relaxation and tension release score	Item 3 _____ + Item 10	_____ =	_____
d. Challenge and achievement score	Item 4 _____ + Item 11	_____ =	_____
e. Social score	Item 5 _____ + Item 12	_____ =	_____
f. Appearance score	Item 6 _____ + Item 13	_____ =	_____
g. Competition score	Item 7 _____ + Item 14	_____ =	_____

Total Score _____

4. Determine your total score by adding each of the previous seven scores. Write your total score in the bottom blank.
5. Use Chart 23.2 to determine your rating on each score.

CHART 23.2 Physical Activity Questionnaire Rating Scale

Classification	Each of Seven Scores	Total Score
Excellent	9–10	63–70
Good	7–8	50–62
Fair	6	42–49
Poor	4–5	30–41
Very Poor	3 or less	29 or less

REFERENCES

Appengeller, O. "What Makes Us Run?" Editorial, *New England Journal of Medicine* 305(1983):578.

Corbin, C. B., ed. A Textbook of Motor Development. 2d ed. Dubuque, IA: Wm. C. Brown Publishers, 1980.

Corbin, C. B. "Self-Confidence of Women in Sports." In *Clinics in Sports Medicine: Women in Sports,* edited by W. M. Walsh, Philadelphia: W. B. Saunders, 1984.

*Corbin, C. B., and R. Lindsey. *The Ultimate Fitness Book.* New York: Leisure Press, 1984.

Friedman, M., and R. H. Rosenman. *Type A Behavior and Your Heart.* New York: A. A. Knoph, 1974.

*Glasser, W. *Positive Addiction.* New York: Harper and Row, 1976.

Harris, L., and Associates. *The Perrier Study: Fitness in America.* New York: Great Waters of France, 1979.

Little, J. C. "The Athlete's Neurosis: A Deprivation Crisis." In *Psychology of Running,* edited by M. H. Sacks and M. L. Sacks, Champaign, IL: Human Kinetics, 1981.

Magill, R. *Motor Learning* 2d ed. Dubuque, IA: Wm. C. Brown Publishers, 1980.

Research and Forecasts, Inc. *The Miller Lite Report on American Attitudes toward Sports.* Milwaukee: Miller Brewing Company, 1983.

Riddle, P. K. "Attitudes, Beliefs, Behavioral Intentions and Behaviors of Women and Men toward Regular Jogging." *Research Quarterly for Exercise and Sports* 51(1980):663.

Rossman, J. R. "Participant Satisfaction with Employees Recreation." *Journal of Physical Education, Recreation and Dance* 54(1983):60.

Slava, S., D. R. Laurie, and C. B. Corbin. "The Long-Term Effects of a Conceptual Physical Education Program." *Research Quarterly for Exercise and Sports* 55(1984):161.

24
PLANNING YOUR EXERCISE PROGRAM

CONCEPT 24

In order to get maximal benefits from exercise,

it is essential

that a regular progressive program be planned

to meet the specific needs

of the individual. *

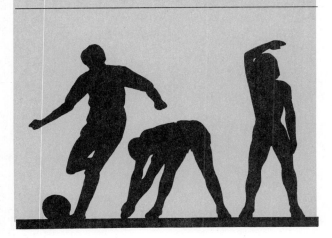

INTRODUCTION

There is no single exercise program best suited to all people. In planning an exercise program it is important to consider your own unique needs and interests. Five steps to fitness program development are presented within this concept to aid you in your planning.

THE FACTS

There are five steps that should be considered in planning your personal exercise program.

Step 1—Identify your personal physical fitness needs.
If you have no medical problems, the first step in program planning is to test your physical fitness on each of the health-related components. Information concerning self-testing and physical fitness rating standards are presented in Labs 6C (cardiovascular fitness); Labs 7A and 7B (strength); Lab 8 (muscular endurance); Lab 9 (flexibility); Labs 10A and 10B (body composition); Labs 16A and 16B (posture and care of the back); and Lab 11 (skill-related physical fitness).

    Fill out the physical fitness profile charts in Lab 24 (Charts 24.1 and 24.2, pages 254–55). These charts will help you identify your fitness strengths and weaknesses. This information can be used to help you select activities for your personal exercise program.

Step 2—Select the activities for your personal fitness program, including those that build all components of physical fitness.
Exercise is an excellent way to achieve physical fitness and one means of attaining good health. However, not all physical activities and exercises are good for developing physical fitness. Once you know what your fitness needs are, make sure you are aware of the facts on which kinds of exercise may best meet your personal needs.

    To be sure that the exercises you select are safe, consult Concepts 4, 17, and 25. To be sure that the activities you select are done often enough (frequency), hard enough (intensity), and long enough (time) to build all parts of fitness, consult Concepts 5, 6, 7, 8, 9, and 10. Information concerning different exercise programs is included in Concepts 12, 13, 14, 15, and 16. The tables that summarize the specific fitness values of different activities will be especially valuable as you try to decide which exercise programs are best for your personal needs (see Tables 12.2 on page 93, 15.1 on page 118, 15.2 on page 119, and 15.3 on page 124).

    After reviewing these tables, write down all of the activities you currently do on a regular basis. Next, write down a list of activities (new ones) that would be especially good for developing those components of fitness in which you need improvement. Use Chart 24.3 on page 255 to write down the activities you plan to do.

Include activities from each of the following three areas: (1) activities you currently do; (2) new activities for specific aspects of fitness; and (3) activities you especially enjoy doing. It is important to include activities that build all parts of fitness, but also to include some activities that you simply enjoy doing. The best program in the world is not good unless you do it. If you don't enjoy it, you won't do it. You may want to check Concept 23 to get some ideas for making exercise more enjoyable.

Remember, no single activity can meet all of your needs. Make sure you select exercise to build each of the physical fitness components.

Step 3—Write it down. Make up a personal weekly exercise schedule.

You are more likely to do your exercise program if you write it down. A sample exercise schedule for a young adult is shown here. Chart 24.4 on page 256 provides you with a chart just like the sample. Using the chart, write out a weekly personal exercise schedule. Be sure you give a specific day and time for each of the activities you listed in step 2.

Step 4—Do it.

Regularity is one of the keys to the success of an exercise program. A "hit or miss" program may turn into no program at all. From the beginning, set aside a specific time and place for your activity. Place a high priority on your exercise time. Don't allow anything to interrupt your exercise schedule. Build your exercise into your daily routine; make it as much a habit as taking a bath or eating regular meals. It is recommended that some form of exercise be done five to six days a week; three days should be the minimum.

Step 5—Periodically evaluate and modify your program.

The weekly program you wrote down in step 5 may be an excellent one. However, as time goes by, your needs, interests, and other factors change. For this reason, you should periodically evaluate and revise your personal program. If you become bored with certain activities, you may wish to drop them and add other new and interesting activities. Changes in the weather, the availability of facilities, and personal schedules may all require program changes. Each time you change your program, follow steps 1 through 4. It is not necessary to do the same program forever; the key is to have a program that meets your current needs and interests.

Warm-Up and Cool-Down Activities

Calf stretcher
toe touch
leg hug
side stretch
two-minute walk

Special Exercises

sit-ups (bent knee)
pectoral stretch
Billigs' exercise
contract-relax routine
before bed when I am tense

Daily Schedules
(List the activities and times of day for each activity.)

Monday

7:00 a.m. "Special exercises"
5:30 p.m. Warm-up
racquetball

Tuesday

7:00 a.m. "Special exercises"
12:30 p.m. Walk after lunch
5:30 p.m. Weight training
(30 minutes)

Wednesday

7:00 a.m. "Special exercises"
5:30 p.m. Warm-up
racquetball

Thursday

7:00 a.m. "Special exercises"
12:30 p.m. Walk after lunch
5:30 p.m. Weight training
(30 minutes)

Friday

7:00 a.m. "Special exercises"
12:30 p.m. Walk after lunch

Saturday

afternoon - walk or swim
Weight training
(30 minutes)

Sunday

"Special exercises" when I get up.
Other exercise if I have no other
plans.
Tennis if I can find a partner
I may take lessons.

Program Evaluation
(Fill in after trying out your program.)

This seems to be working
pretty well. I find I usually
walk rather than swim because
it is inconvenient to go to the pool.
I am taking tennis lessons.

25
EXERCISE AND THE CONSUMER

CONCEPT 25

Caveat Emptor (Let the Buyer Beware)

is a good motto

for the consumer seeking advice or a program

for developing or maintaining fitness.

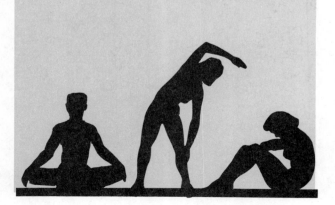

INTRODUCTION

People have always searched for the fountain of youth and the "easy," the "quick," and the "miraculous" route to health and happiness. This search has included the area of physical fitness, especially exercise and weight loss. Because of the popularity of these two subjects, the mass media have made it possible to convey as much *misinformation* as information. All people should seek the truth to protect their health as well as their pocket books. This concept discusses some myths and separates fact from fancy (also review Concepts 17 and 18 regarding drugs and supplements).

TERMS

A.M.A.—Abbreviation for the American Medical Association.

E.C.G.—Abbreviation for the electrocardiograph test of heart function.

F.D.A.—Abbreviation for the Food and Drug Administration: A federal agency that recommends and enforces government regulations regarding certain foods and drugs.

Panacea—A cure-all, a remedy for all ills.

Passive—A type of exercise in which no voluntary muscle contraction occurs; some outside force moves the body part with no effort by the person.

Tonus—The most frequently misused and abused term in fitness vocabularies. It is "the resistance (tension) developed in a muscle as a result of passive stretch of a muscle. Tonus can not be determined by palpation or inspection of a muscle and has little or nothing to do with the voluntary strength of a muscle" (DeLateur 1982).

THE FACTS

Exercise has many benefits, but is not a panacea.

There are many benefits of exercise, many of which have been described throughout this book. However, some media accounts would have you believe the impossible. Those who contemplate beginning a fitness or weight-reducing program are reminded of the following items:

1. The most satisfactory way to lose weight is a combination of caloric reduction and exercise.
2. Exercise will *not* change the size of bony structures (e.g., ankles).
3. Exercise will *not* change the size of glands (e.g., breasts) (however, chest/bust girth may be increased by strengthening chest muscles).

4. Exercise does *not* break up fatty deposits, though it does burn calories and thus fat will eventually be burned.
5. Exercise does *not ensure* good posture or good health, but it does help attain or maintain these attributes.
6. There is *no* such thing as "effortless exercise."

Passive exercise is not effective in weight reduction, spot reduction, increasing strength, or increasing endurance.

Passive exercise or devices come in a variety of forms.

1. *Rolling machines*—These ineffective wooden or metal rollers, operated by an electric motor, roll up and down the body part to which they are applied. They do *not* remove, break up, or redistribute fat.
2. *Vibrating belts*—These wide canvas or leather belts may be designed for the chin, hips, thighs, or abdomen. Driven by an electric motor, they jerk back and forth causing loose tissue of the body part to shake. They do *not* have any beneficial effect on fitness, fat, or figure, and they are potentially harmful if used on the abdomen (especially if used by women during pregnancy, menstruation, or while an I.U.D. is in place). They might also aggravate a back problem.
3. *Vibrating tables and pillows*—Contrary to advertisements, these passive devices will not improve posture, trim the body, reduce weight, or develop muscle "tonus." For some people, vibration can help induce relaxation.
4. *Motor-driven cycles and rowing machines*—Like all mechanical devices that "do the work" for the individual, these motor-driven machines are *not* effective in a fitness program. They may help increase circulation, and some devices may even help maintain flexibility, but they are not as effective as active exercise. *Nonmotorized* cycles and rowing machines are very good equipment for use in a fitness program.
5. *Massage*—Whether done by a masseur or by a mechanical device, massage is passive, requiring no effort on the part of the individual. It can help increase circulation, induce relaxation, help prevent or loosen adhesions, and serve other therapeutic uses when administered in the clinical setting for medical reasons, but massage has *no* useful role in a physical fitness program and will not alter your shape.
6. *Electrical muscle stimulators*—These devices, when applied to a muscle, cause the muscle to contract involuntarily. In the hands of qualified medical personnel, muscle stimulators are valuable therapeutic devices. They should never be used by the layperson and have *no* place in a reducing or fitness program. They can help prevent atrophy in a patient who is unable to move, and they may decrease spasticity and contracture, but they will *not* change your figure/physique. These devices can be harmful and may induce heart attacks, may complicate gastrointestinal, orthopedic, kidney, and other disorders, and may aggravate epilepsy, hernias, and varicose veins.
7. *Weighted belts*—Claims have been made that these belts reduce waists, thighs, and hips when worn for several hours under the clothing. In reality, they do none of these things and have been reported to cause actual physical harm. When used in a progressive resistance program, wristlet, anklet, or laced-on weights can help produce an overload and, therefore, develop strength or endurance.
8. *Inflated, constricting, or nonporous garments*—These garments include rubberized inflated devices ("sauna belts" and "sauna shorts") and garments that are airtight plastic or are rubberized. Evidence indicates that their girth-reducing claims are *unwarranted*. If exercise is performed while wearing such garments, the exercise, *not* the garment, may be beneficial. You can *not* squeeze fat out of the pores *nor* can you melt it!
9. *Figure wrapping*—Some reducing salons, gyms, or clubs advertise that wrapping the body in bandages soaked in a "magic solution" will cause a permanent reduction in body girth. This so-called "treatment" is pure quackery. Tight, constricting bands can temporarily indent the skin and squeeze body fluids into other parts of the body, but the skin or body will regain its original size within minutes or hours. This practice may be dangerous to your health; at least one fatality has resulted.

Exercise, even of an active nature, is not effective in promoting physical fitness unless it meets the appropriate threshold of training.

Some popular literature suggests that only a few minutes of exercise a day is necessary to develop total physical fitness. Research, however, indicates that total fitness (cardiovascular fitness, strength, muscular endurance, flexibility, and desirable body composition) can be attained only through considerable effort. As mentioned previously, exercise must be of sufficient frequency (daily or every other day), intensity and time (at least fifteen to thirty minutes *each* day you exercise) for it to be effective. Programs that "promise" complete fitness but do not meet the necessary levels for frequency, intensity, and time of exercise should be strongly questioned.

Sauna, steam, and whirlpool baths are not effective in weight reduction nor in the prevention and cure of colds, arthritis, bursitis, backaches, sprains, and bruises.

The effect of such baths is largely psychological, although some temporary relief from aches and pains may result from the heat. The same relief, though, can be had by sitting in a tub of hot water at home. Sauna and steam baths are potentially dangerous for the elderly and persons suffering from diabetes, heart disease, or high blood pressure. They should not be used within an hour after eating or while under the influence of alcohol or such drugs as anticoagulants, stimulants, hypnotics, narcotics, or tranquilizers.

Contrary to some claims, Hatha Yoga is not a good program for developing physical fitness.

Some advocates of Hatha Yoga claim that regular practice of the asanas (positions) will bring about improved flexibility, grace, serenity, relaxation, sleep, vitality, endurance, circulation, strength and firmness of muscles, strength of vital organs and glands, taut, smooth skin, ideal body weight, recovery, alertness, clarity of mind; even cure arthritis, the common cold, diabetes, gall stones, menstrual disorders, piles, and maintain good vision and hearing.

There is no scientific evidence to support most of these claims. Hatha Yoga will not help you lose weight, trim inches, remove flab, improve endurance, maintain proper circulation, strengthen glands and organs, or improve complexion. Neither will it cure diseases.

Hatha Yoga is considered useful for improving flexibility, although some of the positions are contraindicated (see Concept 7). Hatha Yoga is also useful in reducing stress reactions and in neuromuscular relaxation. In some cases, it may be effective in lowering blood pressure in hypertensives. If a person has very weak muscles to begin with, mild strengthening and muscular endurance may develop from assuming and holding the positions.

DMSO (dimethyl sulfoxide) should not be used for muscular soreness or strains and sprains sustained during exercise.

DMSO is an industrial solvent that has been widely used since the 1940s. However, athletes, fitness buffs, and arthritics have been using it for aches and pains. The Food and Drug Administration has approved it for humans only for the treatment of a bladder problem, and even that use has been questioned. A controlled study has shown that it is ineffective in tendonitis, yet the superstitious belief in its healing power persists. The short-term side effects of DMSO when absorbed through the skin include disturbed vision, headache, nausea, diarrhea, and burning on urination. Long-term effects include clouding of the eye lens and allergic reactions. Until researchers can establish the efficacy of its use, DMSO should *not* be applied to the skin.

You can usually tell the difference between an expert and a quack because a quack does not use scientific methods.

Some of the ways to identify quacks, frauds, and rip-offs is to look for these clues:

1. They do not use the scientific method of controlled experimentation that can be verified by other scientists.
2. To a large extent, they use testimonials and anecdotes to support their claims rather than scientific methods.
3. They advise you to buy something you would not otherwise have bought.
4. They have something to sell.
5. They claim *everyone* can benefit from the product or service they are selling.
6. They promise "quick," "miraculous" results.
7. They may claim there is a conspiracy against them by "bureaucrats," "organized medicine," the F.D.A., the A.M.A., and other experts and governmental bodies.
8. Their credentials may be irrelevant to the area in which they claim expertise.
9. They use scare tactics, such as "if you don't do this, you will die of a heart attack"; or they may switch to being a sympathetic friend who wants to share with you a "new discovery."
10. They may quote from a scientific journal or other legitimate source, but they misquote or quote out of context to mislead you; or they mix a little bit of truth with a lot of fiction.
11. They may cite research or quote from individuals or institutions that have questionable reputations for scientific truth.
12. They may claim it is a "new discovery" (usually it is said to have originated in Europe).
13. The product or organization name is often similar to that of a famous person or creditable institution (e.g., the Mayo Diet had no connection with the Mayo clinic).

Getting rid of cellulite does not require a special diet or device, as some books and advertisements insist.

Cellulite is ordinary fat with a fancy name. You do not need a special treatment, a special device, or special anything to get rid of it. Fat is fat. To decrease fat, eat fewer calories and exercise more.

"Spot reducing," or losing fat from a specific location on the body, is not possible. It is a fallacy.

When you exercise, calories are burned and fat is recruited from all over the body in a genetically determined pattern. You can not selectively exercise, bump, vibrate, or squeeze the fat from a particular spot. If you were flabby to begin with, local exercise could strengthen the local muscles, causing a change in the contour and the girth of that body part. But exercise affects the muscles, not the fat on that body part. General aerobic exercises are the most effective for burning fat, but you cannot control where the fat comes off.

The consumer who plans to purchase equipment should keep in mind certain guidelines to get the most for the money.

The following suggestions will help you select equipment:

1. Unless you are wealthy or just like to collect gadgets, but there is no need to buy a lot of exercise equipment. A complete fitness program can be carried out with *no* equipment. If you learn to depend upon equipment, you may eventually feel like you cannot exercise unless you are at home or at a gym.
2. If you do not like jogging or swimming, and you hate calisthenics, then the minimal equipment you may want to consider is a bicycle (regular or stationary), treadmill, or rowing machine for cardiovascular fitness; and a set of weights, pulleys, or isokinetic device for strength and endurance.
3. Consult an expert if you want to know if a product is effective. Individuals with college or university degrees in physical education, physical therapy, corrective therapy, and exercise physiology should be able to give you good advice.
4. Buy from a well-established, reputable company that will not disappear overnight and will back up warranties.

It is not necessary to join a club, spa, or salon to develop fitness, but if you are considering joining such an establishment, make your choice with care.

The consumer should observe these precautions before becoming a member of a club, spa, or salon.

1. Do not expect "miraculous" results as advertised.
2. Be prepared to haggle over prices and to resist a very hard sell for a long-term contract.
3. Choose a no-contract, pay-as-you-go establishment if possible. Otherwise, choose the shortest term contract available.

4. If there is a contract, read the fine print carefully and look for:
   a. the interest rate;
   b. "confession of judgment" clauses waiving your right to defend yourself in court;
   c. noncancelable clauses;
   d. "holder-in-due-course" doctrines allowing the establishment to sell your note to a collection agency;
   e. a waiver of the establishment's liability for injury to you on the premises.
5. Consult with an independent expert if you have questions about the programs offered by the establishment.
6. Do not accept diets, drugs, or food supplements from the club. Your physician will prescribe these if they are needed.
7. You do not have to conform to the program they suggest for you. Do not perform dangerous exercises, passive exercises, or participate in fraudulent "treatments." Choose only those activities that meet the criteria explained in this book.
8. Refuse to be pestered by solicitations for new members.
9. Make a trial visit to the establishment during the hours when you would normally expect to use the facility to determine if it is open, if it is overcrowded, if the equipment is available, if the attendants are selling rather than assisting, and if you would enjoy the company of the other patrons.
10. Determine the qualifications of the personnel, especially the individual responsible for programming you. Are they an expert as defined previously?
11. Make certain it is a well-established facility that will not disappear overnight.
12. Check its reputation with the Better Business Bureau.
13. Investigate the programs offered by the Y, local colleges and universities, and municipal park and recreation departments. These agencies often have excellent fitness classes at lower prices than commercial establishments and usually employ qualified personnel. For weight loss, investigate franchised clubs, such as Weight Watchers or Tops, or affiliate with a hospital-based program.

LAB RESOURCE MATERIALS
(FOR USE WITH LAB 25, PAGE 257)

CHART 25.1 Exercise Evaluation*

	Yes	No
1. Is the article or book written by an expert as defined in Concept 25?	☐	☐
2. Does the exercise employ the overload principle?	☐	☐
3. Does it employ the progression principle?	☐	☐
4. Does it employ the F.I.T. principle?	☐	☐
5. Does it employ the principle of specificity?	☐	☐
6. Is it a safe exercise?	☐	☐
7. Is it an "active" exercise in which your own muscles contract?	☐	☐
8. Are the benefits claimed for the exercise reasonable?	☐	☐
9. Are the authors trying to help you (rather than selling a product)?	☐	☐
10. Do they refrain from using terms such as "quick," "miraculous," "tone," "remove fat," "new discovery," or other gimmick words?	☐	☐

*If in doubt, you may seek an expert's opinion on some of these questions.

REFERENCES

Barrett, S. *The Health Robbers*. Philadelphia: George F. Stickley Co., 1980.

Bennet, W., and Gurin, J. *The Dieter's Dilemma*. New York: Basic Books, 1982.

Berland, T., and Editors of *Consumer Guide*. *Rating the Diets*. Skokie, IL: *Consumer Guide*, 1974.

Consumer Union, *Health Quackery*. Orangeburg, NY: Consumer Reports Books, 1980.

Delateur, B. J. "Therapeutic Exercise to Develop Strength and Endurance" in *Krusen's Handbook of Physical Medicine and Rehabilitation*, edited by Kotlke, Stillman, and Lehman. 3d ed. Philadelphia: W. B. Saunders Co., 1982.

*Herbert, V., and S. Barrett. *Vitamins and Health Foods: The Great American Hustle*. Philadelphia: George F. Stickley Co., 1981.

Kuntzleman, C. T., and Editors of *Consumer Guide*. *Rating the Exercises*. New York: William Morrow and Company, Inc., 1978.

Lindsey, R. "Figure Wrapping: Would You Believe It?" *Fitness for Living* (1972).

Lindsey, R. *The Reducing Racket*. Unpublished book manuscript.

Maryland Center for Public Broadcasting. *Consumer Survival Kit: No Sweat*. Owings Mills, MD: Maryland Center for Public Broadcasting.

Percy, E. C., and J. D. Carson. "The Use of DMSO in Tennis Elbow and Rotator Cuff Tendonitis: A Double Blind Study." *Medicine and Science in Sports and Exercise* 13(1981):215.

Pollock, M. L., J. H. Wilmore, and S. M. Fox. *Health and Fitness through Physical Activity*. New York: John Wiley and Sons, 1978.

Romero, J. A., T. L. Sanford, R. V. Schroeder, and T. D. Fahey. "The Effect of Electrical Stimulation of Normal Quadriceps on Strength and Girth." *Medicine and Science in Sports and Exercise* 14(1982):194.

"The Truth about DMSO." *Harvard Medical School Health Letter* VI(1981).

THE LABS

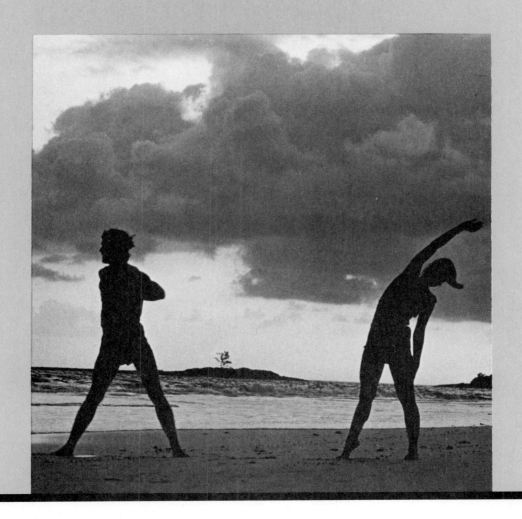

LAB 1

A PHYSICAL ACTIVITY
QUESTIONNAIRE

NAME _____ SECTION _____ DATE _____

PURPOSE

The purposes of this laboratory are:

1. To evaluate your feelings concerning physical activity.
2. To determine the specific reasons why you do or do not participate in regular physical activity.

PROCEDURE

1. Read each of the fourteen items in the physical activity questionnaire, Chart 1.1 shown here or in the Lab Resource Materials for Concept 1 on page 6.
2. After each statement, check one box indicating whether you strongly agree, agree, disagree, or strongly disagree with it. If you are unsure of your answer, check "undecided."
3. When all fourteen items have been answered, use the scoring procedure in Chart 1.1 to score the physical activity questionnaire.

RESULTS

1. After you have determined seven different physical activity questionnaire scores and a total score, use Chart 1.2, also in the Lab Resource Materials for Concept 1, to determine your rating for each score.
2. Check your rating for each of the seven reasons for exercising and your total score here.

	Ex	Good	Fair	Poor	VP
Health and fitness	☐	☐	☐	☐	☐
Fun and enjoyment	☐	☐	☐	☐	☐
Relaxation and tension release	☐	☐	☐	☐	☐
Challenge and achievement	☐	☐	☐	☐	☐
Social	☐	☐	☐	☐	☐
Appearance	☐	☐	☐	☐	☐
Competition	☐	☐	☐	☐	☐
Total Score	☐	☐	☐	☐	☐

Read Concept 1 before completing this section. The seven scores on the physical activity questionnaire should reflect your reasons for participating in physical activity.

1. Do you think that the scores on which you were rated "excellent" or "good" accurately reflect the reasons why you might do regular exercise? Explain.

2. Do you think that the scores on which you were rated "poor" or "very poor" might be reasons why you would avoid physical activity? Explain.

3. Those who are physically active should score high on the total score. Is your total score a good reflection of your overall attitude about physical activity? Explain.

CHART 1.1 The Physical Activity Questionnaire

The term "physical activity" in the following statements refers to all kinds of activities, including sports, formal exercises, and informal activities, such as jogging and cycling. Check your answers first, and then read the directions for scoring, found in the Lab Resource Materials for Concept 1 on page 7.

	Strongly Agree	Agree	Undecided	Disagree	Strongly Disagree	Score
1. Doing regular physical activity can be as harmful to health as it is helpful.	☐	☐	☐	☐	☐	_____
2. One of the main reasons I do regular physical activity is because it is fun.	☐	☐	☐	☐	☐	_____
3. Participating in physical activities makes me tense and nervous.	☐	☐	☐	☐	☐	_____
4. The challenge of physical training is one reason why I participate in physical activity.	☐	☐	☐	☐	☐	_____
5. One of the things I like about physical activity is the participation with other people.	☐	☐	☐	☐	☐	_____
6. Doing regular physical activity does little to make me more physically attractive.	☐	☐	☐	☐	☐	_____
7. Competition is a good way to keep a game from being fun.	☐	☐	☐	☐	☐	_____
8. I should exercise regularly for my own good health and physical fitness.	☐	☐	☐	☐	☐	_____
9. Doing exercise and playing sports is boring.	☐	☐	☐	☐	☐	_____
10. I enjoy taking part in physical activity because it helps me to relax and get away from the pressures of daily living.	☐	☐	☐	☐	☐	_____
11. Most sports and physical activities are too difficult for me to enjoy.	☐	☐	☐	☐	☐	_____
12. I do not enjoy physical activities that require the participation of other people.	☐	☐	☐	☐	☐	_____
13. Regular exercise helps me look my best.	☐	☐	☐	☐	☐	_____
14. Competing against others in physical activities makes them enjoyable.	☐	☐	☐	☐	☐	_____

LAB 2

PHYSICAL FITNESS

NAME _____   SECTION _____   DATE _____

Read Concept 2 before completing this lab.

PURPOSE

The purposes of this laboratory session are:

1. To help you identify different components of physical fitness. It is hoped that, through participation, you can begin to see the differences between the various aspects of physical fitness, especially the differences between health-related and skill-related physical fitness.
2. To help you to gain insight into the importance of various components of physical fitness and to help you evaluate them.

PROCEDURE

Perform all of the physical fitness stunts described in Chart 2.1 in the Lab Resource Materials for Concept 2 on pages 13–15. Record your results in the appropriate blank opposite each item.

RESULTS

The stunts you tried are *not* good tests of fitness, but attempting the stunts may help you see that fitness is not just one thing; it is many different things. Circle the numbers of the skill-related and health-related items you passed.

Skill-related   1   2   3   4   5   6

Health-related   7   8   9   10   11

CONCLUSIONS AND IMPLICATIONS

To really test your fitness, you will need to do many of the tests presented later in this text. Therefore, you may be especially interested in testing yourself in those areas in which you did not do well on various stunts. For your own well-being, you should want to do well in health-related fitness.

How did you do on the health-related fitness stunts?

Were you surprised or disappointed in your performance? Explain.

How did you do on the skill-related fitness stunts?

Were you surprised or disappointed in your performance? Explain.

LAB 3

HYPOKINETIC DISEASES
AND CONDITIONS

NAME _____ SECTION _____ DATE _____

Read Concept 3 before completing this lab.

PURPOSE

The purpose of this lab is to help you determine the extent to which hypokinetic diseases and conditions have a direct effect on your life at the present time.

PROCEDURE

1. Answer each of the questions in Chart 3.1 shown here and in the Lab Resource Materials for Concept 3.
2. Determine the extent to which hypokinetic diseases or conditions directly affect your life by scoring each question on Chart 3.1.

CHART 3.1 Incidence of Hypokinetic Diseases and Conditions

Listed here are various hypokinetic diseases and conditions. In the column beside each condition or disease, place a check (✔) if you possess it, if one of your close relatives possesses it, or if one of your close friends possesses it. Close relatives are the four or five people you consider to be closest to you, whether parents, brothers, sisters, grandparents, spouse, or children. Close friends are the four or five nonrelatives you care about most. You need not live close to the individual to classify him or her as a close friend or relative.

The Hypokinetic Disease or Condition	Self	Close Relative	Close Friend
1. Heart disease	☐	☐	☐
2. High blood pressure	☐	☐	☐
3. Back pain or problems	☐	☐	☐
4. Overfat or obese	☐	☐	☐
5. Ulcer	☐	☐	☐
6. Diabetes	☐	☐	☐
7. Insomnia	☐	☐	☐
8. Depression	☐	☐	☐
9. Type A personality	☐	☐	☐
Column Totals	_____	_____	_____

RESULTS

What is your own personal hypokinetic disease score? _____

What is the hypokinetic disease score of your relatives? _____

What is the hypokinetic disease score of your friends? _____

CONCLUSIONS AND IMPLICATIONS

How would you interpret the significance of these scores?

LAB 4A

PHYSICAL ACTIVITY READINESS

NAME _____ SECTION _____ DATE _____

Read Concept 4 before completing this lab.

PURPOSE

The purpose of this lab is to help you determine your physical readiness for participation in a program of regular exercise.

PROCEDURE

1. Read the directions on "The PAR-Q and You" form shown here or in the Lab Resource Materials for Concept 4.
2. Answer each of the seven questions on the form.
3. If you answered yes to one or more of the questions, follow the directions in the lower left hand corner of the PAR-Q regarding medical consultation.
4. If you answered no to all seven questions, follow the directions at the lower right hand corner of the PAR-Q.
5. Note: It is important that you answer all questions honestly. The PAR-Q is a scientifically and medically researched preexercise selection device. It complements exercise programs, exercise testing procedures, and the liability considerations attendant with such programs and testing procedures. PAR-Q, like any other preexercise screening device will misclassify a small percentage of prospective participants, but no preexercise screening method can entirely avoid this problem.

RESULTS

Circle the number of yes answers that you had.   0   1   2   3   4   5   6   7

CONCLUSIONS AND IMPLICATIONS

Based on the answers to the PAR-Q, should you seek medical consultation before beginning or modifying your exercise program? Why or why not?

PHYSICAL ACTIVITY READINESS QUESTIONNAIRE (PAR-Q)*
A Self-administered Questionnaire for Adults

PAR Q& YOU

PAR-Q is designed to help you help yourself. Many health benefits are associated with regular exercise, and the completion of PAR-Q is a sensible first step to take if you are planning to increase the amount of physical activity in your life.

For most people physical activity should not pose any problem or hazard. PAR-Q has been designed to identify the small number of adults for whom physical activity might be inappropriate or those who should have medical advice concerning the type of activity most suitable for them.

Common sense is your best guide in answering these few questions. Please read them carefully and check the ☑ YES or NO opposite the question if it applies to you.

YES NO

☐☐ 1. Has your doctor ever said you have heart trouble?

☐☐ 2. Do you frequently have pains in your heart and chest?

☐☐ 3. Do you often feel faint or have spells of severe dizziness?

☐☐ 4. Has a doctor ever said your blood pressure was too high?

☐☐ 5. Has your doctor ever told you that you have a bone or joint problem such as arthritis that has been aggravated by exercise, or might be made worse with exercise?

☐☐ 6. Is there a good physical reason not mentioned here why you should not follow an activity program even if you wanted to?

☐☐ 7. Are you over age 65 and not accustomed to vigorous exercise?

If You Answered

YES to one or more questions

If you have not recently done so, consult with your personal physician by telephone or in person BEFORE increasing your physical activity and/or taking a fitness test. Tell him what questions you answered YES on PAR-Q, or show him your copy.

programs
After medical evaluation, seek advice from your physician as to your suitability for:
● unrestricted physical activity, probably on a gradually increasing basis.
● restricted or supervised activity to meet your specific needs, at least on an initial basis. Check in your community for special programs or services.

NO to all questions

If you answered PAR-Q accurately, you have reasonable assurance of your present suitability for:
● A GRADUATED EXERCISE PROGRAM - A gradual increase in proper exercise promotes good fitness development while minimizing or eliminating discomfort.
● AN EXERCISE TEST - Simple tests of fitness (such as the Canadian Home Fitness Test) or more complex types may be undertaken if you so desire.

postpone
If you have a temporary minor illness, such as a common cold.

* Developed by the British Columbia Ministry of Health. Conceptualized and critiqued by the Multidisciplinary Advisory Board on Exercise (MABE).
Reference: PAR-Q Validation Report, British Columbia Ministry of Health, May, 1978.
* Produced by the British Columbia Ministry of Health and the Department of National Health & Welfare.

THE WARM-UP AND
COOL DOWN

NAME _____   SECTION _____   DATE _____

Read Concept 4 before completing this lab.

PURPOSE

The purpose of this lab is to familiarize you with a sample group of exercises which can be used as a warm-up or cool down for aerobic types of workout.

PROCEDURE

Perform the exercises described in Concept 4 on page 29.

RESULTS

1. In which of the stretches did you feel the most tightness?

	None	Moderate	Severe
Calf stretcher	☐	☐	☐
Toe touch	☐	☐	☐
Leg hug	☐	☐	☐
Side stretch	☐	☐	☐
Cardiovascular warm-up	☐	☐	☐

2. Did you notice an increase in heart rate during the cardiovascular warm-up? Yes _____   No _____

Do you think that the sample warm-up and cool down program is adequate for the activities you plan to do as part of your exercise program? Yes ____ No ____ Explain.

Does the sport or activity you plan to do involve vigorous use of muscles not stretched by this program? Yes ____ No ____ If so, what muscles or body parts will need special attention?

Read Concept 14 and consider those stretching exercises for your warm-up and cool down.

LAB 6A

COUNTING THE PULSE
(HEART RATE)

NAME _____ SECTION _____ DATE _____

Read Concept 6 before completing this lab.

PURPOSE

The purpose of this lab is to learn to count the pulse at two different locations: the carotid artery on the side of the neck and the radial artery near the wrist.

PROCEDURE

1. Practice counting the number of pulses felt for a given period of time at both the carotid and radial locations (see the Lab Resource Materials for Concept 6 on page 42 for directions on counting the pulse). Use a clock or watch to count for 15, 30, and 60 seconds. To establish your heart rate in beats per minute, multiply the fifteen-second count by four, and multiply your thirty-second count by two.
2. Practice locating your carotid and radial pulses quickly. This is important when trying to count your pulse after exercise. Counting pulse after exercise will be necessary in Labs 6B and 6C.
3. Practice counting the pulse of another person using both the wrist and carotid locations (do not use your thumb).

RESULTS

Record the various pulse counts you have taken in the spaces provided here.

Carotid Pulse Count (Self)   Heart Rate Per Minute

_____ 15 seconds × 4 _____

_____ 30 seconds × 2 _____

_____ 60 seconds × 1 _____

Carotid Pulse Count (Partner)   Heart Rate Per Minute

_____ 15 seconds × 4 _____

_____ 30 seconds × 2 _____

_____ 60 seconds × 1 _____

Radial Pulse Count (Self)   Heart Rate Per Minute

_____ 15 seconds × 4 _____

_____ 30 seconds × 2 _____

_____ 60 seconds × 1 _____

Radial Pulse Count (Partner)   Heart Rate Per Minute

_____ 15 seconds × 4 _____

_____ 30 seconds × 2 _____

_____ 60 seconds × 1 _____

CONCLUSIONS AND IMPLICATIONS

1. Which pulse did you find easiest to locate on yourself?
   (circle one)   Carotid   Radial

2. Which pulse did you find easiest to locate on your partner?
   (circle one)   Carotid   Radial

3. Which of the two methods of counting pulse do you think you would prefer to use when counting heart rate? Why?

LAB 6B

THE CARDIOVASCULAR
THRESHOLD OF TRAINING

NAME _____ SECTION _____ DATE _____

Read Concept 6 before completing this lab.

PURPOSE

The purposes of this laboratory session are:

1. To understand the threshold of training and target zone concepts.
2. To establish a personal minimal cardiovascular threshold of training.
3. To establish a personal target zone for cardiovascular fitness.
4. To determine the specific jogging speed necessary to elevate your heart rate to threshold of training and target zones.

PROCEDURE

To determine your cardiovascular fitness threshold and target heart rates, you will use your age and your resting heart rate.

1. Find your threshold of training and target zone on Chart 6B.1 in the Lab Resource Materials for Concept 6 on page 42 and record it in the results section.
2. Select a partner.
3. One partner should run a quarter-mile, then the other partner should count her or his heart rate at the end of the run (use carotid pulse). Try to run at a rate that you think will keep the rate of the heart above the threshold of training and in the target zone. Use fifteen-second pulse counts and multiply by four to get heart rate in beats per minute (bpm). Record the bpm in the results section.
4. Repeat, alternating roles, the second person running, and the first person counting heart rate. Record the results.
5. Repeat the test so each person runs a second time. Record the results.

RESULTS

What is your threshold of training (from Chart 6B.1)? _____ bpm

What is your target zone (from Chart 6B.1)? _____ bpm

What was your heart rate for the first run? (15 sec.) $\times$ 4 = _____ bpm

What was your heart rate for the second run? (15 sec.) $\times$ 4 = _____ bpm

How fast do you have to run to get your heart rate above threshold and into the target zone? Check the following.

First run speed just right ☐   Faster than the second run ☐

Faster than the first run ☐   Slower than the second run ☐

Slower than the first run ☐   Second run speed just right ☐

Do you achieve the cardiovascular threshold in the course of a normal day? Yes ____   No ____

What would you suggest for yourself as a regular (3–5 times per week) cardiovascular exercise program? Explain.

LAB 6C

EVALUATING CARDIOVASCULAR FITNESS

NAME _____ SECTION _____ DATE _____

Read Concept 6 before completing this lab.

PURPOSE

The purposes of this laboratory are:

1. To acquaint you with several methods for evaluating cardiovascular fitness.
2. To help you evaluate and rate your own cardiovascular fitness.

PROCEDURE

Perform one or more of the three cardiovascular fitness tests described in the Lab Resource Materials for Concept 6 on pages 43–44. Determine your ratings on the test(s) using the rating charts provided.

RESULTS

Record the information obtained from taking the cardiovascular fitness test(s) (one or more) in the space provided.

Twelve-Minute Run

Distance _____ miles

The Step Test

Heart Rate _____ bpm

The Bicycle Test

Workload _____ kpm

Heart Rate _____ bpm

Weight _____ lbs.

Weight in kg _____

(Weight in lbs. $\div$ 2.2)

ml/O_2/kg _____

Rating _____   Rating _____   Rating _____

CONCLUSIONS AND IMPLICATIONS

If you took more than one test, were the ratings for each similar? Yes ____ No ____ If so, were the ratings what you expected them to be?

If not, which rating do you think is really the best indicator of your cardiovascular fitness? Explain.

If you took only one test, do you think your rating is really representative of your cardiovascular fitness? Yes ____ No ____ Explain.

Is your cardiovascular fitness what you think it ought to be? Yes ____ No ____ Explain.

LAB 7A

EVALUATING ISOTONIC STRENGTH

NAME _____   SECTION _____   DATE _____

Read Concept 7 before completing this lab.

PURPOSE

The purpose of this lab is to evaluate the strength of four muscle groups and the power of one muscle group using self-testing stunts.

PROCEDURE

1. Attempt the stunt groups found on in the Lab Resource Materials for Concept 7 on pages 52–54 in any order, starting with the stunt in each grouping that you believe is the most difficult one that you are likely to pass. If you can pass it, try the next most difficult one in that same group, etc. If you cannot pass it, try the next lower stunt, etc.
2. Give yourself the score of the highest difficult stunt that you can pass in each group.
3. Record your scores and your rating in the results section of this report.
4. When you have attempted all of the tests, perform the isotonic exercises in Concept 13.

RESULTS

Record your score for each part of the test and then total all scores.

Best score, test I   _____

Best score, test II   _____

Best score, test III   _____

Best score, test IV   _____

Best score, test V   _____

Total score   _____

Find your total score on the rating chart (Chart 7A.1 in the Lab Resource Materials for Concept 7).
Rating _____

What muscle groups are involved in each of the tests?

Test I _____

Test II _____

Test III _____

Test IV _____

Test V _____

CONCLUSIONS AND IMPLICATIONS

Explain what the tests told you about the strength (or power) of those muscles, and suggest some exercises you might do to correct any strength deficiencies.

LAB 7B

EVALUATING ISOMETRIC STRENGTH

NAME _____ SECTION _____ DATE _____

Read Concept 7 before completing this lab.

PURPOSE

The purpose of this lab is to evaluate the isometric strength of three muscle groups.

PROCEDURE

All individuals will be tested on four isometric strength tests: right-hand grip strength, left-hand grip strength, back strength, and leg strength. Testing procedures are found on page 54 of the Lab Resource Materials for Concept 7. Measurements are made with dynamometers. If time permits, three measures on each test should be taken and the best score recorded in the results section of this report.

RESULTS

Isometric strength scores:

Grip strength (right)   Grip strength (left)   Back strength   Leg strength

_____   _____   _____   _____

Total score = _____ (Sum of four figures)

   To determine strength per pound of body weight, divide the *total score* by the body weight.

Strength per lb. of wt. _____

   Check your rating on isometric strength using Chart 7B.1 in the Lab Resource Materials for Concept 7. Note that there are different charts for men and women.

	Ex	VG	Fair	Poor	VP
Right grip	☐	☐	☐	☐	☐
Left grip	☐	☐	☐	☐	☐
Back strength	☐	☐	☐	☐	☐
Leg strength	☐	☐	☐	☐	☐
Total score	☐	☐	☐	☐	☐
Per lb./wt.	☐	☐	☐	☐	☐

Which hand is the strongest? Right _____ Left _____ What is your explanation for this?

Do you need to perform strength exercises (regularly)? Yes _____ No _____ Explain.

What isometric exercises would you choose to correct any deficiencies found today?

What other muscle groups might also need isometric strength exercises?

LAB 8

EVALUATING MUSCULAR ENDURANCE

NAME _____ SECTION _____ DATE _____

Read Concept 8 before proceeding with this lab.

PURPOSE

The purpose of this laboratory session is to evaluate the muscular endurance of two muscle groups.

PROCEDURE

1. Perform the sitting tucks and chins or bent arm hang tests described in the Lab Resource Materials for Concept 8 on page 58.
2. When not being tested, perform muscular endurance exercises in Concept 13 using a light weight and many repetitions.
3. Record your tests scores in the results section. Determine and record your rating from Charts 8.1 and 8.2 in the Lab Resource Materials for Concept 8.

RESULTS

Record your scores below.

Sitting tucks _____ Chins _____ Hang _____ (seconds)

Check your ratings below.

	Ex	VG	Fair	Poor	VP
Sitting tucks	☐	☐	☐	☐	☐
Chins	☐	☐	☐	☐	☐

For Those Who Cannot Do a Chin

Hang ____

Making progress toward a chin ____

Do you need to regularly perform muscular endurance exercises? Yes ____ No ____ Explain.

What muscular endurance exercises do you think you need to perform regularly?

LAB 9
EVALUATING FLEXIBILITY

NAME _____   SECTION _____   DATE _____

Read Concept 9 before completing this lab.

PURPOSE

The purpose of this laboratory session is to evaluate your flexibility in several joints.

PROCEDURE

1. Take the flexibility tests as outlined on pages 66–67 of the Lab Resource Materials for Concept 9.
2. Record your scores in the results section.
3. Use Chart 9.1 in the Lab Resource Materials for Concept 9 to determine your rating on both of the flexibility tests, then record your rating in the results section.

RESULTS

	Test 1	Test 2	Test 3 Right up	Left up
What were your flexibility scores?	_____	_____	_____	_____
Record your flexibility ratings.	_____	_____	_____	_____

Do any of these muscle groups need stretching:

	Yes	No
Back of the thighs and knees (hamstrings)	☐	☐
Calf muscles	☐	☐
Lower back (lumbar region)	☐	☐
Front of right shoulder	☐	☐
Back of right shoulder	☐	☐
Front of left shoulder	☐	☐
Back of left shoulder	☐	☐
Most of the body	☐	☐

Note: Read Concept 14 and Lab 14 for exercises to improve your flexibility.

Discuss your current flexibility and your flexibility needs for the future.

LAB 10A

EVALUATING BODY FATNESS

NAME _____   SECTION _____   DATE _____

Read Concept 10 before completing this lab.

PURPOSE

The purposes of this laboratory session are:

1. To determine your percent body fat using skinfold measurements.
2. To learn to use skinfold calipers to make skinfold measurements.

PROCEDURE

1. Read the directions for using skinfold calipers and for making skinfold measurements on pages 75–78 in the Lab Resource Materials for Concept 10.
2. If possible, observe a demonstration of the proper procedures for measuring skinfolds at each of the different body locations. For men use the chest, abdominal, and thigh skinfolds. For women use the triceps, the iliac crest, and the thigh locations.
3. If possible have an expert make the appropriate skinfold measurements on you.
4. Work with a partner (if possible). Take several measurements on your partner at each of the different skinfold locations. Allow your partner to make the appropriate measurements on you.
5. Record each of the measurements in the results section. Add the three skinfold measurements together. Locate the sum of your three skinfolds on the appropriate chart in the Lab Resource Materials for Concept 10 (Chart 10A.1 for males and Chart 10A.2 for females). Look for the sum of your skinfolds in the column under your age, and find your percent body fat in the left-hand column of the chart.
6. Rate your fatness using Chart 10A.3 in the Lab Resource Materials for Concept 10.
7. If different types of calipers are available to you, practice making measurements with each type so that comparisons of results can be made.
8. Remember that body composition measurements are confidential information. Care should be taken not to discuss another person's results. Results are intended to be useful information to the people being tested. Take the skinfold testing seriously.

RESULTS

Write your skinfold measurements in the blanks on the following page. In some cases, all measurements may not be possible. Provide results for the tests you were able to complete. List the name of the caliper used.

Males

Measurement by Partner #1

Chest _____ mm

Abdominal _____ mm

Thigh _____ mm

Sum _____

Percent Body Fat _____

Rating _____

Caliper Used _____

Measurement by the Instructor (if possible)

Chest _____ mm

Abdominal _____ mm

Thigh _____ mm

Sum _____

Percent Body Fat _____

Rating _____

Caliper Used _____

Females

Measurement by Partner #1

Tricep _____ mm

Iliac Crest _____ mm

Thigh _____ mm

Sum _____

Percent Body Fat _____

Rating _____

Caliper Used _____

Measurement by the Instructor (if possible)

Tricep _____ mm

Iliac Crest _____ mm

Thigh _____ mm

Sum _____

Percent Body Fat _____

Rating _____

Caliper Used _____

CONCLUSIONS AND IMPLICATIONS

If you did more than one assessment of fatness, were the results consistent? Yes ____ No ____ Explain.

Is your fatness (percent body fat) what you would like it to be? Yes ____ No ____ Explain.

What do you think you will need to do in the future to obtain or maintain a desirable level of body fatness?

LAB 10B

DETERMINING "DESIRABLE" BODY WEIGHT

NAME _____   SECTION _____   DATE _____

Read Concept 10 and complete Lab 10A before doing this lab.

PURPOSE

The purposes of this laboratory session are:

1. To determine "desirable" weight.
2. To compare two different methods for determining "desirable" body weight.

PROCEDURE

1. Measure percent of body fat (see Lab 10A), height (without shoes), and weight (with indoor clothing and shoes).
2. Determine your frame size (small, medium, or large) using the following procedure. With a tape, measure the smallest girth of your wrist just above the styloid process (boney bump on wrist). Pull the tape snugly (but not tight enough to indent the skin) around the wrist as you measure. Look up your frame size on Chart 10B.1 in the Lab Resource Materials for Concept 10 on page 78.
3. Determine your "desirable" weight. Locate your height in inches on the left and your frame size across the top. Find the "desirable" weight for your height and your frame size. Men are to use Chart 10B.2 and women are to use Chart 10B.3, both of which are in the Lab Resource Materials for Concept 10 on page 79.
4. Determine your "desirable" weight using a different procedure. Locate your actual body weight on the left and your percent body fat (from lab 10A) across the top. Find the "desirable" weight for your weight and body fat percent. Men are to use Chart 10B.4; women are to use Chart 10B.5. Both charts are also in the Lab Resource Materials for Concept 10.

RESULTS

Record your scores below:

Percent body fat _____

Weight (indoor clothes) _____ lbs.

Height (without shoes) _____ inches

Frame size   small _____ medium _____ large _____

"Desirable" weight (Chart 10B.2 or 10B.3) _____ lbs.

"Desirable" weight (Chart 10B.4 or 10B.5) _____ lbs.

Is your "desirable" weight as determined from the height-weight chart what it should be? Yes _____ No _____

Is your "desirable" weight as determined from percent body fat what it should be? Yes _____ No _____

Is there a discrepancy between your answers? Yes _____ No _____

Using both "desirable" weights, what body weight do you feel you should maintain for the rest of your life?

_____ lbs. Explain.

LAB 11

EVALUATING SKILL-RELATED PHYSICAL FITNESS

NAME _____   SECTION _____   DATE _____

Read Concept 11 before completing this lab.

PURPOSE

The purpose of this lab is to help you evaluate your own skill-related fitness, including agility, balance, coordination, power, speed, and reaction time. This information may be of value in planning your personal fitness program and in deciding which sports may be best, based on your own skill-related fitness.

PROCEDURE

1. Read the directions for each of the skill-related fitness tests presented on pages 83–86 of the Lab Resource Materials for Concept 11.
2. Take as many of the tests as possible, given the time and equipment available.
3. Be sure to warm up before and to cool down after the tests.
4. It is alright to practice the test before trying them. However, you should decide ahead of time which trial you will use to test your skill-related fitness.
5. After completing the tests, write your scores in the appropriate places in the results section.
6. Determine your rating for each of the tests from the rating charts on pages 84–86 of the Lab Resource Materials for Concept 11.

RESULTS

Place a check in the box for each of the tests you completed.

Agility (Illinois run)   ☐

Balance (Bass test)   ☐

Coordination (stick test)   ☐

Power (vertical jump)   ☐

Reaction time (stick drop test) ☐

Speed (three-second run)   ☐

Record your score and rating (from Charts 11.1–11.6 in the Lab Resource Materials) in the following spaces.

	Score	Rating	
Agility	_____	_____	(Chart 11.1, page 84)
Balance	_____	_____	(Chart 11.2, page 84)
Coordination	_____	_____	(Chart 11.3, page 85)
Power	_____	_____	(Chart 11.4, page 85)
Reaction Time	_____	_____	(Chart 11.5, page 85)
Speed	_____	_____	(Chart 11.6, page 86)

Discuss your strengths and weaknesses in skill-related fitness. How do you account for your strengths and what can you do to eliminate your weaknesses?

Certain sports require different components of skill-related fitness. Which sports seem best suited for you, given your skill-related fitness? Why?

LAB 12A

JOGGING/RUNNING

NAME _____ SECTION _____ DATE _____

Read Concept 12 before completing this lab.

PURPOSE

The purposes of this laboratory session are:

1. To give you an opportunity to experience one type of jogging program that can be used to develop and maintain cardiovascular fitness.
2. To acquaint you with basic jogging techniques.

PROCEDURE

1. Work with a partner and evaluate each other on jogging techniques. Make notes on Chart 12A.1, describing any problems in your technique.
   a. Stand twenty yards in front of your partner while he/she jogs toward you; watch his/her arm and leg swing and foot placement.
   b. Jog along ten yards behind your partner while he/she is jogging and watch for arm and leg swing and foot placement.
   c. Stand ten yards to one side as your partner jogs past you; watch for body position and foot placement.
2. Using proper jogging technique, jog for fifteen minutes at your own individual cardiovascular threshold of training. (Determine your threshold of training using Chart 6B.1, page 42.)

RESULTS

What is your cardiovascular target zone heart rate? _____ bpm

What was your heart rate after your fifteen-minute jog? _____ bpm

During your fifteen-minute jog, did you reach your threshold of training? Yes ____ No ____

With the help of a partner, note on Chart 12A.1 any problems in technique. Read the information on jogging in Concept 12, page 92, before evaluating your partner's jogging technique.

CHART 12A.1 Jogging Technique

Source of Problem	Severity of Problem	
	None	Needs Work
Foot placement		
Length of stride		
Arm movement		
Body position		

CONCLUSIONS AND IMPLICATIONS

Do you have any jogging problems? Yes _____ No _____

Do you feel that you can solve any jogging problems you have? Yes _____ No _____ Explain.

Do you think that jogging is a good type of exercise for you? Yes _____ No _____ Explain.

Do you think that you will include jogging in your exercise program for use in later life? Yes _____ No _____ Explain (if different from answer above).

LAB 12B

AEROBIC EXERCISE

NAME _____ SECTION _____ DATE _____

Read Concept 12 before completing this lab.

PURPOSE

The purposes of this laboratory session are:

1. To give you an opportunity to experience an aerobic exercise program that is particularly good for developing cardiovascular fitness and aiding in fat reduction.
2. To familiarize you with an exercise program that can be continued as part of your normal life's pattern.

PROCEDURE

1. Select a sample program for some form of aerobic exercise and try it out. It can be earning points by Cooper's Aerobics Chart (page 90), trying the sample calisthenics program (pages 90–91), or performing a sample of any of the other forms of aerobic exercise discussed in Concept 12. For example, you may want to try a sample dance aerobic program, jumping rope, or a circuit weight program.

   If you would like to repeat this lab more than once doing a different activity each time, space is provided in the results section for four descriptions.

RESULTS

Name the activity in which you participated and briefly describe and evaluate your experience.

Activity name _____

Time spent _____ minutes

Description and evaluation

Activity name _____

Time spent _____ minutes

Description and evaluation

Activity name _____

Time spent _____ minutes

Description and evaluation

Activity name _____

Time spent _____ minutes

Description and evaluation

CONCLUSIONS AND IMPLICATIONS

Did you like the aerobic activity you performed? Yes ____   No ____

Do you think you would choose to make these activities part of your regular exercise program?

Yes ____   No ____   Explain.

If you did more than one aerobic activity, which one did you most enjoy? _____

Why?

Of all the aerobic activities discussed in Concept 12, which ones do you think you would be most likely to include in your regular exercise program?

LAB 13

WEIGHT TRAINING
FOR STRENGTH

NAME _____ SECTION _____ DATE _____

Read Concepts 7 and 13 before proceeding with this lab.

PURPOSE

1. To give you an opportunity to experience a sample weight training program.
2. To acquaint you with a strength program that can be continued throughout your life.
3. To give you an opportunity to experiment with free weights and weight machines.

PROCEDURE

1. Read Concepts 7 and 13 to learn about strength and weight training.
2. Perform the exercises in Chart 13.1. Choose either the exercises listed in the free weight column, or if you have machines, perform those listed in the weight machine column. If you have both free weights and machines available, choose one or the other, but not both. Use the weight amount listed in the final columns. (The names and numbers of the exercises shown in Chart 13.1 correspond with the detailed exercises shown in Concept 13 on pages 99–104.)
3. Use three sets of six repetitions with the load suggested. Note: This is only a "get acquainted" program and is not suitable for adoption as your regular program. (Follow the guidelines in Concept 7 to develop your own program to fit your individual needs.)

CHART 13.1 Sample Weight Training Program

Free Weight Exercise		Weight Machine Exercise		Suggested Weight	
Name	**Number**	**Name**	**Number**	**Men**	**Women**
shoulder shrug	1	hamstring curl	9	40	30
military press	2	bench press	6	50	40
half squat	3	leg press	3	60	40
biceps curl	4	biceps curl	1	40	30
triceps curl	5	triceps curl	5	25	15
toe raises	6	ankle press	7	60	40
pull to chin	7	seated rowing	2	30	30

RESULTS

Which program did you choose? _____

List the muscles you exercised by choosing this program.

How long did it take you to complete the program? _____ minutes

CONCLUSIONS AND IMPLICATIONS

Were the weights suggested too heavy for you? Yes ____ No ____

Were the weights suggested too light for you? Yes ____ No ____

Briefly give your reaction to weight training as a potential program for you to use to develop your own fitness (strength or endurance).

LAB 14

STRETCHING EXERCISES

NAME _____   SECTION _____   DATE _____

Read Concept 14 before performing this lab. Also review Concept 9.

PURPOSE

The purposes of this laboratory session are:

1. To give you an opportunity to experience different flexibility exercises.
2. To acquaint you with a flexibility program that can be continued throughout your life.
3. To help you distinguish between the types of flexibility exercises.

PROCEDURE

1. Review the stretching exercises in Concept 14 on pages 112–16.
2. Perform each of the exercises to your threshold (or slightly below if you have not been exercising regularly). See Concept 9 for your threshold level.

RESULTS

List the exercises that you found difficult to perform.

Which exercises would you include in your stretching program?

Explain.

LAB 15A

SPORTS FOR PHYSICAL FITNESS

NAME _____   SECTION _____   DATE _____

Read Concept 15 before completing this lab.

PURPOSE

The purpose of this lab is to explore the use of different sports as a part of your personal physical fitness program.

PROCEDURE

1. On Chart 15A.1 check any of the ten most popular sports in America in which you especially like to participate.
2. Also on Chart 15A.1 check the sports in which you feel you are skilled (ones in which you have enough skill to enjoy playing a game without more lessons).
3. Perform, in or out of class, two or three different sports, each for thirty to sixty minutes.
4. On Chart 15A.2 in the results section list the sports you played.
5. Check the fitness parts in which you think you improved by playing the sport. Refer to Table 15.1, page 118.

RESULTS

CHART 15A.1 Sports Interests and Proficiencies

Sports	Check If Interested	Check If Proficient
Bowling	☐	☐
Tennis	☐	☐
Basketball	☐	☐
Softball	☐	☐
Baseball	☐	☐
Golf	☐	☐
Volleyball	☐	☐
Football	☐	☐
Frisbee	☐	☐
Table Tennis	☐	☐
Others (write in)		
_____	☐	☐
_____	☐	☐

CHART 15A.2 Fitness Benefits

Benefit	Sport _____	Sport _____	Sport _____
Cardiovascular fitness	☐	☐	☐
Flexibility	☐	☐	☐
Body leanness	☐	☐	☐
Strength	☐	☐	☐
Muscular endurance	☐	☐	☐

CONCLUSIONS AND IMPLICATIONS

Which sports do you feel you might actually include in your exercise program for a lifetime?

Why did you choose them?

LAB 15B

PREPLANNED
AND ANAEROBIC EXERCISE
PROGRAMS

NAME _____   SECTION _____   DATE _____

Read Concept 15 before completing this lab.

PURPOSE

The purposes of this laboratory session are:

1. To give you an opportunity to experience an exercise program that is either preplanned or anaerobic in nature.
2. To familiarize you with an exercise program that can be continued as part of your normal life's pattern.

PROCEDURE

1. Select a sample preplanned or aerobic program as presented in Concept 15 and try it out. As an alternative, you may want to try a dance exercise or aqua dynamics program with which you are familiar.
2. In the results section, briefly describe the program you chose to do.
3. You may want to repeat this lab more than once, doing a different activity each time. Space is provided in the results section should you choose to try more than one preplanned or anaerobic activity.

RESULTS

List the activity you tried in the space provided and briefly discuss what you did during that exercise period.

Activity name _____

Time spent _____ minutes

Description

Activity name _____

Time spent _____ minutes

Description

Activity name _____

Time spent _____ minutes

Description

Activity name _____

Time spent _____ minutes

Description

CONCLUSIONS AND IMPLICATIONS

Did you enjoy the activity you performed? Yes _____ No _____

Do you think you would choose to make this activity part of your regular exercise program?

Yes _____ No _____ Why or why not?

If you did more than one preplanned or anaerobic program, which one did you like best? _____

Why?

Of all of the preplanned and anaerobic exercise programs, which ones do you think you would be most likely to include as a part of your own personal exercise program?

LAB 16A

CARE OF THE BACK

NAME _____   SECTION _____   DATE _____

Read Concept 16 before completing this lab.

PURPOSE

The purposes of this laboratory session are:

1. To determine if you have some muscle imbalance.
2. To learn exercises suitable for preventing or correcting lordosis and preventing or alleviating low back pain.

PROCEDURE

1. Secure a partner and administer the muscle tests to each other. (Details appear on page 133 of the Lab Resource Materials for Concept 16.) Record results of tests in the results section of this laboratory.
2. Determine your rating by circling your score on Chart 16A.1.
3. Under the direction and supervision of the instructor, perform the following exercises described in Concept 16, numbers 9–16 and 19. For the purposes of this lab, two or three repetitions of each exercise will be adequate.

RESULTS

1. On test 1, was there evidence that you have shortened lumbar and/or hip flexor muscles?

   Yes ____   No ____

2. a. On test 2, was there evidence that you have short hamstrings? Yes ____   No ____

      Right ____   Left ____

   b. Was there evidence of short lumbar and/or hip flexor muscles? Yes ____   No ____

3. On test 3, was there evidence that you have short hip flexors? Yes ____   No ____   Right ____   Left ____

4. Did you have difficulty performing any of the exercises? Yes ____   No ____

   If so, which ones?

5. What was your overall rating from Chart 16A.1?

CHART 16A.1 Rating for Back ''Health''

Rating	Number of Tests Passed
Good	3
Fair	2
Poor	0–1

CONCLUSIONS AND IMPLICATIONS

If you had difficulty with any of the exercises, explain why. If you had no difficulty, how do you account for it?

What specific exercises might help correct your muscle imbalance?

LAB 16B
POSTURE

NAME _____ SECTION _____ DATE _____

Read Concept 16 before completing this lab.

PURPOSE

The purposes of this laboratory session are as follows:

1. To learn to recognize postural deviations and thus become more posture conscious.
2. To determine your posture limitations in order that a preventive and corrective program might be instituted.

PROCEDURE

1. Wear as little clothing as possible (bathing suits are recommended) and remove shoes and socks.
2. Work in groups of two or three, with one person acting as the "subject" while partners serve as "examiners"; alternate roles.
   a. Stand by a vertically hung plumb line.
   b. Use Chart 16B.1 found in the Lab Resource Materials for Concept 16 on page 134. Check any deviations and indicate their severity as follows: 0—none; 1—slight; 2—moderate; 3—severe.
   c. Total the score and determine your posture rating from Chart 16B.2 in the Lab Resource Materials.
3. If time permits, perform the following ten exercises from Concept 16: 1–8; 18, 19.

RESULTS

Record your posture score. _____

Record your posture rating. _____

CONCLUSIONS AND IMPLICATIONS

Were you aware of the deviations that were found? Yes ____   No ____

List the deviations that were moderate or severe.

What program will you follow to build or maintain good posture? List specific exercises from Concept 16 that you need to practice to correct each deviation you have identified.

If you were checked as having some of the symptoms of scoliosis, see your instructor for a more thorough examination and possible referral to a physician.

LAB 17

CONTRAINDICATED EXERCISES

NAME _____   SECTION _____   DATE _____

Read Concept 17 before performing this lab.

PURPOSE

To experience some good exercises that can accomplish the purpose of some of the "bad" exercises.

PROCEDURE

1. In your textbook, turn to Concept 17 and look at the pictures of the "bad" exercises. Then look up the "good" exercises (listed in the column labeled "good" alternative exercises in Table 17.1 on page 140).
2. For each "bad" exercise listed in Table 17.1, there is one (or more) good alternative to accomplish the same purpose, but without harm to the individual. Perform the "good" exercises listed.

RESULTS

1. List the names of the "bad" exercises that you have used in the past.

   _____   _____   _____
   _____   _____   _____
   _____   _____   _____
   _____   _____   _____

2. List the "good" exercises you have used in the past.

   _____   _____   _____
   _____   _____   _____
   _____   _____   _____
   _____   _____   _____

CONCLUSIONS AND IMPLICATIONS

List the names of the exercises that you will use as alternatives in the future.

LAB 18A

NUTRITION AND
ACTIVITY ASSESSMENT

NAME _____ SECTION _____ DATE _____

Read Concept 18 before proceeding with this lab.

PURPOSE

1. To determine your average daily caloric intake.
2. To determine your average daily caloric output.
3. To determine the nutritional quality of your weekly diet.
4. To predict the effect of your weekly caloric balance on your weight.

PROCEDURE

1. a. Record your daily intake of food and beverages on the diet record form (Chart 18A.1) on page 147 in the Lab Resource Materials for Concept 18 (duplicate as many copies as necessary) for at least seven consecutive days. Indicate the name of the food, the amount or size of serving, the number of calories (see Appendix B).
   b. Place one check mark in one square (in the column labeled nutrition) for each serving of each food group for each day.
   c. Total the number of calories consumed each day.
2. a. Use the activity record form (Chart 18A.2), also located in the Lab Resource Materials for Concept 18, to record the number of minutes and hours you spent in activity each day for the same consecutive seven days. Duplicate as many copies as necessary.
   b. Compute the number of calories used by referring to Appendix C. Multiply the number of minutes by the number of calories (per minute per pound) times your weight in pounds.

RESULT

Summarize as follows:

Caloric input: Average number of calories consumed per day
                   $7 \sqrt{\text{week's total}}$ _____

Caloric output: Average number of calories burned per day
                   $7 \sqrt{\text{week's total}}$ _____

Caloric surplus: Difference between input and output ($+$ or $-$)   _____

1. If one pound of fat is equivalent to 3,500 calories, how long will it take you to gain ($+$) or lose ($-$) one pound if you continue these dietary and activity habits? (surplus or deficit $\sqrt{3,500}$) _____ days.

2. Did you eat the recommended number of servings of the four food groups each day? Yes ____ No ____
    Or over the 7 days, did you eat the total recommended servings of each food group? Yes ____ No ____

3. Based on these results, what should you do about your nutrition and activity?

LAB 18B

EXERCISE FOR CALORIC EXPENDITURE

NAME _____   SECTION _____   DATE _____

Read Concept 18 and perform Lab 18A before performing this lab.

PURPOSE

1. To experience an exercise period that will expend as many calories as are consumed at lunch.
2. To relate caloric consumption (eating) with caloric expenditure (exercise).

PROCEDURE

1. From Chart 18A.1, record the foods you consumed at lunch on the first day recorded on your diet record. (If you did not eat lunch on that day, use the record for day 2.) Also record the number of calories for each food item. Copy this data on the chart below.

Lunch Food—Day 1	Calories	Check Off

2. From Appendix C select one or more activities and perform them until you have expended enough calories to equal the lunch item with the fewest calories. When you have done that, check off that item on the list, then continue to exercise until another food item has been equaled in caloric output and check that item off, until all have been checked off or until the period is ended.
3. To determine the number of calories expended (in number 2), multiply the hours or fractions of hours, times the number of calories, times the body weight. If you wish to convert the caloric cost of an exercise into minutes rather than hours, divide the calories-per-hour-per-pound by sixty to obtain calories-per-minute-per-pound.

RESULTS

1. How many calories were you able to expend ("burn") in this exercise period? _____
2. Were you able to expend enough calories to burn off your lunch? Yes _____ No _____

CONCLUSIONS AND IMPLICATIONS

Do you feel that you exercise enough each day to expend the calories you consume each day?

Yes ____   No ____

Do you believe that exercise alone is the method you could use to balance your caloric input and output?

Yes ____   No ____

Explain your answer.

LAB 19A

EVALUATING YOUR STRESS LEVEL

NAME _____ SECTION _____ DATE _____

Read Concept 19 before proceeding with this lab.

PURPOSE

The purpose of this laboratory is to help you evaluate your current stress level. Research shows that when people are stressed, they are more susceptible to certain diseases. Some stress-related diseases include heart disease, ulcers, allergy, hypertension, and insomnia. People with high stress levels need to recognize the causes and effects of stress and need to consider ways of avoiding, coping with, or reducing stress. Exercise and relaxation are important therapeutic techniques.

PROCEDURE

1. Look at the list of stressful life events in Table 19A.1 shown here or in the Lab Resource Materials for Concept 19. Circle the score opposite each event that seems to be true for you.
2. Add up all the circled numbers. Record your score.
3. Look up your rating on Chart 19A.1.
4. Interpret your score by answering the questions below.

CHART 19A.1 Rating Scale for Stressful Life Events

Rating	Score	Implication for Illness
Low stress	150 or less	This indicates that a person has a 35% chance of getting a stress-related disease in the next two years.
Moderate stress	151–300	51% chance of getting a stress illness in the next two years.
High stress	301 or higher	80% chance of getting a stress illness in the next two years.

RESULTS

Record your score on the test _____

What is your rating? _____

CONCLUSIONS AND IMPLICATIONS

What does your stress score suggest in terms of possible future illnesses?

Do you feel that you need to do anything to reduce your stress level? Yes ＿＿ No ＿＿ Explain.

TABLE 19A.1 Stressful Life Events*

Event	Score	Event	Score
Death of spouse	100	Son/daughter leaves home	29
Divorce	73	Trouble with in-laws	29
Marital separation	65	Outstanding achievement	28
Jail term	63	Spouse begins work	26
Death of close family member	63	Start or finish school	26
Personal injury/illness	53	Change in living conditions	25
Marriage	50	Revision of personal habits	24
Fired from work	47	Trouble with boss	23
Marital reconciliation	45	Change in work hours, conditions	20
Retirement	45	Change in residence	20
Change in family member's health	44	Change in schools	20
Pregnancy	40	Change in recreational habits	19
Sex difficulties	39	Change in church activities	19
Addition to family	39	Change in social activities	18
Business readjustment	39	Mortgage/loan under $10,000	18
Change in financial status	38	Change in sleeping habits	16
Death of close friend	37	Change in number of family gatherings	15
Change in number of marital arguments	35	Change in eating habits	15
Mortgage/loan over $10,000	31	Vacation	13
Foreclosure of mortgage/loan	30	Christmas season	12
Change in work responsibilities	29	Minor violation of law	11

*This test is adapted from the Social Readjustment Scale devised by Thomas Holmes and Richard Rahe. Used by permission.

LAB 19B
RESPONSE TO STRESS

NAME _____ SECTION _____ DATE _____

Read Concept 19 before proceeding with this lab.

PURPOSE

The purposes of this laboratory session are as follows:

1. To observe and compare the effects of a variety of physical and emotional stressors.
2. To determine the amount of time required to recover from the stressors.

PROCEDURE

(You may work with or without a partner)

1. Determine your resting heart rate by counting your pulse for thirty seconds, and record on the chart provided.
2. Next, you will be exposed to a stressor by your instructor.*
3. Immediately after the stressor is applied, count your heart rate for thirty seconds and record.
4. Three minutes or more will be allowed for recovery, and then another stressor will be applied.
5. Continue to record your thirty-second pulse after each stressor.

*Note: Instructor should refer to the Instructor's Manual.

RESULTS

Resting heart rate: Self ____bpm   Partner ____ bpm

Record stressors and thirty-second heart rates on the chart that follows.

Stressor	Heart Rate	
	Self	Partner
1. _____	_____	_____
2. _____	_____	_____
3. _____	_____	_____
4. _____	_____	_____
5. _____	_____	_____

Graph your own heart rate on the following graph by drawing a line across each bar at the level of your heart rate. Then darken the bar with a pen or felt marker.

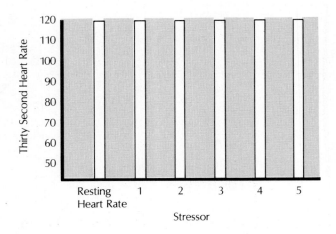

CONCLUSIONS AND IMPLICATIONS

Indicate which type of stressor affected your heart rate most by checking the appropriate blank.
Emotional ____ Physical ____
Did you react more to the stressor than did your partner? Yes ____ No ____
Could your present (last twenty-four hours) physical or emotional state affect the way you responded today?
Yes ____ No ____
Explain.

Could your previous experiences affect the way you responded to these stressors? Yes ____ No ____
Explain.

LAB 19C

EVALUATING NEUROMUSCULAR TENSION

NAME _____ SECTION _____ DATE _____

Read Concept 19 before proceeding with this lab.

PURPOSE

The purpose of this laboratory session is to learn to recognize signs of excess tension in yourself and in others by symptomatic mannerisms and by manually testing ability to relax. If time permits, perform the relaxation exercises in Concept 19 before executing the lab.

PROCEDURE

1. Choose a partner. Designate one partner as the subject and the other as the tester. Alternate roles.
2. The subject should lie supine in a comfortable position and try to consciously relax as described in Concept 19. This may be done alone, or the instructor may wish to direct the entire group in this procedure.
3. The tester should kneel beside the subject's right hand and remain very still and quiet while the subject is concentrating.
4. After five minutes have elapsed, the tester should observe the subject for signs of tension according to the procedures outlined on page 155 of the Lab Resource Materials for Concept 19.
5. Record your relaxation rating in the results section of this report. (Use Chart 19C.2 in the Lab Resource Materials for Concept 19.)

RESULTS

What is your tension score? _____
What is your relaxation rating? _____

CONCLUSIONS AND IMPLICATIONS

Were you aware of your own tensions? Yes ____ No ____
Was it more difficult to relax than you expected? Yes ____ No ____
Did your awareness of your partner make it more difficult to concentrate? Yes ____ No ____
Can you concentrate on your breathing without altering its rhythm? Yes ____ No ____

Could you learn to consciously release muscular tension with additional practice? Yes ____ No ____

Could you learn to release tension while sitting or standing with your eyes open? Yes ____ No ____

Do you think your score today is typical of your normal tension level? Yes ____ No ____

What implications does this concept have for you in terms of your daily life (e.g., sleeping, studying, taking exams, performing on stage, etc.).

LAB 19D

RELAXING TENSE MUSCLES

NAME _____   SECTION _____   DATE _____

Read Concept 19 before completing this lab.

PURPOSE

To learn how to relax tense muscles.

PROCEDURE

(*Note:* You will need your textbook to do this lab.)

Part I
Perform each of the exercises in the box in Concept 19, page 152.

Part II

1. Sit in a chair or lie on your back in a quiet, nondistracting atmosphere while you are learning this relaxation technique (later you will want to be able to use the technique in public, everyday situations, while you are at work, or any time you are under stress.) Get as comfortable as possible.
2. Do the contract-relax routine for relaxation in Concept 19, page 153. Contract the muscles to a moderate level of tension (do not use maximum contractions) as you inhale for five to seven seconds. Study where you are feeling the tension. Try to keep the tension isolated to the designated muscle group without allowing it to spill over to other muscles. Use the dominant side of body first; repeat on the nondominant side.
3. Next, release the tension completely, instantly relaxing the muscles, and exhale. Extend the feeling of relaxation throughout your muscles for twenty to thirty seconds before contracting again. Think of relaxing expressions like "warm," "calm," "peaceful," and "serene."
4. If time permits, you should practice each muscle group two to five times (until tension is gone) before going on to the next group. In a class situation, you may have time for only one trial. For home practice, do the routine twice a day for fifteen minutes.

Did you find the relaxation exercises relaxing? Yes ＿＿ No ＿＿

Do you think you would find them useful as part of your normal daily routine? Yes ＿＿ No ＿＿ Explain.

Did you find the contract-relax exercise routine relaxing? Yes ＿＿ No ＿＿

Do you think you would find them useful as part of your normal daily routine? Yes ＿＿ No ＿＿

Explain.

LAB 21

ASSESSING HEART DISEASE RISK FACTORS

NAME _____ SECTION _____ DATE _____

Read Concept 21 before completing this lab.

PURPOSE

The purpose of this lab is to assess your risk of developing coronary heart disease.

PROCEDURE

1. Complete the ten questions on the heart disease risk factor questionnaire (shown here or on page 164 in the Lab Resource Materials for Concept 21) by circling the answer that is most appropriate for *you*.
2. Look at the top of the column for each of your answers. In the space provided at the right of each question, write down the number of risk points for that answer.
3. Determine your unalterable risk score by adding the risk points for questions 1, 2, and 3.
4. Determine your alterable risk score by adding the risk points for questions 4 through 10.
5. Determine your total heart disease risk score by adding the scores obtained in steps 3 and 4.
6. Look up your risk ratings on Chart 21.1 (page 165 in the Lab Resource Materials for Concept 21).

RESULTS

Write your risk scores and risk ratings in the appropriate blanks below.

	Score	**Rating**
Unalterable risk	_____	_____
Alterable risk	_____	_____
Total heart disease risk	_____	_____

CONCLUSIONS AND IMPLICATIONS

The higher your score on the heart disease risk questionnaire, the greater your heart disease risk. Which of the risk factors do you need to try to control to reduce your risk of heart disease? Why?

Heart Disease Risk Factor Questionnaire*

Circle the appropriate answer to each question.

			Risk Points			
		1	**2**	**3**	**4**	**Score**
Unalterable Factors						
1.	How old are you?	30 or less	31–40	41–54	55+	_____
2.	Do you have a history of heart disease in your family?	none	grandparent with heart disease	parent with heart disease	more than one with heart disease	_____
3.	What is your sex?	female		male		_____
					Total Unalterable Risk Score	_____
Alterable Factors						
4.	What is your percent of body fat?	F = 17%↓ M = 14%↓	22%↓ 17%↓	27%↓ 19%↓	28%↑ 20%↑	_____
5.	Do you have a high-fat diet?	no	slightly high in fat	above normal in fat	eat a lot of meat, fried and fatty foods	_____
6.	What is your blood pressure? (systolic or upper score)	120↓	121–135	136–155	155↑	_____
7.	Do you have other hypokinetic diseases?	no	ulcer	diabetes	both	_____
8.	Do you exercise regularly?	4–5 days a week	3 days a week	less than 3 days a week	no	_____
9.	Do you smoke?	no	cigar or pipe	less than 1/2 pack a day	more than 1/2 pack a day	_____
10.	Are you under much stress?	less than normal	normal	slightly above normal	quite high	_____
					Total Alterable Risk Score	_____
					Grand Total Risk Score	_____

*Adapted from Stone, W. J. CAD Risk Factor Scoring Scale. *Tempe, Arizona: State University, 1984.*

LAB 22

PHYSICAL ACTIVITY
FOR A LIFETIME

NAME _____ SECTION _____ DATE _____

Read Concept 22 before performing this lab.

PURPOSE

The purposes of this laboratory session are:

1. To estimate your fitness needs twenty years from now.
2. To plan a program for your use twenty years from now.
3. To determine the difference in exertion for your current program and your program for later life.

PROCEDURE

1. Assume that your age is twenty years more than it is today. Look up your cardiovascular threshold of training for that specific age. Estimate your resting heart rate (it tends to go up as you get older and less fit). Record it in the results section.
2. Estimate what exercise would make you reach the cardiovascular threshold of training for a person of your assumed age. Think of a person you know (perhaps a parent) as you plan the program. Write this exercise down in the results section and note the rate (for example, one mile in seven minutes).
3. List three flexibility exercises and three strength or muscular endurance exercises that you think you should be performing (list only those you really think you could do at that age). Record this in the results section.
4. Perform the cardiovascular exercise for fifteen minutes and do the flexibility and strength-muscular endurance exercises.

RESULTS

What age have you assumed? _____ years

What will be your cardiovascular target zone at the age you have assumed? _____ bpm

What exercise(s) would you do to get your heart rate above the level noted for the age you have assumed?

List three flexibility exercises you would do at the age you have assumed.

Exercise	Repetitions
1. _____	_____
2. _____	_____
3. _____	_____

List three strength or muscular endurance exercises you would do at the age you have assumed.

Exercise		**Repetitions**
1. _____		_____
2. _____		_____
3. _____		_____

CONCLUSIONS AND IMPLICATIONS

How much easier for you were these exercises than the exercises in your own program?

Do you really think you will be fit enough to do the listed exercises at the age you have assumed?
Yes ____ No ____ Could your parent of the same sex or a relative of an age similar to the one you have assumed do the exercises you have selected? Yes ____ No ____ Why or why not?

At the age you have assumed, do you expect to be more or less fit than the typical person at that age?
More Fit ____ Average ____ Less Fit ____ Explain.

Could you help a person of the age you have assumed plan an exercise program? Yes ____ No ____ Explain.

LAB 23

A PHYSICAL ACTIVITY QUESTIONNAIRE: A REEVALUATION

NAME _____ SECTION _____ DATE _____

Read Concept 23 before performing this lab.

PURPOSE

The purpose of this laboratory session is to help you to detect any change in feelings about physical activity that may have developed from the time you completed questionnaire 1 (Concept 1) to the completion of questionnaire 2 (Concept 23).

PROCEDURE

1. Read each of the fourteen items in the physical activity questionnaire shown here or on page 175 of the Lab Resource Materials for Concept 23.
2. After each statement, check one box indicating whether you strongly agree, agree, disagree, or strongly disagree with it. If you are unsure of your answer, check undecided.
3. When all fourteen items have been answered, use the procedures on page 176 to score the physical activity questionnaire.

RESULTS

After scoring your test, write your rating in the chart provided for each scale of the questionnaire under rating 2. Then look up your rating from the first time you took the test (Chart 1.1) and record that under rating 1. Check whether your score increased ($+$), decreased ($-$), or stayed the same.

	Rating 1	Rating 2	$+$	Same	$-$
Health and fitness	_____	_____	____	____	____
Fun and enjoyment	_____	_____	____	____	____
Relaxation and tension release	_____	_____	____	____	____
Challenge and achievement	_____	_____	____	____	____
Social	_____	_____	____	____	____
Appearance	_____	_____	____	____	____
Competition	_____	_____	____	____	____
Total Score	_____	_____	____	____	____

Discuss any changes in your feelings about physical activity between questionnaire 1 and questionnaire 2. If changes occurred, how do you account for them?

If changes did not occur, why?

CHART 23.1 The Physical Activity Questionnaire

The term "physical activity" in the following statements refers to all kinds of activities, including sports, formal exercises, and informal activities, such as jogging and cycling. Check your answers first, and then read the directions for scoring, found in the Lab Resource Materials for Concept 23 on page 176.

	Strongly Agree	Agree	Undecided	Disagree	Strongly Disagree	Score
1. Doing regular physical activity can be as harmful to health as it is helpful.	☐	☐	☐	☐	☐	_____
2. One of the main reasons I do regular physical activity is because it is fun.	☐	☐	☐	☐	☐	_____
3. Participating in physical activities makes me tense and nervous.	☐	☐	☐	☐	☐	_____
4. The challenge of physical training is one reason why I participate in physical activity.	☐	☐	☐	☐	☐	_____
5. One of the things I like about physical activity is the participation with other people.	☐	☐	☐	☐	☐	_____
6. Doing regular physical activity does little to make me more physically attractive.	☐	☐	☐	☐	☐	_____
7. Competition is a good way to keep a game from being fun.	☐	☐	☐	☐	☐	_____
8. I should exercise regularly for my own good health and physical fitness.	☐	☐	☐	☐	☐	_____
9. Doing exercise and playing sports is boring.	☐	☐	☐	☐	☐	_____
10. I enjoy taking part in physical activity because it helps me to relax and get away from the pressures of daily living.	☐	☐	☐	☐	☐	_____
11. Most sports and physical activities are too difficult for me to enjoy.	☐	☐	☐	☐	☐	_____
12. I do not enjoy physical activities that require the participation of other people.	☐	☐	☐	☐	☐	_____
13. Regular exercise helps me look my best.	☐	☐	☐	☐	☐	_____
14. Competing against others in physical activities makes them enjoyable.	☐	☐	☐	☐	☐	_____

LAB 24

PLANNING YOUR PERSONAL EXERCISE PROGRAM

NAME _____ SECTION _____ DATE _____

Read Concept 24 before completing this lab.

PURPOSE

The purpose of this lab is to plan a personal fitness program using the five steps outlined in Concept 24.

PROCEDURE

Answer the questions and fill in the tables following the five steps outlined below.

1. Identify Your Personal Fitness Needs

In Chart 24.1, darken the boxes of your self-test rating for each of the tests you have taken. (Refer to the appropriate rating charts to determine your ratings.) If you did not take a test, darken the "no result" box.

In Chart 24.2, darken one box for each component of fitness. Make only *one* rating for each by combining ratings from Chart 24.1. If you took more than one test for a particular fitness component, use your own judgment in determining your single ratings. Use ratings 1–3 for cardiovascular fitness, 4–5 for strength, 6 for muscular endurance, 7 for strength, and 8 for fatness. Make only one rating for skill-related fitness using ratings 9–14 from Chart 24.1. Make only one rating for fitness of the back and posture using ratings 15–16 from Chart 24.1. Connect the darkened boxes to create your own personal fitness profile.

The completed profile will give you important information for planning your program. You should be especially careful to include exercise for the components of fitness for which you have low ratings.

2. Select Activities

Fill in Chart 24.3. In the top part of the chart, list the activities you currently do on a regular basis that you would like to continue. In the middle section, write down some new activities that would be especially good for developing fitness in the areas in which you have a weakness or special need (see Chart 24.2). Finally, in the bottom section of the chart, list some new activities you would especially like to try because you enjoy them (even if they do not meet your special fitness needs). After each, note the component of fitness developed by the activity. You should have at least one activity for each of the health-related fitness components.

3. Write Down a Personal Schedule

Fill in Chart 24.4. For each day of the week, write down the activities you plan to do on that particular day. Select the activities from Chart 24.3. A special place at the top of the chart is provided for your warm-up and cool-down activities. In this section, write down the activities you will do to warmup and cool down each day. (You do not need to list these each day on the daily schedules. Another section is provided at the top of the chart for "special exercises" that you may do on a regular basis.) These may include exercises for the back, or just a set of calisthenics or exercises you plan to do. Once you list these activities in the "special exercise section," you need only refer to them in your daily schedule as "special exercises," rather than writing them on each day's schedule.

4. Try It Out

Actually perform your program for at least one week and for several weeks if possible. You may perform the exercises for one or more days of the program during class time.

5. Evaluate and Modify Your Program

After you have tried your program, either in class or on your own, evaluate it. Note your comments in the appropriate section of Chart 24.4. *Remember, even the best program needs periodic evaluation and modification.*

CHART 24.1 Ratings for Fitness Self-Tests

Rating Chart	Rating					
	Excellent	Very Good	Marginal	Poor	Very Poor	No Results
1. Twelve-Minute Run Chart 6C.1, page 43	☐	☐	☐	☐	☐	☐
2. Step Test Chart 6C.2, page 44	☐	☐	☐	☐	☐	☐
3. Bicycle Test Chart 6C.3, page 45	☐	☐	☐	☐	☐	☐
4. Isotonic Strength Chart 7A.1, page 54	☐	☐	☐	☐	☐	☐
5. Isometric Strength Chart 7B.1, page 55	☐	☐	☐	☐	☐	☐
6. Muscular Endurance Chart 8.1, page 58	☐	☐	☐	☐	☐	☐
7. Flexibility Chart 9.1, page 67	☐	☐	☐	☐	☐	☐
8. Fatness Rating Chart 10A.3, page 78	☐	☐	☐	☐	☐	☐
9. Agility Chart 11.1, page 84	☐	☐	☐	☐	☐	☐
10. Balance Chart 11.2, page 84	☐	☐	☐	☐	☐	☐
11. Coordination Chart 11.3, page 85	☐	☐	☐	☐	☐	☐
12. Power Chart 11.4, page 85	☐	☐	☐	☐	☐	☐
13. Reaction Time Chart 11.5, page 85	☐	☐	☐	☐	☐	☐
14. Speed Chart 11.6, page 86	☐	☐	☐	☐	☐	☐
15. Fitness of the Back Chart 16A.1, page 133	☐	☐	☐	☐	☐	☐
16. Posture Chart 16B.1, page 134	☐	☐	☐	☐	☐	☐

CHART 24.2 A Profile of Personal Fitness

Rating Chart	Rating				
	Ex	**VG**	**Fair**	**Poor**	**VP**
Cardiovascular	☐	☐	☐	☐	☐
Endurance	☐	☐	☐	☐	☐
Strength	☐	☐	☐	☐	☐
Flexibility	☐	☐	☐	☐	☐
Fat Control	☐	☐	☐	☐	☐
Skill-Related Fitness	☐	☐	☐	☐	☐
Posture and Fitness of the Back	☐	☐	☐	☐	☐

CHART 24.3 Personal Physical Activities

Current Activities
(List activities in which you currently participate.)

Activity	Fitness Components Developed by Activity	
1. _____	_____	_____
2. _____	_____	_____
3. _____	_____	_____
4. _____	_____	_____
5. _____	_____	_____

New Activities for Fitness
(List new activities for meeting fitness needs.)

Activity	Fitness Components Developed by Activity	
1. _____	_____	_____
2. _____	_____	_____
3. _____	_____	_____
4. _____	_____	_____
5. _____	_____	_____

New Activities Just for Fun
(List new activities that you think you might especially enjoy, but that may not be good for developing fitness.)

Activity

1. _____
2. _____
3. _____

CHART 24.4 A Weekly Exercise Schedule

Warm-Up and Cool-Down Activities	Special Exercises
Daily Schedules (List the activities and times of day for each activity.) **Monday**	**Tuesday**
Wednesday	**Thursday**
Friday	**Saturday**
Sunday	**Program Evaluation** (Fill in after trying out your program.)

LAB 25

EXERCISE AND THE CONSUMER

NAME _____ SECTION _____ DATE _____

Read Concept 25 before completing this lab.

PURPOSE

To practice evaluating exercises found in popular literature.

PROCEDURE

1. Read a popular book or magazine and find an exercise that claims to improve your health, fitness, figure, or posture.
2. Use Chart 25.1 to evaluate the exercise (or program). Check yes or no for each item. Then record your scores in the result section.

CHART 25.1 Exercise Evaluation*

	Yes	No
1. Is the article or book written by an expert as defined in Concept 25?	☐	☐
2. Does the exercise employ the overload principle?	☐	☐
3. Does it employ the progression principle?	☐	☐
4. Does it employ the F.I.T. principle?	☐	☐
5. Does it employ the principle of specificity?	☐	☐
6. Is it a safe exercise?	☐	☐
7. Is it an "active" exercise in which your own muscles contract?	☐	☐
8. Are the benefits claimed for the exercise reasonable?	☐	☐
9. Are the authors trying to help you (rather than selling a product)?	☐	☐
10. Do they refrain from using terms such as "quick," "miraculous," "tone," "remove fat," "new discovery," or other gimmick words?	☐	☐

If in doubt, you may seek an expert's opinion on some of these questions.

RESULTS

1. Give the program you are evaluating one point for a "yes" answer on questions 1, 8, 9, and 10.
   _____ (Score 1)
2. Give the program one point for a "no" answer on questions 2, 3, 4, 5, 6, and 7. _____ (Score 2)
3. Total of score 1 and score 2. _____ (Total score)

CONCLUSIONS AND IMPLICATIONS

1. A high score 1 total (3 or 4) in the results section indicates that the authors of the program know what they are talking about.
2. A high score 2 total (5 or 6) indicates that the program is consistent with good exercise theory.
3. A high total score (8 to 10) suggests that the program is sound for at least some aspects of fitness.

Using this information, write an assessment here of the program from the book or magazine you read.

APPENDIX A

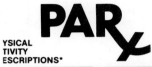

PAR$_x$

PHYSICAL ACTIVITY PRESCRIPTIONS*

PAR$_x$ is a checklist of medical conditions requiring that a degree of precaution and/or special advice be considered for adults undertaking physical activities. Three categories are provided, and conditions are grouped by system or otherwise as appropriate. Comments under Special Prescriptive Conditions/Advice are general, since details and alternatives require clinical judgment in each individual instance.

ABSOLUTE CONTRAINDICATIONS	RELATIVE CONTRAINDICATIONS	SPECIAL PRESCRIPTIVE CONDITIONS/ ADVICE		System
• Permanent restriction, or temporary restriction until condition is treated, stable, and/or past acute phase.	• Highly variable. Value of exercise testing and/or program may exceed risk. Activity may be restricted. • Desirable to maximize control of condition. • Direct or indirect medical supervision of exercise program may be desirable.	• Individualized prescriptive advice generally appropriate: • limitations imposed and/or • special exercises prescribed • May require medical following and/or initial medical supervision in exercise program.		Comments
☐ aortic aneurysm (dissecting) ☐ aortic stenosis (severe) ☐ congestive heart failure ☐ crescendo angina ☐ myocardial infarction (acute) ☐ myocarditis (active or recent) ☐ pulmonary or systemic embolism — acute ☐ thrombophlebitis ☐ ventricular tachycardia and other dangerous dysrhythmias (e.g. multi-focal ventricular activity)	☐ aortic stenosis (moderate) ☐ subaortic stenosis (severe) ☐ marked cardiac enlargement ☐ supraventricular dysrhythmias (uncontrolled or high rate) ☐ ventricular ectopic activity (repetitive or frequent) ☐ ventricular aneurysm ☐ hypertension — untreated or uncontrolled severe (systemic or pulmonary)	☐ aortic (or pulmonic) stenosis — mild angina pectoris and other manifestations of coronary insufficiency (e.g. post-acute infarct) ☐ cyanotic heart disease ☐ shunts (intermittent or fixed) ☐ conduction disturbances • complete AV block • left BBB • Wolff-Parkinson-White syndrome ☐ dysrhythmias — controlled ☐ fixed rate pacemakers	• clinical exercise test may be warranted in selected cases, for specific determination of functional capacity and limitations and precautions (if any). • slow progression of exercise to levels based on test performance and individual tolerance. • consider individual need for initial conditioning program under medical supervision (indirect or direct)	Cardio-vascular
		☐ intermittent claudication	progressive exercise to tolerance	
		☐ hypertension: systolic 160-180; diastolic 105+	progressive exercise; care with medications (serum electrolytes; post-exercise syncope; etc.)	
☐ acute infectious disease (regardless of etiology)	☐ subacute/chronic/recurrent infectious diseases (e.g. malaria, others)	☐ chronic infections	variable as to condition	Infections
	☐ uncontrolled metabolic disorders (diabetes, thyrotoxicosis, myxedema)	☐ renal, hepatic & other metabolic insufficiency ☐ obesity (25-50+ pounds overweight)	variable as to status dietary moderation, and initial light exercises with slow progression (walking, swimming, cycling)	Metabolic
	☐ complicated pregnancy (e.g. toxemia, hemorrhage, incompetent cervix, etc.)	☐ advanced pregnancy (late 3rd trimester)	taper off intensity near term	Pregnancy
		☐ chronic pulmonary disorders ☐ obstructive lung disease ☐ asthma ☐ "exercise-induced asthma"	special relaxation and breathing exercises; breath control during endurance exercises to tolerance; avoid polluted air; avoid hyperventilation during exercise	Lung
		☐ anemia — severe (< 10 Gm/dl) ☐ electrolyte disturbances	control preferred; exercise as tolerated	Blood
		☐ hernia	minimize straining and isometrics; strengthen abdominal muscles	Hernia
		☐ convulsive disorder not completely controlled by medication	minimize exercise in hazardous environments and/or exercising alone (e.g. swimming, mountain climbing, etc.)	CNS
		☐ low back conditions (pathological, functional) ☐ arthritis—acute (infective, rheumatoid; gout) ☐ arthritis — subacute ☐ arthritis—chronic (osteoarthritis and above conditions) ☐ orthopedic	avoid forced extreme flexion, extinsion, and violent twisting, correct posture, proper back exercises treatment, plus judicious blend of rest, splinting and gentle movement progressive increase of active exercise therapy maintenance of mobility and strength; endurance exercises to minimize joint trauma (e.g. cycling, swimming, etc.) highly variable and individualized	Musculo-skeletal
		☐ antianginal ☐ antiarrhythmic ☐ antihypertensive ☐ anticonvulsant ☐ beta-blockers ☐ digitalis preparations ☐ diuretics ☐ ganglionic blockers ☐ others	NOTE: consider underlying condition. Potential for: exertional syncope, electrolyte imbalance, bradycardia, dysrhythmias, impaired coordination and reaction time, heat intolerance. May alter resting and exercise ECG's and exercise test performance.	Medications
		☐ post-exercise syncope ☐ heat intolerance ☐ temporary minor illness	moderate program; prolong cool-down with light activities postpone until recovered	Other

PHYSICAL ACTIVITY RECOMMENDATIONS

Provided as a physician checklist or patient handout

PHYSICAL ACTIVITY RECOMMENDATIONS

If you have been cleared by your physician for unrestricted activity and/or a progressive exercise program, these key points may be of assistance to you.

☐ Components of a balanced exercise program (the 3S's)
  • Strength — arms, shoulders, back, abdomen and legs
  • Suppleness — stretch and relaxation of body and limbs
  • Stamina — endurance fitness through aerobic activities (large muscle action that increases the heart rate)

☐ Progression — slow and easy; gradually increase the volume and vigor of your activities over several weeks.

☐ Warm-up and cool-down — quiet entry and exit of a few minutes each, such as with calisthenics and light activities.

☐ FITT is a guide to your Stamina (endurance) activities.

FREQUENCY	INTENSITY	TIME	TYPE
3 to 5 times per week	Work up to and sustain a target heart rate (for your age) during exercise	Once your body is accustomed to exercise, attempt to keep moving for at least 15 minutes (even if it means slowing down a little)	Any endurance exercise — walking, jogging, swimming, cycling, skipping, vigorous ball games, ski touring, etc.

☐ Pulse count is a good method to assess your response to aerobic exercises. Count for 10 seconds *immediately* after stopping your activity. Have your physician or exercise professional show you how to count your pulse. The chart below is age-adjusted. Be content to work at the lower FIT START heart rate initially until your condition improves, then slowly increase the intensity of your activity until your heart rate is reaching the KEEP FIT level. Remember, enter and exit your activity gently.

FIT START

AGE	HEART RATE
20 - 29	118
30 - 39	112
40 - 49	106
50 - 59	100
60 - 69	94

Progress Slowly →

KEEP FIT

AGE	HEART RATE
20 - 29	146 - 164
30 - 39	138 - 156
40 - 49	130 - 148
50 - 59	122 - 140
60 - 69	116 - 132

Derived from the "Half-As-Much" approach, B.C. Department of Health

* REFER TO SPECIAL PUBLICATIONS FOR ELABORATION AS REQUIRED.

MAJOR REFERENCES FOR PAR$_x$ CHART:
1. Fox, S.M. III, Naughton, J.P., and Haskell, W.C. Physical Activity and the Prevention of Coronary Heart Disease. Ann. Clin. Res. 3: 404-432, 1971.
2. American College of Sports Medicine. Guidelines for Graded Exercise Testing and Exercise Prescription. Lea and Febiger. 1975.
3. Committee on Exercise and Physical Fitness. Evaluation for Exercise Participation — The Apparently Healthy Individual. JAMA 219: 900-01, 1972.
4. Cooper, K.H. Guidelines in the Management of the Exercising Patient. JAMA 211: 1663-67, 1970.
5. Licht, S. Theraputic Exercise Volume III. Waverly Press, 1965.
6. Recommendations and Guidelines of the Canadian Heart Foundation for Exercise Testing and Exercise Programmes for Improving Cardiopulmonary and General Physical Fitness. 1975.

PAR-X
Physical Activity Readiness Examination

Par-X is the medical complement to Par-Q, the Physical Activity Readiness Questionnaire. Please refer to "Guide To Use" below.

NAME

ADDRESS

BIRTHDATE		SEX	TELEPHONE
S.I. No.		MEDICAL No.	

PAR-Q

	No	Yes	Comments / Additional History
Q1 Heart Trouble	☐	☐	
Q2 Chest Pain	☐	☐	
Q3 Dizziness	☐	☐	
Q4 Blood Pressure	☐	☐	
Q5 Musculoskeletal	☐	☐	
Q6 Other reason	☐	☐	
Q7 Over 65 Years	☐	☐	
Medications (relevant)	☐	☐	

ACTIVITY LEVEL

	L	M	H
Job	☐	☐	☐
Leisure	☐	☐	☐

Fitness Program
- ☐ Regular
- ☐ Sporadic
- ☐ None

ACTIVITY INTERESTS

- ☐ Recreation
- ☐ Sports
- ☐ Fitness Program
- ☐ Other

PHYSICAL EXAM

Ht. _____ Wt. _____ BP / (/)

- ☐ Cardiovascular
- ☐ Respiratory
- ☐ Musculoskeletal
- ☐ Other

TESTS AS INDICATED

- ☐ ECG
- ☐ Exercise Test
- ☐ X-Ray   ☐ Hemoglobin   ☐ Urinalysis
- ☐ Other

STATUS

PLAN

Recommend	☐ Unrestricted Activity
	☐ Progressive Exercise Program
Prescribe	☐ Avoid _____
	☐ Add _____
	☐ Medically Supervised Program
	☐ Physiotherapy _____
	☐ Further Investigation
	☐ Exercise Contraindicated
	☐ Indefinite ☐ Temporary

The tear-off tab below is made available for use at the discretion of the Physician.

PHYSICAL ACTIVITY READINESS

Based upon a current review of health status, _____

_____ is considered suitable for:

- ☐ Unrestricted Activity
- ☐ Progressive Exercise Program
  - ☐ with no restrictions/special exercises
  - ☐ with avoidance of _____

    _____
  - ☐ with addition of _____

    _____
- ☐ Only a medically supervised exercise program until further medical clearance
- ☐ Physiotherapy

Special Concerns (if any):

_____ M.D.

_____ 19 _____
(Date)

Further Information:
- ☐ Attached
- ☐ To Be Forwarded
- ☐ Available Upon Request

GUIDE TO USE

Most adults are able to readily participate in physical activity and fitness programs. PAR-Q by itself is adequate for the majority of adults. However, some may require a medical evaluation and specific advice (exercise prescription).

PAR-X is an exercise-specific checklist for clinical use for persons with positive responses to PAR-Q or when further evaluation is otherwise warranted. In addition, PAR-X can serve as a permanent record. Its use is self explanatory.

Following evaluation, generally a PLAN is devised for the patient by the examining physician. To assist in this, three additional sections are provided:

- PHYSICAL ACTIVITY RECOMMENDATIONS (overleaf) with selected advice and pointers for most adults who are suited to participate in any activity and/or a progressive exercise conditioning program.

- PHYSICAL ACTIVITY PRESCRIPTIONS (PAR$_x$ overleaf) is a chart-type checklist of conditions requiring special medical consideration and management.

- PHYSICAL ACTIVITY READINESS form (to right) is an optional tear-off tab for verifying clearance, restrictions, etc., or for making a referral.

PAR-Q, PAR-X and PAR$_x$ were developed by the British Columbia Department of Health. They were conceptualized and critiqued by the Multidisciplinary Advisory Board on Exercise (MABE). Translation, reproduction and use of each in its entirety is encouraged.

REPRINTED FROM B.C. MEDICAL JOURNAL – Vol. 17, No. 11, November, 1975 Courtesy B.C. Ministry of Health & Dept. of National Health & Welfare

CALORIE GUIDE TO COMMON FOODS*

Beverages

Coffee (black)	3
Coke (12 oz.)	137
Hot chocolate, milk (1 cup)	247
Lemonade (1 cup)	100
Limeade, diluted to serve (1 cup)	110
Soda, fruit flavored (12 oz.)	161
Tea (clear)	3

Breads and Cereals

Bagel (1 half)	76
Biscuit (2″ × 2″)	135
Bread, Pita (1 oz.)	80
Bread, raisin (½″ thick)	65
Bread, rye	55
Bread, white enriched (½″ thick)	64
Bread, whole wheat (½″ thick)	55
Bun (hamburger)	120
Cereals, cooked (½ cup)	80
Corn flakes (1 cup)	96
Corn Grits (1 cup)	125
Corn muffin (2½″ diam.)	103
Crackers, graham (1 med.)	28
Crackers, soda (1 plain)	24
English muffin (1 half)	74
Macaroni, with cheese (1 cup)	464
Muffin, plain	135
Noodles (1 cup)	200
Oatmeal (1 cup)	150
Pancakes (1–4″ diam.)	59
Pizza (1 section)	180
Popped corn (1 cup)	54
Potato chips (10 med.)	108
Pretzels (5 small sticks)	18
Rice (1 cup)	225
Roll, plain (1 med.)	118
Roll, sweet (1 med.)	178
Shredded wheat (1 med. biscuit)	79
Spaghetti, plain cooked (1 cup)	218
Tortilla (1 corn)	70
Waffle (4½″ × 5″)	216

Dairy Products

Butter, 1 pat (1½ tsp.)	50
Cheese, cheddar (1 oz.)	113
Cheese, cottage (1 cup)	270
Cheese, cream (1 oz.)	106
Cheese, Parmesan (1 tbsp.)	29
Cheese, Swiss natural (1 oz.)	105
Cream, sour (1 tbsp.)	31
Dairy Queen Cone (med.)	335
Frozen custard (1 cup)	375
Frozen yogurt, vanilla (1 cup)	180
Ice cream, plain (prem.) (1 cup)	350
Ice cream soda, choc. (large glass)	455
Ice milk (1 cup)	184
Ices (1 cup)	177
Milk, chocolate (1 cup)	185
Milk, half-and-half (1 tbsp.)	20
Milk, malted (1 cup)	281
Milk, skim (1 cup)	88
Milk, skim dry (1 tbsp.)	28
Milk, whole (1 cup)	166
Sherbet (1 cup)	270
Whipped topping (1 tbsp.)	14
Yogurt (1 cup)	150

Desserts and Sweets

Cake, angel (2″ wedge)	108
Cake, chocolate (2″ × 3″ × 1″)	150
Cake, plain (3″ × 2½″)	180
Chocolate, bar	200–300
Chocolate, bitter (1 oz.)	142
Chocolate, sweet (1 oz.)	133
Chocolate, syrup (1 tbsp.)	42
Cocoa (1 tbsp.)	21
Cookies, plain (1 med.)	75
Custard, baked (1 cup)	283
Doughnut (1 large)	250
Gelatin, dessert (1 cup)	155
Gelatin, with fruit (1 cup)	170
Gingerbread (2″ × 2″ × 2″)	180
Jams, jellies (1 tbsp.)	55
Pie, apple (1/7 of 9″ pie)	345
Pie, cherry (1/7 of 9″ pie)	355
Pie, chocolate (1/7 of 9″ pie)	360
Pie, coconut (1/7 of 9″ pie)	266
Pie, lemon meringue (1/7 of 9″ pie)	302
Sugar, granulated (1 tsp.)	27
Syrup, table (1 tbsp.)	57

*Reprinted with permission from R. Lindsey and A. Whitley. *Fitness for Health, Figure/Physique, Posture.* Dubuque, IA: William C. Brown Publishers, 1983.

Fruit

Apple, fresh (med.)	76
Applesauce, unsweetened (1 cup)	184
Avocado, raw (½ peeled)	279
Banana, fresh (med.)	88
Cantaloupe, raw (½, 5″ diam.)	60
Cherries (10 sweet)	50
Cranberry sauce, unsweetened (1 tbsp.)	25
Fruit cocktail, canned (1 cup)	170
Grapefruit, fresh (½)	60
Grapefruit, juice, raw (1 cup)	95
Grape juice, bottled (½ cup)	80
Grapes (20–25)	75
Nectarine (1 med.)	88
Olives, green (10)	72
Olives, ripe (10)	105
Orange, fresh (med.)	60
Orange juice, frozen diluted (1 cup)	110
Peach, fresh (med.)	46
Peach, canned in syrup (2 halves)	79
Pear, fresh (med.)	95
Pears, canned in syrup (2 halves)	79
Pineapple, crushed in syrup (1 cup)	204
Pineapple (½ cup fresh)	50
Prune juice (1 cup)	170
Raisins, dry (1 tbsp.)	26
Strawberries, fresh (1 cup)	54
Strawberries, frozen (3 oz.)	90
Tangerine (2½″ diam.)	40
Watermelon, wedge (4″ × 8″)	120

Meat, Fish, Eggs

Bacon, drained (2 slices)	97
Bacon, Canadian (1 oz.)	62
Beef, hamburger chuck (3 oz.)	316
Beef, pot pie	560
Beef steak, sirloin or T-bone (3 oz.)	257
Beef and vegetable stew (1 cup)	185
Chicken, fried breast (8 oz.)	210
Chicken, fried (1 leg and thigh)	305
Chicken, roasted breast (2 slices)	100
Chili, without beans (1 cup)	510
Chili, with beans (1 cup)	335
Egg, boiled	77
Egg, fried	125
Egg, scrambled	100
Fish and Chips (2 pcs. fish; 4 oz. chips)	275
Fish, broiled (3″ × 3″ × ½″)	112
Fish stick	40
Frankfurter, boiled	124
Ham (4″ × 4″)	338
Lamb (3 oz. roast, lean)	158
Liver (3″ × 3″)	150

Luncheon meat (2 oz.)	135
Pork chop, loin (3″ × 5″)	284
Salmon, canned (1 cup)	145
Sausage, pork (4 oz.)	510
Shrimp, canned (3 oz.)	108
Tuna, canned (½ cup)	185
Veal, cutlet (3″ × 4″)	175

Nuts and Seeds

Cashews (1 cup)	770
Coconut (1 cup)	450
Peanut butter (1 tbsp.)	92
Peanuts, roasted, no skin (1 cup)	805
Pecans (1 cup)	752
Sunflower seeds, (1 tbsp.)	50

Sandwiches
(2 slices of bread—plain)

Bologna	214
Cheeseburger (small McDonald's)	300
Chicken salad	185
Egg salad	240
Fish Filet (McDonald's)	400
Ham	360
Ham and cheese	360
Hamburger (small McDonald's)	260
Hamburger, Burger King Whopper	600
Hamburger, Big Mac	550
Hamburger (McDonald's Quarter Pounder)	420
Peanut butter	250
Roast Beef (Arby's Regular)	425

Sauces, Fats, Oils

Catsup, tomato (1 tbsp.)	17
Chili sauce (1 tbsp.)	17
French dressing (1 tbsp.)	59
Margarine (1 pat)	50
Mayonnaise (1 tbsp.)	92
Mayonnaise-type (1 tbsp.)	65
Vegetable, sunflower, safflower oils (1 tbsp.)	120

Soup, Ready to Serve

Bean (1 cup)	190
Beef noodle	100
Cream	200
Tomato	90
Vegetable	80

Vegetables

Alfalfa sprouts (½ cup)	19
Asparagus (6 spears)	22
Bean sprouts (1 cup)	37
Beans, green (1 cup)	27
Beans, lima (1 cup)	152
Beans, navy (1 cup)	642
Beans, pork and molasses (1 cup)	325
Broccoli, fresh cooked (1 cup)	60
Cabbage, cooked (1 cup)	40
Cauliflower (1 cup)	25
Carrot, raw (med.)	21
Carrots, canned (1 cup)	44
Celery, diced raw (1 cup)	20
Coleslaw (1 cup)	102
Corn, sweet, canned (1 cup)	140
Corn, sweet (med. ear)	84
Cucumber, raw (6 slices)	6
Lettuce (2 large leaves)	7
Mushrooms, canned (1 cup)	28
Onions, french fried (10 rings)	75
Onions, raw (med.)	25
Peas, field (½ cup)	90
Peas, green (1 cup)	145
Pickles, dill (med.)	15
Pickles, sweet (med.)	22
Potato, baked (med.)	97
Potato, french fried (8 stick)	155
Potato, mashed (1 cup)	185
Radish, raw (small)	1
Sauerkraut, drained (1 cup)	32
Spinach, fresh, cooked (1 cup)	46
Squash, summer (1 cup)	30
Sweet pepper (med.)	15
Sweet potato, candied (small)	314
Tomato, cooked (1 cup)	50
Tomato, raw (med.)	30

APPENDIX C
CALORIES PER MINUTE
IN ACTIVITY

(Approximate Number of Calories Used Per Pound of Body Weight)

Activity	Calories Per Minute Per Pound
Daily Activities	
Lying	
Sleeping	.0066
Resting	.0079
Sitting	
Quietly; reading	.0080
Viewing T.V.; conversing; hand sewing; eating	.0116
Writing	.0120
Typing (manual)	.0166
Driving a car	.0150
Playing piano	.0150
Standing	
Dressing; undressing; grooming	.0133
Cooking; dishwashing; ironing	.0150
Household tasks (cleaning, dusting, sweeping, etc.)	.0200
Singing	.0190
Washing clothes	.0190
Showering	.0230
Making bed	.0270
Exercise and Sports	
Archery	.0340
Basketball	.0470
Bicycling (level) 5.5 mph	.0330
(uphill)	.0410
(downhill)	.0180
Bowling	.0440
Calisthenics	.0330
Dancing (moderately)	.0270
(vigorously)	.0460
Football	.0670
Golf	.0360
Squash; racquetball	.0690
Table tennis	.0260
Tennis	.0460
Walking slowly (level)	.0183
(uphill)	.0560

Note: For a complete listing of foods, the reader is referred to: *Nutritive Value of Foods,* U.S. Department of Agriculture, Washington, D.C., Home and Gardens Bulletin, No. 72. (Available in most libraries, university bookstores, and Home Economics departments).

INDEX

Abdomen, protruding, 22
Abdominal stretch, 138–39
Achilles tendon, 26, 27, 111, 112, 116
Acquired aging, 166
Activity records, 148
Adaptation to stress, 149
Adolescence, fitness of, 166
Adolescent, activity for, 167
Aerobic
    activities, involvement of children, 117
    activities, popularity among adults, 89
    dance, 92, 118
    exercise, 36, 38, 88–93, 219
    lab, 219
    points chart, 90
Age and hypokinetic disease, 163
Agility, 10, 13
    evaluating, 83, 215
    rating scale, chart, 84
Aging
    acquired, 166, 168
    process, 168
    time-dependent, 166
Alarm reaction, 149
A.M.A. (American Medical Association), 180
American College of Sports Medicine
    guidelines, 27
Anabolic steroids, 46, 51
Anaerobic exercise, 36, 38, 41, 88, 124–25
    achieving fitness through, 124
    lab, 227
Anemia, 37
Angina pectoris, 16, 17
Ankle press, 104
Anorexia nervosa, 71, 72
Antagonistic muscles, 46
Antagonist-stretch, 60, 62, 64
Anxiety, 149
Appetite
    and exercise, 75
    thermostat (appestat), 75
Aquadynamics, 93, 119
Arm
    circling, 121
    and leg-lift, 122
    press in doorway, 108
    stretch, 115
Arteries, 37
Arteriosclerosis, 16, 17, 37
Arthritis, 63, 140
Assisted-stretch, 60, 64, 65
Astrand-Ryhming bicycle test, 41, 43, 44
    lab, 201
Atherosclerosis, 3, 16, 17, 18, 19, 37
Athlete's heart, 17
Autogenic relaxation training, 151
Automation, 2, 4

B₁₅ (pangamic acid), 145
Baby fat, 75
Back
    ache, 65, 112, 126–34
        causes of, 158
    arching, 138, 139
    care of, 126–34
    lab, 229
    pain, 4, 20–22
    -to-wall test, 133
    weakness, testing for, 133
Backpacking, 92
Balance, 10, 13, 82
    bass test of dynamic, 84, 215
    evaluating, 84
Ballistic
    ballet bar stretch, 139
    stretch, 60, 61, 62
Baseball, 117
Basketball, 93, 117
Bass test of dynamic balance, 84, 215
    rating scale, chart, 84
Belts, weighted, 181
Bench press, 104
Bent
    arm hang, 58
        rating scale, 59
    arm lift, 127
    knee let-down, 95
    leg stretcher, 129
Biceps curl, 100, 102
Bicycling, 89, 117, 118
Bilateral transfer, 50
Billig's exercise, 113, 114
Biofeedback, autogenic training, 153
Blood fat levels, 18
Blood lipids, 162
Blood pressure, 162
    diastolic, 162
    systolic, 162
Blood sugar, 144
Body composition, 8, 15, 69–81
Body fatness, 8, 15
    assessment, 70
    controlling, 72, 75
    evaluating, 75
    exercise and, 72, 75
    hypokinetic disease, 163
    lab, 211
    location of, 70
    measuring, 71
    reduction of, 73
    mechanics, 156–61
    target zone for, 73
    threshold of training, 73
Bone degeneration, 23
Bow exercise, 110
Bowling, 117–18
Breakfast, 144
Bulemia, 71, 72

Caffeine, 146
Calcium, 143

Calf
    muscles, 112
    stretcher, 29, 116
Calisthenics, 117
    isotonic, 94–98
    sample program, 90
Caloric
    balance, 69, 75
    count, 75
    expenditure, 72, 73, 74
    intake, 71, 72, 75
Calorie, 69
Calories, 143–44
    in common foods, 261
    expended in activities, 74, 259, 264
    lab, 237
Camping, 118
Capillaries, 37
Carbohydrates, 143, 145
Carbohydrate loading, 145
Cardiovascular
    cool down, 30
    warm-up, 29
Cardiovascular fitness, 8, 14, 15, 36–45, 88, 92, 93, 118
    evaluation, 41, 43
    lab, 201
    threshold of training, lab, 199
Catharsis, 172, 174
Caveat emptor, "let the buyer beware," 180
Cellulite, 182
Cellulose, 142
Center of gravity, 156
Chest push, 105
Children's participation in sports and activities, 117–18
Chins, 58
Choice of exercises and activities, 6
Cholesterol, 18, 144
Chronic fatigue, 149
Circuit overload training, 89
Cold weather exercise, 140
Collateral circulation, 16
Commercial establishments, 141
Concentric contractions, 46
Congestive heart failure, 16, 17
Continuous exercise, 88
Contraction
    concentric, 46
    isotonic, 46
Contract-relax exercise routine, 153
Contraindicated exercise, lab, 233
Cool-down exercise, 26, 28
    for an aerobic workout, 29
    lab, 195
Cooper, Kenneth, 89
Coordination, 10, 14, 82
    evaluating, 84, 215
    rating scale, chart, 85

Coping strategies, tension, 151
Coronary
    circulation, 37
    occlusion, 16, 17
    thrombosis, 16
Coronary Collateral Circulation Theory, 19
Coronary heart disease, 17
    cholesterol, risk factor, 144
    theories of, 17–20
Cotton mouth, 144
Crash diets, 71
Creative activity, 12
Creeping obesity, 75
Cross-country skiing, 92
Cross-education, 50
Cureton, Thomas, 91
Curls, 107
Cycles and rowing machines, 181
Cycling, 89

Dance aerobics, 92, 118
Dance exercise, 119
Dancercise, 92
Deep knee bends, 139
Dehydration, 136, 140, 143
Depression, 23
    benefits of exercise, 175
Desirable weight, lab, 213
Diabetes, 23, 140
Diastolic blood pressure, 162
Diet, 69, 72, 73, 75, 143–48
    crash, 71, 146
    fad, 145
    hypokinetic disease, 163
    record chart, 146
Discs
    herniated, 137
    ruptured, 156
    slipped, 158
DMSO (dimethyl sulfoxide), 182
Double heel kick, 14
Double-jointedness, 60
Double leg-lift, 138
Double progressive system, 49
Drugs
    effect of and exercise, 141
Duration of exercise, 41
Dynamic posture
    lifting and carrying, 159
    pushing and pulling, 160
    saving energy, 161
Dysmenorrhea, 60, 65

Eccentric contraction, 46
    exercise, 49
ECG, electrocardiogram, 180
Effective lifting, 12
EKG, 43
Electrical muscle stimulators, 181
Emotional storm, 16, 20
Employee fitness programs, 4, 12

Endurance
  dynamic, 56
  events, 145
  muscular, 56–59
  static, 56
Environmental conditions, 30
Epiglottis, 136
Epinephrine, 141
Erythrocytes, 37
Exercise
  activity neurosis, 5
  aerobic, 36, 38, 88–93
  allergy to, 141
  anaerobic, 36, 38, 41, 88,
    124–25
  attitudes, 4
  benefits, 146
  calisthenics, 90
  cautions, 136–42
  competitive experience, 5
  consumer, 180–84
    lab, 257
  continuous, 88
  dance, 119
  dangers/contraindications,
    5
  definition, 2
  eccentric (negative), 49
  employee fitness, 4
  enjoyment of, 5, 12, 172–76
  equipment, harmful, 137
  facts and statistics, 3–6
  and fat loss, 72–73
  frequency, 34
  good health, 17
  harmful, 140
  ignorance of the facts, 3
  importance in industry, 4
  induced anaphylaxis, 141
  intensity, 35
  intermittent, 88
  lifetime, 166–69
  minimal amount, 28
  misconceptions, 3, 4
  most popular, 5
  nutrition, 143–48
  optimal amount, 28
  passive, 181
  physical appearance, 5
  pregnancy, 141
  preparing for, 26–32
  program planning, 177–79
  proper dress for, 27
  proper footwear for, 27
  psychological benefits, 174
  reasons for exercising, 4–5
  reasons for not exercising, 4
  regular, 12, 17, 18, 20, 23,
    75
  social experience of
    involvement, 5
  target zones, 28
  time, 35
  value of, 4
  women in, 4
Exercise programs
  lab, 253
  preplanned, 117, 118–24
Exercises
  endurance, 94–110
  relaxation, 152
  strength, 94–110
  stretching, 111–16
  water, 93

Fartlek, 124
Fat
  calories per gram, 144
  children, 75
  control, 72
  loss, 73, 75, 76
  reduction, 73
Fatigue
  chronic, 149
  physiological, 149
  psychological, 149, 151
Fatness
  body fatness assessment, 70
  rating scale, chart, 78
Fats, 18, 143, 144
F.D.A. (Food and Drug
    Administration), 180
Fibrin, 16
Fibrin Deposit Theory, 19
Fight or flight response, 2
Figure wrapping, 181
Fist squeeze, 105
FIT (frequency, intensity,
    time), 34
Fitness, physical
  decrease in, 3
  definition, 3
  lab, 189
  skill-related, 82–86
  sports, 82
Fitness target zones, 33–35, 47
Flexed arm hang
  rating scale, chart, 59
Flexibility, 8, 14, 60–68
  exercises, advantages, 64
  fitness target zone, 63
  influences of age and sex,
    65
  lab, 209
  rating scale, 67
  sample exercises, 112
  spine, 128
  stunt, 67
  tests, 66
  threshold of training, 63
Food and Drug Administration,
    180
Food and Nutrition Board, 143
Food groups, 143, 144
Foot defects, 157
Foot lift, 107
Forward lunge, 97
Four-minute hop, 15
Frame size
  rating chart, 78
Free weights, 94
Frequency, 34, 38, 41, 47
Fun and competition, 173

Glucose, 145
Gluteal
  lift, 132
  pinch, 110
Glycogen stores, 145

Half squat, 99
Hamstring
  curl, 104
  stretches, 116
Hamstrings, 62, 111, 113, 116
Handball, 93
Hatha Yoga, 182
Head, forward, 156
Health clubs, 141, 183
Health definition, 11
Health foods, 145

Health-related fitness
  and aerobic exercise, 88
  components, 11
  terms, 8
Heart attack, 3, 17
Heart disease, 3, 17–20
  rating scale, chart, 165
  risk factor questionnaire,
    164
  lab, 247
  theories of, 17–20
Heart muscle, 18, 36
Heart rate, 39
  formula for calculating
    target, 40
  lab, 197
  maximal, 40
  resting, 36
  working, 40
Heat stress, 140
Heel walking, 137
Hemoglobin, 36, 37
Heredity, 163
Herniated disc, 156
High blood pressure, 3
High density lipoprotein
    (HDL), 19
Hiking, 92
Honey, 145
Hurdler's stretch, 137
Hyperextended knees, 156
Hypertension, 16, 17, 162
  lower back, 137
  neck, 137
  neuromuscular, 149, 151
Hypertrophy of muscle, 46, 50
Hyperventilation, 136
Hypoglycemia, 145
Hypokinetic disease, 2, 3, 11,
    16–25
  definition, 3
  lab, 191–92
  risk factors, 162–65

Iliopsoas, 116
  Illinois agility run, 115, 130
  stretcher, 115, 130
Imagery (self-hypnosis), 153
Inactivity, 17, 20, 75
  excuses for, 168
Inoculation against stress, 153
Insomnia, 23, 140
Intensity, 34, 35, 38, 41, 47
Intermittent exercise, 88
Interval training program,
    124–25
Isokinetic exercise, 49
Isokinetics, 47–48
Isometric exercise, 47, 48, 94
  harmful, 137
  lab, 205
  strength evaluation, 54
Isotonic exercise, 47, 48, 94
  calisthenics, 94
  contraction, 46
  exercises, 94–95
  lab, 203
  strength evaluation, 52

Jack spring, 13
Jacobson's progressive
    relaxation method,
    151
Jazzercise, 92

Jogging, 92, 118
  for cardiovascular fitness,
    140
  injuries, 112
  lab, 217
Joint mobility, 63

Kennedy, John F., 12
Kilogram, 143
Knee
  bends, deep, 139
  extension, 104
  injury, 137
  pull-down, 139
  raising, 120
  -to-chest
    exercise, 130
    test, 133
  -to-nose touch, 98
Kneeling leg extensions, 98
Kyphosis, 127, 136, 156

Lateral bending, 121
Lateral neck flexion, 128
Lateral trunk
  exercise, 128
  stretcher, 114
Lat pull-down, 103
Laxity, 62
Leanness, assessment, 70
Leg
  extension exercise, 96, 106,
    109
  hug, 29, 113
  -lift, supine, 133
  -lift, double, 138
  over, tuck, 123
  press, 102, 108
  side raises, 97
  -up exercise, 131
Lifetime sport, 117, 118, 173
Lifting and carrying, 159
Ligaments, 62
Linear motion, 156
Lipid, 116
Lipid Deposit Theory, 18
Lipoprotein, 16, 18–19
Loafer's Heart Theory, 20
Long arch, foot, 137
Long jump, 13
Lordosis, 16, 21, 112, 113, 115,
    128, 129–30
Low back pain, 3, 22, 126
Low density lipoproteins
    (LDL), 19
Lower leg-lift, 97
Lower leg stretcher, 112
Lumbar, 136
Lumbar lordosis, 156
Lumbar muscles, 62

Making weight, 143, 146
Massage, 153, 181
Maximal heart rate, 39
Maximal oxygen uptake, 36,
    41, 43
Mechanics, body, 156–61
Medical examination, 27
Meditation, Transcendental,
    151
Menstrual cramps
    (dysmenorrhea), 60,
    65, 113
Mental illness, 12
Mental practice, 172, 174

M.E.T., 69, 72
Migraine, 140
Military press, 99
  in doorway, 107
Milk, 140
Minerals, 143
Modified push-up, 122
Muscle
  biopsies, 47
  -bound, 51
  bulk, 50
  cardiac, 46
  cramps, 113
  definition, 46, 50
  fast twitch, 47
  fatigue, 21
  skeletal, 46
  slow twitch, 47
  smooth, 46
  soreness, 49
  spasm, 19
  tension, 158
Muscular endurance, 8, 15,
    56–59, 94
  fitness target zone, 57
  four-minute hop, 15
  lab, 207
  program for developing, 57
  rating scale, chart, 58
  sample isotonic exercise for,
    95–98
  threshold of training, 56, 57
Muscle fitness, 20–22
  of children, 21
Muscle imbalance, 133, 137
Muscle soreness, 111
Muscular tension, evaluating,
    155
Musculoskeletal problems, 22
Myofascial pain syndrome, 62,
    150

Neck
  aches, 158
  extension exercise, 129
  flexion, lateral, 128
  hyperextension, 139
  pull, 106
  rotation, 115
  stretch, 152
Negative (eccentric) exercise,
    49
Neuromuscular hypertension,
    149
  lab, 243
Nutrition and exercise, 143–48
  lab, 235

Obesity, 3, 23, 69, 71
  childhood, 75
  creeping, 75
  fear of, 71, 72
Occupations, stressful, 150
One-foot balance, 13
One-leg stretcher, 113
Optimum health, 11
Orthopedic problems, 65
Osteoporosis, 23
Overfat, 69, 71
  schoolchildren, 75
Overhead pull, 106
Overlearning, 172, 174
Overload principle, 33, 47
Overtraining, 141
Overweight, 69, 71
Oxygen Pump Theory, 18
Oxygen uptake, maximal, 36

Panacea, 180
Pangamic acid, (B_{15}), 145
Paper ball bounce, 14
Paper drop, 13
Paralysis by analysis, 172, 173
Parasympathetic dominance,
    20
Parasympathetic nervous
    system, 16
PAR-Q (Physical Activity
    Readiness
    Questionnaire), 26, 27
  lab, 193
PAR-X (Physical Activity
    Readiness
    Examination), 26, 27
Passive exercise, 180
Peak experience, 5
Pectoral stretcher, 114
Pelvic tilt, 110, 130, 131
Phospholipids, 18
Physical activity
  adults, 167–69
  challenge, 5
  children, 166–67
  good health, 17
  lifetime, lab, 249
  mental health benefits, 4,
    12
  personalized, 173
  physical health benefits, 11
  questionnaire, 6, 175
    lab, 187, 251
  reasons for exercising, 4–5
  reasons for not exercising, 4
  sense of personal
    accomplishment, 5
  surveys, 3
Physical Activity Readiness
    Examination, 26
Physical Activity Readiness
    Questionnaire, 26
Physical appearance, 5
Physical fitness, 8–15
  definition, 3
  facts, 11
  ignorance of the facts, 3
  lab, 189
  meeting unexpected
    emergencies, 12
  misconceptions, 3
  skill-related, 82–86
  stunts, 12
  value, 4
Physiological fatigue, 149
Plough, 138
Plough shear, 138
Plyometrics, 48, 49
PNF
  exercise, 62
  stretching, 61
Posture, 126–34, 156
  comparison of bad and
    good, 157
  dynamic, 159–61
  evaluation, chart, 134
  lab, 231
  poor, 157
  rating scale, chart, 134
Power, 10, 13, 82
  evaluating, 85, 215
  rating scale, chart, 85
PRE, 46, 47, 48, 94
Preevent meal, 145
Pregnancy and exercise, 141

Preplanned exercise programs,
    117, 118–24
  achieving fitness through,
    119
  lab, 227
  problems, 119
Press up, high leg, 15
Program planning, lab, 253
Progression, principle of, 34
Progressive resistance exercise
    (PRE), 46, 47, 48, 94
Protective Protein Theory, 18
Protein needs, 144
Proteins, 143
Psychological fatigue, 149, 151
Ptosis, abdominal, 131
Pull-to-chin, 101
Pull-ups
  chinning, 96
  modified, 95
Pulmonary emphysema, 140
Pulse, 39, 42
  carotid, 39, 42
  lab, 197
  radial, 42
Pushing and pulling, 160
Push-ups
  bent-knee, 95
  full-length, 95
  modified, 122
Pyriformis syndrome, 136

Quack devices, 33
Quackery, fitness, 180–84
Quadriceps stretch, 139
Qualified personnel
  commercial establishments,
    141
Quick energy boosts, 145

Racquetball, 93
Reaction time, 10, 13, 82
  evaluation, 85, 215
  rating scale, chart, 85
Reciprocal innervation, 62
Recommended daily allowance
    (RDA), 143
Recreational sports skills, 118
Referred pain, 16, 21, 22, 156
Rehabilitation
  heart patients, 140
Referred pain, 16, 21, 22, 156,
    158
Regular exercise, 12, 17, 18,
    20, 23, 75, 163
Relaxation, 5, 149–55
  autogenic training, 151
  biofeedback, 153
  contract-relax routine, 153
  exercises, 152
  Jacobson's method, 151
  lab, 245
  techniques, 151
  three Rs of, 151
Repetitions, 47
Respiratory system, 37
Resting heart rate, 36
Rhythmic aerobics, 92
Risk factors, 16, 162
  lab, 247
Rolling machines, 181
Rope jumping, 92
Rounded shoulders, 127, 156
Rowing machines, 183
Royal Canadian XBX and 5BX
    programs, 120
  sample program, 120–23

Run and half knee bends, 123
Runner's high, 92
Running, lab, 217
Ruptured disc, 156

Salt tablets, 140
Saturated fats, 18
Sauna belts and shorts, 181
Sciatica, 136, 156
Scoliosis, 21, 156
Seated rowing, 102
Sedentary living, 3
  heart disease, 17
Shin and quadriceps stretch,
    139
Shin splints, 65, 116, 140
Shin stretcher, 8
Shoulder
  lift, 152
  shrug, 99
  pull, 105
  stand, bicycle, 138
Side leg raises, 97, 122
Side stretch, 29
Sitting
  stretcher, 112
  toe touch, 116
  tucks, 58, 97
Sit-ups, 121, 132
  bent-knee, 96
  hands-behind-head, 138
  reverse, 96
Skill analysis, 172
Skill learning, 174
Skill proficiency in sports, 173
Skill-related fitness, 82–86
  athletes, 83
  components, 11
  emergency situations, 82
  enjoying leisure time, 83
  evaluating, 83
  health related fitness, 82
  lab, 215
  skill specificity, 83
  terms, 10
  work efficiency, 82
Skinfold
  calipers, 70, 75
  locations for men, 78
  locations for women, 78
  measurement, 70, 75
Slim, 58
Slimming wheel, 137
Slipped disc, 158
Smoking, 163
Soccer, 93
Softball, 118
Somatotype, 69
Spasm cycle, 22
Specificity, principle of, 34, 47
Specificity of training, 34, 47,
    48
Speed, 10, 14, 82
  evaluation, 86, 215
  rating scale, chart, 86
Speed play, 124
Spinal alignment, poor, 132
Sports, 117–18
  continuous, 93
  contribution to health, 118
  fitness benefits, 82, 118
  lab, 225
  lifetime, 117, 118
  recreational, skills, 118
  team, 117
  ten most popular, 118

Spot reducing fallacy, 183
Standing toe touch, 139
Static endurance, 56, 57
Static muscle stretching, 28
Stationary leg change, 98
Step test, 41, 43, 44
    lab, 201
Steroids, 141
Stick drop test, 85
Stick test of coordination, 84
Straight arm lift, 127
Straight leg back flattener, 131
Strength, 8, 15, 46–55
Strengthening
    sample isotonics program,
        95–98
Strength evaluations
    isometric, 55
        lab, 205
    isotonic, 52
        lab, 203
Strength training
    guidelines, 50
    fallacies, 51
    lab, 221
Stress, 20, 163
    lab, 241
Stress, tension, and relaxation,
    149–55
Stressful occupations, 150
    life events, 154
        lab, 239
Stressor, 149
Stretching exercises, 111–16
    ballistic-, 60, 61, 62, 111
    guidelines, 111
    high-risk, 137
    lab, 223
    PNF, 61, 111
    side, 29
    static-, 61, 62, 111
    therapeutic, 113

Stroke, 3
Supine leg-lifts, 133
Supplement to diet, 145
Swimming, 93, 117, 118
Sympathetic dominance, 20
Sympathetic nervous system,
    16
Systolic blood pressure, 162

Target zones, 33–35
    aerobic exercise, 38
    heart rate, 41
        chart, 42
Tennis, 117, 118
Tension, 5, 149–55
    contract exercise, 152
    coping strategies, 151
    muscle, 158
    muscular evaluation, 155
Tension-relaxation
    rating scale, chart, 155
Threshold of training, 28,
        33–35, 38, 41, 47, 56
Tiptoe exercise, 137
Toe raise, 101
Toe touch, 14, 29, 139
    sitting, 116, 120
Tonus, 180
Total fitness, 11
Training
    interval, 124–25
    overtraining, 141
    strength, 50
Transfer of, 50

Transcendental Meditation
    (TM), 151
Triceps curl, 100, 103
Triceps extension, 109
Trigger points, 62, 65
    cervical, 128, 129
    myofascial, 137, 150
    in neck, 115
Triglycerides, 18
Trunk curl, 131
Trunk lift
    lower, 98
    upper, 98
Trunk stretch, 152
Trunk swing, 152
Twelve-minute run, 41, 43
    lab, 201
Type A behavior, 23
    personality, 163

Ulcer, 23
Underwater weighing, 70
Upper back lift, 97

Waist pull, 109
Walking, 93, 117, 118
Wall seat, 108
Wall slide, 132
Wand exercise, 116, 117
Warm-up
    aerobic, 29
    cardiovascular, 29
    exercises, 26–28
    lab, 195

Water exercises, 93
Weather, 30
Weight
    control, 69–81, 140
    { desirable, men, chart, 79
    { desirable, women, chart, 79
    losing gimmicks, 140
    loss and gain, 72
    loss programs, 75
    watchers, 184
Weight training, 94
    lab, 221
    machines, 102
Weights, homemade, 94
Whirlpool baths, 182
Working heart rate, 40
Workweek, average, 2
World Health Organization, 11

XBX and 5BX, 119
    Royal Canadian programs,
        120
    sample programs, 120–23

Yoga, Hatha, 182